T0362007

MR Imaging of the Foot and Ankle

Editor

MARY G. HOCHMAN

MAGNETIC RESONANCE IMAGING CLINICS OF NORTH AMERICA

www.mri.theclinics.com

Consulting Editors
SURESH K. MUKHERJI
LYNNE S. STEINBACH

February 2017 • Volume 25 • Number 1

ELSEVIER

1600 John F. Kennedy Boulevard • Suite 1800 • Philadelphia, Pennsylvania, 19103-2899

http://www.mri.theclinics.com

MRI CLINICS OF NORTH AMERICA Volume 25, Number 1
February 2017 ISSN 1064-9689, ISBN 13: 978-0-323-49653-7

Editor: John Vassallo (j.vassallo@elsevier.com)
Developmental Editor: Meredith Clinton

© **2017 Elsevier Inc. All rights reserved.**

This periodical and the individual contributions contained in it are protected under copyright by Elsevier, and the following terms and conditions apply to their use:

Photocopying
Single photocopies of single articles may be made for personal use as allowed by national copyright laws. Permission of the Publisher and payment of a fee is required for all other photocopying, including multiple or systematic copying, copying for advertising or promotional purposes, resale, and all forms of document delivery. Special rates are available for educational institutions that wish to make photocopies for non-profit educational classroom use. For information on how to seek permission visit www.elsevier.com/permissions or call: (+44) 1865 843830 (UK)/ (+1) 215 239 3804 (USA).

Derivative Works
Subscribers may reproduce tables of contents or prepare lists of articles including abstracts for internal circulation within their institutions. Permission of the Publisher is required for resale or distribution outside the institution. Permission of the Publisher is required for all other derivative works, including compilations and translations (please consult www.elsevier.com/permissions).

Electronic Storage or Usage
Permission of the Publisher is required to store or use electronically any material contained in this periodical, including any article or part of an article (please consult www.elsevier.com/permissions). Except as outlined above, no part of this publication may be reproduced, stored in a retrieval system or transmitted in any form or by any means, electronic, mechanical, photocopying, recording or otherwise, without prior written permission of the Publisher.

Notice
No responsibility is assumed by the Publisher for any injury and/or damage to persons or property as a matter of products liability, negligence or otherwise, or from any use or operation of any methods, products, instructions or ideas contained in the material herein. Because of rapid advances in the medical sciences, in particular, independent verification of diagnoses and drug dosages should be made.

Although all advertising material is expected to conform to ethical (medical) standards, inclusion in this publication does not constitute a guarantee or endorsement of the quality or value of such product or of the claims made of it by its manufacturer.

Magnetic Resonance Imaging Clinics of North America (ISSN 1064-9689) is published quarterly by Elsevier Inc., 360 Park Avenue South, New York, NY 10010-1710. Months of issue are February, May, August, and November. Business and Editorial Offices: 1600 John F. Kennedy Blvd., Ste. 1800, Philadelphia, PA 19103-2899. Customer Service Office: 3251 Riverport Lane, Maryland Heights, MO 63043. Periodicals postage paid at New York, NY and additional mailing offices. Subscription prices are $380.00 per year (domestic individuals), $661.00 per year (domestic institutions), $100.00 per year (domestic students/residents), $420.00 per year (Canadian individuals), $861.00 per year (Canadian institutions), $545.00 per year (international individuals), $861.00 per year (international institutions), and $275.00 per year (international and Canadian students/residents). International air speed delivery is included in all *Clinics* subscription prices. All prices are subject to change without notice. **POSTMASTER:** Send address changes to *Magnetic Resonance Imaging Clinics*, Elsevier Health Sciences Division, Subscription Customer Service, 3251 Riverport Lane, Maryland Heights, MO 63043. Customer Service (orders, claims, online, change of address): Elsevier Health Sciences Division, Subscription **Customer Service, 3251 Riverport Lane, Maryland Heights, MO 63043. Tel:1-800-654-2452 (U.S. and Canada); 314-447-8871 (outside U.S. and Canada). Fax: 314-447-8029. E-mail: journalscustomer service-usa@elsevier.com (for print support); journalsonlinesupport-usa@elsevier.com (for online support).**

Reprints. For copies of 100 or more of articles in this publication, please contact the Commercial Reprints Department, Elsevier Inc., 360 Park Avenue South, New York, NY 10010-1710. Tel.: 212-633-3874; Fax: 212-633-3820; E-mail: reprints@elsevier.com.

Magnetic Resonance Imaging Clinics of North America is covered in the *RSNA Index of Imaging Literature, MEDLINE/PubMed (Index Medicus),* and *EMBASE/Excerpta Medica.*

Contributors

CONSULTING EDITORS

SURESH K. MUKHERJI, MD, MBA, FACR
Department of Radiology, Michigan State
University, East Lansing, Michigan

LYNNE S. STEINBACH, MD, FACR
Professor of Radiology and Orthopaedic
Surgery, Department of Radiology
and Biomedical Imaging, University of
California, San Francisco, San Francisco,
California

EDITOR

MARY G. HOCHMAN, MD, MBA
Staff Radiologist, Section Chief
Emeritus–Musculoskeletal Imaging and
Intervention, Department of Radiology, Beth
Israel Deaconess Medical Center, Assistant
Professor, Harvard Medical School, Boston,
Massachusetts

AUTHORS

WON C. BAE, PhD
Assistant Professor, Radiology Service,
Veterans Affairs San Diego Healthcare System,
San Diego, California; Department of
Radiology, Musculoskeletal Imaging Research
Laboratory, University of California, San Diego,
La Jolla, California

DANIEL BAUMFELD, MD
Department of Surgery, Orthopedics and
Traumatology, Federal University of Minas
Gerais (UFMG), Belo Horizonte, Minas Gerais,
Brazil

JENNY T. BENCARDINO, MD
Professor of Radiology and Orthopedic
Surgery, Department of Radiology, New York
University School of Medicine, New York
University Hospital for Joint Diseases,
New York, New York

CHING-DI CHANG, MD
Department of Radiology, Kaohsiung Chang
Gung Memorial Hospital, Chang Gung
University College of Medicine, Kaohsiung
City, Taiwan

YVONNE CHEUNG, MD, MS
Associate Professor, Department of Radiology,
Dartmouth-Hitchcock Medical Center,
Lebanon, New Hampshire

CHRISTINE B. CHUNG, MD
Professor, Radiology Service, Veterans Affairs
San Diego Healthcare System, San Diego,
California; Department of Radiology,
Muskuloskeletal Imaging Research
Laboratory, University of California, San Diego,
La Jolla, California

JULIA CRIM, MD
Professor, Department of Radiology, University
of Missouri, Columbia, Missouri

KIRSTEN ECKLUND, MD
Assistant Professor, Department of
Radiology, Harvard Medical School,
Boston Children's Hospital, Boston,
Massachusetts

MARY G. HOCHMAN, MD, MBA
Staff Radiologist, Section Chief
Emeritus–Musculoskeletal Imaging and
Intervention, Department of Radiology, Beth
Israel Deaconess Medical Center, Assistant
Professor, Harvard Medical School, Boston,
Massachusetts

JEFFREY KAYE, MD
Fellow, Department of Radiology, New
England Baptist Hospital, Tufts University
School of Medicine, Boston,
Massachusetts

GRACE MANG YUET MA, MD
Department of Radiology, Ohio State
University Wexner Medical Center, Columbus,
Ohio

SAMUEL D. MADOFF, MD
Staff Radiologist, Department of Radiology,
New England Baptist Hospital, Tufts University
School of Medicine, Boston,
Massachusetts

**EDGAR LEONARDO MARTINEZ-SALAZAR,
MD**
Division of Musculoskeletal Imaging and
Intervention, Department of Radiology,
Massachusetts General Hospital, Harvard
Medical School, Boston,
Massachusetts

EOGHAN McCARTHY, MD
Division of Musculoskeletal Imaging,
Department of Radiology, Jefferson Medical
College, Thomas Jefferson University,
Philadelphia, Pennsylvania

TIMOTHY M. MEEHAN, MD
Division of Musculoskeletal Imaging and
Intervention, Department of Radiology,
Massachusetts General Hospital, Harvard
Medical School, Boston,
Massachusetts

WILLIAM B. MORRISON, MD
Chief, Division of Musculoskeletal Imaging,
Department of Radiology, Jefferson Medical
College, Thomas Jefferson University,
Philadelphia, Pennsylvania

CAIO NERY, MD
Department of Orthopedics and Traumatology,
UNIFESP - Federal University of São Paulo,
Albert Einstein Jewish Hospital, São Paulo,
Brazil

JOEL S. NEWMAN, MD
Staff Radiologist, Department of Radiology,
New England Baptist Hospital, Clinical
Professor, Tufts University School of Medicine,
Boston, Massachusetts

PHILIP ROBINSON, MBChB, MRCP, FRCR
Musculoskeletal Centre X-Ray Department,
Chapel Allerton Hospital, Leeds, United
Kingdom

ZEHAVA SADKA ROSENBERG, MD
Professor of Radiology and Orthopedic
Surgery, Department of Radiology, New York
University School of Medicine, New York
University Hospital for Joint Diseases,
New York, New York

THUMANOON RUANGCHAIJATUPORN, MD
Faculty of Medicine, Department of Diagnostic
and Therapeutic Radiology, Faculty of
Medicine, Ramathibodi Hospital, Mahidol
University, Rachathewi, Bangkok, Thailand

EDWARD SELLON, MBBS, MRCS, FRCR
Musculoskeletal Centre X-Ray Department,
Chapel Allerton Hospital, Leeds, United
Kingdom

CAROLYN M. SOFKA, MD, FACR
Associate Attending Radiologist, Department
of Radiology and Imaging, Hospital for Special
Surgery, Associate Professor of Radiology,
Weill Cornell Medical College, New York,
New York

MONICA TAFUR, MD
Clinical Fellow, Joint Department of Medical
Imaging, University of Toronto, Toronto,
Ontario, Canada

MARTIN TORRIANI, MD, MMSc
Division of Musculoskeletal Imaging and
Intervention, Department of Radiology,
Massachusetts General Hospital, Harvard
Medical School, Boston, Massachusetts

HILARY UMANS, MD
Albert Einstein College of Medicine, Lenox Hill
Radiology, Imaging and Associates, Bronx,
New York

JIM S. WU, MD
Section Chief, Musculoskeletal Imaging and
Intervention, Department of Radiology, Beth
Israel Deaconess Medical Center, Assistant
Professor, Harvard Medical School, Boston,
Massachusetts

ANDRÉ F. YAMADA, MD
Department of Diagnostic Imaging,
UNIFESP - Federal University of São Paulo,
Department of Radiology, Hospital do
Coração – Hcor, São Paulo, São Paulo, Brazil

ADAM C. ZOGA, MD
Director of Musculoskeletal MRI, Vice Chair
of Radiology for Clinical Practice, Division of
Musculoskeletal Imaging, Department of
Radiology, Jefferson Medical College, Thomas
Jefferson University, Philadelphia,
Pennsylvania

Contents

> There are many challenges involved in obtaining diagnostic MR images of the foot and ankle. The complex anatomy and morphology, with curved and angular structures localized to the periphery of the body, make for an inherent challenge, let alone if an added level of complexity, such as orthopedic instrumentation, is added. This review outlines the technical considerations best designed to produce diagnostic images of the foot and ankle, with an emphasis on the postoperative state, including imaging in the presence of metal.

> Accessory muscles around the ankle are commonly encountered as incidental findings on cross-sectional imaging. Mostly asymptomatic, accessory muscles sometimes mimic mass lesions. They have been implicated as the cause of tarsal tunnel syndrome, impingement of surrounding structures, and chronic pain. Distinguishing these muscles can be challenging, because some travel along a similar path. This article describes these accessory muscles in detail, including their relationships to the aponeurosis of the lower leg. An imaging algorithm is proposed to aid in identification of these muscles, providing a valuable tool in diagnostic accuracy and subsequent patient management.

> MR imaging is ideally suited for characterization of the soft tissue, cartilaginous, and osseous structures of the pediatric ankle. An understanding of the normal MR imaging appearance associated with the dynamic skeletal maturation process will prevent overdiagnosis and unnecessary treatment. In this article, we review the normal MR imaging appearance of the growing ankle as well as several disease processes unique to the pediatric population.

> Acute and chronic ankle inversion injuries are a common source of pain and a diagnostic challenge. Several studies have shown a variety of injury patterns after inversion injury both in acute and chronic settings. Although traditional assessment with

clinical examination and radiographs is generally accepted for inversion injuries, MR imaging is a useful tool to detect occult injuries and in patients with chronic symptoms. This article examines a range of MR imaging findings that may be present in patients with lateral ankle pain following an acute or chronic inversion injury.

Abnormalities of the medial ligaments and posterior tibial tendon can occur because of acute injury or chronic instability or malalignment. Medial ankle injuries may occur because of pronation or supination–external rotation injuries. Deltoid ligament injuries have a significant impact on lateral ankle instability but can be overlooked in patients with lateral ligament injuries. Posterior tibial tendon dysfunction is usually associated with spring ligament or flexor retinaculum injury. Tarsal tunnel syndrome, accessory flexor muscles, and subtalar coalition should be considered as well as ligament and tendon tears in differential diagnosis of chronic medial ankle pain.

Heel pain is common and due to a variety of osseous and soft tissue disorders. Causes of heel pain can be classified by the anatomic structure in which they arise and include disorders of the (1) Achilles tendon, (2) plantar fascia, (3) calcaneus, (4) bursae, (5) nerves in the hindfoot, (6) and heel pad. Although careful history taking and physical examination are important, imaging plays a vital role in the diagnosis and management of heel pain. MR imaging is the best imaging test to assess pain in the heel. This review discusses the common causes of heel pain, focusing on MR imaging appearances.

Following a brief description of the normal anatomy and biomechanics of the midfoot, this article focuses on MR imaging features of common osseous, tendon, and ligament abnormalities that affect the midfoot. Discussion of the anatomy and pathology affecting the Chopart and Lisfranc joint complexes, both of which play important roles in linking the midfoot to the hindfoot and the forefoot respectively, is also included.

The metatarsophalangeal (MTP) joint complex is a weight-bearing structure important to the biomechanics of the standing position, walking, shoe wearing, and sport participation. Acute dorsiflexion injury of the first MTP joint, "turf toe," is common among American football and soccer players. The first and lesser MTP joint complexes can be affected by degenerative or inflammatory arthritis, infarct, and infection. These conditions can lead to plantar plate disruption. Imaging studies help physicians to properly diagnose and treat this condition. This article reviews the anatomy, diagnostic imaging, and clinical management of injury and pathology of the first and lesser MTP joint complexes.

Impingement is a clinical syndrome of chronic pain and restricted range of movement caused by compression of abnormal bone or soft tissue within the ankle joint. It usually occurs following a sprain injury or repetitive microtrauma causing haemorrhage, synovial hyperplasia, and abnormal soft tissue interposition within the joint. MR imaging is particularly valuable in being able to detect not only the soft tissue and osseous abnormalities involved in these syndromes, but also a wide variety of other potential causes of ankle pain and instability that also may need to be addressed clinically.

Soft tissue masses may be encountered in the foot and ankle and may represent true neoplasms, malignant or benign, or other, nonneoplastic entities that mimic musculoskeletal tumors. This article reviews common soft tissue masses encountered in the foot or ankle, highlights their MR imaging appearance, and outlines common pitfalls. Technical considerations for imaging soft tissue masses in the foot and ankle are discussed. On MR imaging, T1-weighted and T2-weighted signal intensity, contrast enhancement characteristics, and lesion location, together with patient demographics, history and physical examination, and findings on radiographs, can be useful in characterizing masses in the foot and ankle.

Abnormalities of the peripheral nervous, vascular, and immune systems contribute to the development of numerous foot and ankle pathologies in the diabetic population. Although radiographs remain the most practical first-line imaging tool, magnetic resonance (MR) is the tertiary imaging modality of choice, allowing for optimal assessment of bone and soft tissue abnormalities. MR allows for the accurate distinction between osteomyelitis/septic arthritis and neuropathic osteoarthropathy. Furthermore, it provides an excellent presurgical anatomic road map of involved tissues and devitalized skin to ensure successful limited amputations when required. Signal abnormality in the postoperative foot aids in the diagnosis of recurrent infection.

MR imaging has an important role in the evaluation of the postoperative foot and ankle. In this article, a variety of operative techniques and postoperative findings in the foot and ankle are described, including tendon and ligament reconstruction, as well as the treatment of tarsal coalition and Morton neuroma. The role of MR imaging in the assessment of complications of foot and ankle surgery is also detailed.

Foot and ankle disorders are common in everyday clinical practice. MR imaging is frequently required for diagnosis given the variety and complexity of foot and ankle anatomy. Although conventional MR imaging plays a significant role in diagnosis, contemporary management increasingly relies on advanced imaging for monitoring therapeutic response. There is an expanding need for identification of biomarkers for musculoskeletal tissues. Advanced imaging techniques capable of imaging these tissue substrates will be increasingly used in routine clinical practice. Radiologists should therefore become familiar with these innovative MR techniques. Many such techniques are already widely used in other organ systems.

MAGNETIC RESONANCE IMAGING CLINICS OF NORTH AMERICA

ISSUE OF RELATED INTEREST

Radiologic Clinics of North America, September 2016 (Vol. 54, No. 5)
Imaging of the Athlete
Adam C. Zoga and Johannes B. Roedl, *Editors*
Available at: www.radiologic.theclinics.com

VISIT THE CLINICS ONLINE!
Access your subscription at:
www.theclinics.com

PROGRAM OBJECTIVE
The goal of Magnetic Resonance Imaging Clinics of North America is to keep practicing physicians up to date with current clinical practice by providing timely articles reviewing the state of the art in patient care.

TARGET AUDIENCE
All practicing physicians and healthcare professionals who provide patient care utilizing findings from Magnetic Resonance Imaging.

LEARNING OBJECTIVES
Upon completion of this activity, participants will be able to:
1. Review best practices and normal variants in MR imaging of the foot and ankle.
2. Discuss MR imaging of common injuries such as Turf Toe, Lisfranc injuries, and impingement, among others.
3. Recognize new techniques in MR imaging of the foot and ankle, as well as pediatric considerations.

ACCREDITATION
The Elsevier Office of Continuing Medical Education (EOCME) is accredited by the Accreditation Council for Continuing Medical Education (ACCME) to provide continuing medical education for physicians.

The EOCME designates this enduring material for a maximum of 15 *AMA PRA Category 1 Credit*(s)™. Physicians should claim only the credit commensurate with the extent of their participation in the activity.

All other health care professionals requesting continuing education credit for this enduring material will be issued a certificate of participation.

DISCLOSURE OF CONFLICTS OF INTEREST
The EOCME assesses conflict of interest with its instructors, faculty, planners, and other individuals who are in a position to control the content of CME activities. All relevant conflicts of interest that are identified are thoroughly vetted by EOCME for fair balance, scientific objectivity, and patient care recommendations. EOCME is committed to providing its learners with CME activities that promote improvements or quality in healthcare and not a specific proprietary business or a commercial interest.

The planning committee, staff, authors and editors listed below have identified no financial relationships or relationships to products or devices they or their spouse/life partner have with commercial interest related to the content of this CME activity:
Won C. Bae, PhD; Daniel Baufield, MD; Jenny T. Bencardino, MD; Ching-Di Chang, MD; Yvonne Cheung, MD, MS; Christine B. Chung, MD; Julia Crim, MD; Kirsten Ecklund, MD; Anjali Fortna; Jeffrey Kaye, MD; Grace Mang Yuet Ma, MD; Samuel D. Madoff, MD; Edgar Leonardo Martinez-Salazar, MD; Eoghan McCarthy, MD; Timothy M. Meehan, MD; William B. Morrison, MD; Caio Nery, MD; Joel S. Newman, MD; Philip Robinson, MBChB, MRCP, FRCR; Zehava Sadka Rosenberg, MD; Thumanoon Ruangchaijatuporn, MD; Edward Sellon, MBBS, MRCS, FRCR; Carolyn M. Sofka, MD, FACR; Lynne S. Steinbach, MD, FACR; Karthik Subramaniam; Megan Suermann; Monica Tafur, MD; Martin Torriani, MD, MMSc; Hillary Umans, MD; John Vassallo; Jim S. Wu, MD; André F. Yamada, MD; Adam C. Zoga, MD.

The planning committee, staff, authors and editors listed below have identified financial relationships or relationships to products or devices they or their spouse/life partner have with commercial interest related to the content of this CME activity:
Mary G. Hochman, MD, MBA has stock ownership in General Electric and Nomir Medical Technologies.

UNAPPROVED/OFF-LABEL USE DISCLOSURE
The EOCME requires CME faculty to disclose to the participants:
1. When products or procedures being discussed are off-label, unlabelled, experimental, and/or investigational (not US Food and Drug Administration [FDA] approved); and
2. Any limitations on the information presented, such as data that are preliminary or that represent ongoing research, interim analyses, and/or unsupported opinions. Faculty may discuss information about pharmaceutical agents that is outside of FDA-approved labelling. This information is intended solely for CME and is not intended to promote off-label use of these medications. If you have any questions, contact the medical affairs department of the manufacturer for the most recent prescribing information.

TO ENROLL
To enroll in the *Magnetic Resonance Imaging Clinics of North America* Continuing Medical Education program, call customer service at 1-800-654-2452 or sign up online at http://www.theclinics.com/home/cme. The CME program is available to subscribers for an additional annual fee of USD 250.

METHOD OF PARTICIPATION

In order to claim credit, participants must complete the following:

1. Complete enrolment as indicated above.
2. Read the activity.
3. Complete the CME Test and Evaluation. Participants must achieve a score of 70% on the test. All CME Tests and Evaluations must be completed online.

CME INQUIRIES/SPECIAL NEEDS

For all CME inquiries or special needs, please contact elsevierCME@elsevier.com.

Foreword

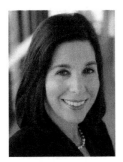

Lynne S. Steinbach, MD, FACR
Consulting Editor

It is with great pride that I introduce this issue of *Magnetic Resonance Imaging Clinics of North America*. I asked the well-respected Dr Mary Hochman from Beth Israel Deaconess Medical Center, Boston to edit this issue and am so pleased with her organization of topics, her choice of authors, and the final product. This work includes articles by the top authorities in the field, bringing the reader up-to-date on MR imaging of the foot and ankle. Many of the authors are world authorities on the subjects that they discuss with multiple peer-reviewed papers and prior books on their subjects, bringing additional updated information to the year 2017. High-quality images and diagrams make it easier for the radiologist to reference and remember these entities.

Specifically, the reader will get information about current technical considerations from Carolyn Sofka, a professor at Hospital for Special Surgery, known for its high-resolution imaging protocols that are provided in table format. Yvonne Cheung from Dartmouth-Hitchcock Medical Center, an author of often-cited articles on accessory muscles, summates this topic with a review of their anatomy and associated problems. Pediatric ankle and foot problems must be differentiated from normal findings, of which there are many variants and mimickers. Grace Ma and Kirsten Ecklund from Ohio State University and Boston Children's Hospital, respectively, elucidate these findings. Timothy Meehan, Edgard Martinez-Salazar, and Martin Torriani from Massachusetts General Hospital show the spectrum of MR findings following ankle inversion injuries, including ligamentous, tendinous, and osseous. Julia Crim, also an author of many books and articles on foot and ankle, currently at the University of Missouri, reviews the normal anatomy and abnormalities that occur on the medial side of the ankle, including deltoid and spring ligament, posterior tibial tendon, tarsal tunnel, and tarsal coalition. Ching-Di Chang from Kaohsiung Chang Gung Hospital in Taiwan and Jim Wu from Beth Israel Deaconess Medical Center, Boston give a synopsis of the various causes and MR findings of heel pain, including disorders of the Achilles tendon, plantar fascia, calcaneus, and some of the neuropathies associated with pain in this area. The well-respected team of Monica Tafur, Zehava Rosenberg, and Jenny Bencardino from New York University discuss MR imaging of the midfoot and disorders that occur at the Chopart and Lisfranc joints. A multinational team of Hilary Umans from Albert Einstein College of Medicine and Lenox Hill Radiology (whom I call the Queen of the Plantar Plate), and Brazilian radiologist, Andrew Yamada, and orthopedic surgeons, Caio Nery and Daniel Baumfeld, elucidate the MR findings and significance of plantar plate disorders, a difficult diagnosis for many radiologists. The group from Chapel Allerton Hospital in Leeds, United Kingdom, which includes Edward Sellon and Philip Robinson, an author of several well-received articles on ankle impingement, discuss impingement and entrapment syndromes of the foot and ankle. Mary Hochman, editor of this issue, and her colleague, Jim Wu, are coauthors of a previous comprehensive review article on musculoskeletal soft tissue tumors. In this volume, they are updating us with a compendium of soft tissue masses in the foot and ankle, many of which are "Aunt Minnies." Adam Zoga and members of his group from Thomas Jefferson University, including William Morrison and Eoghan McCarthy, review the diabetic foot, with an excellent discussion of technical considerations, various findings, and ways to distinguish neuropathic arthropathy and

Magn Reson Imaging Clin N Am 25 (2017) xv–xvi
http://dx.doi.org/10.1016/j.mric.2016.09.005
1064-9689/17/© 2016 Published by Elsevier Inc.

mri.theclinics.com

osteomyelitis. Samuel Madoff and his colleagues from the New England Baptist, including Jeffrey Kaye and Joel Newman, provide the scoop on the much more frequently ordered and challenging area of MR imaging of the postoperative ankle and foot. Last, but not least, the group from UC-San Diego, including Christine Chung, Won Bae, and Thurmanoon Ruangchallatupom, discuss new techniques in MR imaging of the ankle and foot, including their main research focus, ultrashort TE imaging, as well as 3D volume imaging, MR neurography, diffusion-weighted imaging, and newer methods of cartilage evaluation with MR imaging.

Congratulations to our editor and all of the authors for doing an outstanding job on this esteemed issue of *Magnetic Resonance Imaging Clinics of North America*!

Lynne S. Steinbach, MD, FACR
Department of Radiology and Biomedical Imaging
University of California–San Francisco
Box 0628, 505 Parnassus, Suite M392
San Francisco, CA 94143, USA

E-mail address:
lynne.steinbach@ucsf.edu

Preface

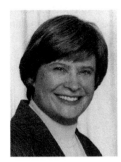

Mary G. Hochman, MD, MBA
Editor

The most recent prior issue of *Magnetic Resonance Imaging Clinics of North America* to address MR imaging of the foot and ankle was published in February 2008. Since that time, our understanding of the MR imaging presentation of anatomy and pathology in the foot and ankle has advanced, new MR imaging technology and techniques have been introduced, and the clinical role of MR imaging of the foot and ankle has expanded. The goal of this issue is to provide a well-illustrated overview of MR imaging of the foot and ankle, including both an accessible introduction for imagers new to the topic and a relevant and timely update for more experienced imagers.

Injuries to the foot and ankle are common, affecting a broad spectrum of patients, and have the potential to be highly debilitating. At the same time, clinicians increasingly recognize the utility of MR imaging for evaluating the symptomatic foot and ankle and are relying more heavily on MR imaging for their clinical problem solving. To meet this need, imagers must have a thorough understanding of the normal and abnormal MR appearance of the foot and ankle and of the clinical context for the imaging findings.

In order to yield accurate diagnoses, MR images must be of high quality, and MR imaging in the foot and ankle presents some special challenges, in both the native foot and ankle and the postoperative setting. To that end, this monograph includes an introductory article on best practice techniques for imaging of the foot and ankle, including a discussion of newer techniques for metal artifact reduction.

Because MR imaging exams are often obtained for especially challenging cases, often without detailed clinical history or provisional clinical diagnoses, a number of the articles here are designed around a regional approach, to aid in the workup of patients who present with pain in a given region, not otherwise specified. Thus, individual articles examine the lateral ankle, including the spectrum of injuries that might be seen following a lateral ankle sprain; the medial ankle, including the deltoid ligaments and other medial-sided structures; hindfoot pain and the imaging features of various abnormalities that give rise to it; the midfoot, an important area that only more recently has gained its deserved attention; and forefoot pain, with a focus on injuries of the plantar plate of the great and lesser MTP joints. For each region, normal anatomy is reviewed; differential causes of regional pain are discussed, and their MR appearance is illustrated.

Several other articles address topics of special interest in the foot and ankle. One article on normal variant accessory muscles is designed to familiarize imagers with these potential pitfalls. Another article describes the normal appearance of the pediatric foot, a topic that can be extremely challenging, even for experienced imagers who are well versed on adult anatomy. Special consideration is given to impingement/entrapment syndromes of the foot and ankle, which can be a source of chronic pain and which rely on an astute imager to appreciate the findings and make the diagnosis. Because soft tissue masses may be encountered either as a presenting symptom or as an incidental finding, one article is dedicated to a review of common benign and malignant masses about the foot and ankle. Given the importance of foot infections as a source of hospital admissions for diabetic patients and the central role MR imaging plays in the workup of infection and neuropathic osteoarthropathy, one article is devoted to MR imaging of pathology of the

Magn Reson Imaging Clin N Am 25 (2017) xvii–xviii
http://dx.doi.org/10.1016/j.mric.2016.09.004
1064-9689/17/© 2016 Published by Elsevier Inc.

diabetic foot. Evaluation of the postoperative foot and ankle can be especially challenging and, thus, one article surveys the various surgical procedures that are performed and demonstrates their imaging appearance. With an eye to the future, a final article addresses new and emerging techniques as they relate to the foot and ankle, to ensure that readers are prepared for future advancements.

In an era when the focus is on the added value being provided by the imager to patient care, in partnership with clinical colleagues, the imager must have a broad and deep understanding of the field and must be able to apply his or her knowledge in a clinically relevant manner in order to facilitate prompt, accurate, and meaningful diagnoses. Moreover, imagers must be prepared to oversee production of diagnostic images and should be prepared to take advantage of new techniques for MR imaging of the foot and ankle.

I hope readers will find this issue a useful resource in their effort to gain a robust and up-to-date understanding of MR imaging of the foot and ankle and to provide effective patient care.

I want to express my deep gratitude to the international experts who generously shared their time, expertise, and love of craft in the preparation of these articles, providing our readers with not only clear and authoritative text, but also remarkable illustrative images. On a personal note, I want to express my sincere thanks to the *Magnetic Resonance Imaging Clinics of North America*'s consulting editors, Drs Suresh Mukherji and Lynne Steinbach, for providing me the opportunity to engage in this endeavor.

Mary G. Hochman, MD, MBA
Musculoskeletal Imaging and Intervention
Department of Radiology
Beth Israel Deaconess Medical Center
Harvard Medical School
330 Brookline Avenue
Boston, MA 02215, USA

E-mail address:
mhochman@bidmc.harvard.edu

Technical Considerations

Best Practices for MR Imaging of the Foot and Ankle

Carolyn M. Sofka, MD

KEYWORDS

- Foot • Ankle • Tendons • Ligaments • Short tau inversion recovery (STIR) • Metal artifact reduction
- Time resolved imaging of contrast kinetics (TRICKS)

KEY POINTS

- MR imaging can be optimized to image the foot and ankle in both the preoperative and the postoperative settings.
- Contrast-enhanced MR angiographic techniques can be used for vascular mapping of the foot and ankle.
- Appropriate MR technique modifications can provide diagnostic image quality even in the setting of metal.

INTRODUCTION

There are many challenges involved in obtaining diagnostic MR images of the foot and ankle. The complex anatomy and morphology, with curved and angular structures localized to the periphery of the body, make for an inherent challenge, let alone if an added level of complexity (orthopedic instrumentation) is added. This review outlines the technical considerations best designed to produce diagnostic images of the foot and ankle, with an emphasis on the postoperative state, including imaging in the presence of metal.

IMAGING THE PREOPERATIVE FOOT AND ANKLE

Non-contrast-enhanced fast spin-echo proton density–weighted sequences have largely become the workhorse in MR imaging of the musculoskeletal system and have been validated against surgical arthroscopic standards.[1–4] A long repetition time (≥3500 milliseconds) and moderate echo time (TE; 28–34 milliseconds) result in differential contrast between articular cartilage and fluid, producing an inherent "arthrographic effect" without the additional complicating diagnostic hindrances that can accompany a direct MR arthrogram (contrast extravasation into the surrounding soft tissues, air bubbles in the joint being confused as intra-articular bodies, and so forth).[5] These standard sequences are used in foot and ankle imaging as well; however, some limitations arise due to the curved anatomy and morphology of structures about the foot and ankle, specifically with regard to ligaments and tendons.

At the author's institution, which mostly sees populations of sports injuries, arthritis, and foot deformities, the default imaging sequences are outlined in **Tables 1–3**. The inherent magnetization transfer properties induced between slices in fast spin-echo, moderate TE imaging, produce relative increased signal intensity from simple fluid. This results in a distinct contrast between higher signal intensity fluid and intermediate signal intensity of articular cartilage, preventing the need to administer

The author has nothing to disclose.
Department of Radiology and Imaging, Hospital for Special Surgery, Weill Cornell Medical College, 535 East 70th Street, New York, NY 10021, USA
E-mail address: sofkac@hss.edu

Magn Reson Imaging Clin N Am 25 (2017) 1–10
http://dx.doi.org/10.1016/j.mric.2016.08.001
1064-9689/17/© 2016 Elsevier Inc. All rights reserved.

Table 1
Suggested protocol for imaging the ankle

	Sagittal IR Inversion Time 150	Sagittal PD	Coronal PD	Axial PD
TR	4000	4500	5000	5000
TE	13–15	25	25	24
ST	3.3	3.0	4.0	3.3
ETL	10	12	12	12
FOV	180	150	110	130
Matrix	256 × 192	512 × 384	512 × 384	512 × 256
NEX	2	2	2	2

Abbreviations: ETL, echo train length; IR, inversion recovery; NEX, number of excitations; PD, proton density; ST, slice thickness (mm); TR, repetition time (ms).

intra-articular or intravenous contrast material for routine anatomic imaging. This noninvasive approach, combined with dedicated surface coils, works to provide optimum image quality[5] (**Fig. 1**).

Dedicated surface coils help to improve spatial resolution and field homogeneity, notably when imaging smaller structures such as the foot and ankle.[6] Either a quadrature (circular polarization) knee coil or an 8-channel phased array dedicated foot and ankle coil are suggested to achieve adequate signal to noise. Images are typically obtained with the foot in neutral position, without excessive dorsiflexion or plantarflexion, although some authors have proposed imaging the foot and ankle in positions that may maximally stress regional tendons and ligaments, such as ballet dancers en pointe, in weight-bearing maximum plantar flexion.[7] Kinematic MR examination has also been explored for the evaluation of ankle ligament integrity.[8]

The magic angle effect, often noted in MR interpretation of the rotator cuff of the shoulder, can contribute to a degree of uncertainty when interpreting images of the foot and ankle, and it is always critical to keep this phenomenon in mind when analyzing the status of ligaments and tendons. The magic angle effect is a phenomenon of MR physics and accounts for signal changes that can be seen in anisotropic tissues, including the ordered collagen bundles that comprise tendons.[9,10] It occurs when the collagen bundle orientation is 55° to the main magnetic field (z-axis). The artifact mimics tendon degeneration in that it is visible on sequences with short TEs such as the T1- and proton density–weighted sequences used commonly when imaging the musculoskeletal system,[11–17] but becomes less apparent on MR sequences with longer TE values (>37 milliseconds) such as T2-weighted and short tau inversion recovery (STIR) images.[9,13,17] When the tendon is oriented at approximately 55° to the main magnetic field, the artifact will be visible in all imaging planes. At the author's institution, we have subjectively found that the addition of axial STIR images positively contributes to the diagnostic interpretation of the status of ankle tendons, and this finding has been independently validated by Srikhum and colleagues.[18] Other ways to minimize

Table 2
Suggested protocol for imaging the midfoot

	Coronal IR Inversion Time 150	Coronal PD	Axial PD	Sagittal PD
TR	4500	4500	4500	5000
TE	16	27	26	25
ST	3.0	2.0	3.0	4.0
ETL	12	14	18	14
FOV	160	150	110	160
Matrix	256 × 192	512 × 320	512 × 320	512 × 256
NEX	2	2	2	2

From approximately the mid subtalar joint to the proximal metatarsals.
Coronal, parallel to the bottom of the foot; Axial, transverse to the longitudinal arch of the foot.

Table 3
Suggested protocol for imaging the forefoot

	Coronal IR Inversion Time 170	Coronal PD	Axial PD	Sagittal PD Lesser Toes	Sagittal PD Hallux
TR	6200	5500	6700	4100	6100
TE	18	25	25	25	25
ST	2.5	2.0	2.8	2.5	1.2
ETL	12	12	16	14	12
FOV	160	120	120	140	140
Matrix	256 × 192	512 × 384	512 × 384	512 × 384	512 × 256
NEX	1	1	1	1	1

From approximately the naviculocuneiform articulation through the toes.
Coronal, parallel to the bottom of the foot; Axial, Transverse to the longitudinal arch of the foot.

this peculiarity include imaging the foot in slight (20°) plantar flexion.[11]

STIR imaging to evaluate for areas of bone marrow edema pattern in the ankle is suggested, especially when contrasted with frequency selective fat-suppressed (usually T2) weighted images. The curved nature of the structures about the foot and ankle combined with the location of the foot and ankle at the periphery of the bore of the magnet, away from isocenter, results in inherent magnetic field inhomogeneities, which become accentuated when using frequency selective fat suppression as opposed to STIR imaging, certainly in the presence of metal.

Obtaining images in the standard 3 planes: axial, sagittal, and coronal, is usually satisfactory for diagnosing most abnormalities about the foot and ankle; however, "coronal" images of the ankle are often somewhat angled, obtained at a plane parallel to the talonavicular joint to optimize visualization of the slightly obliquely oriented major ankle ligamentous stabilizers. This provides a satisfactory plane of imaging for most abnormalities; however, it can often incompletely demonstrate intra-articular abnormality such as an osteochondral lesion (osteochondral fracture, osteochondritis dissecans). In such cases, a true "straight" coronal parallel to the ankle joint (long axis of the tibia) is preferred for more detailed evaluation (**Fig. 2**).

For optimal imaging in the foot, consideration must be paid to targeted fields of view and tailored imaging planes. Moreover, terminology for imaging planes in the foot often varies from institution to institution. In many institutions, planes in the foot are prescribed with respect to the foot itself, with axial oriented perpendicular to the sole of the foot (short axis) and coronal images oriented parallel to the sole of the foot (long axis). In other institutions, planes are prescribed with respect to the body, with axial images oriented both axial to the body and parallel to the sole of the foot, and with coronal images oriented both coronal to the

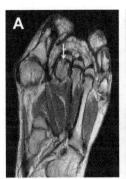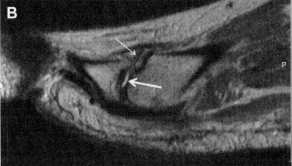

Fig. 1. (*A*) Coronal fast spin-echo (field of view, FOV, 160 mm, 2.0-mm slice thickness) proton density–weighted image of the forefoot demonstrates an acute chondral shearing injury over the second metatarsal head with full-thickness chondral loss (*arrow*). (*B*) Thin sagittal fast spin-echo (FOV 140 mm, 1.5-mm slice thickness) proton density–weighted image of the second toe in the same patient demonstrates the site of the focal chondral shearing injury (*thick arrow*) as well as the displaced chondral fragment in the dorsal joint recess (*thin arrow*).

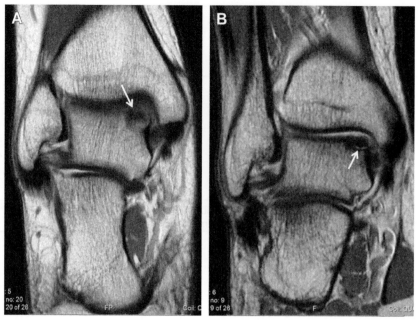

Fig. 2. (A) Oblique coronal fast spin-echo MR image of the ankle (FOV, 110 mm, 4.0-mm slice thickness) obtained at a plane parallel to the talonavicular joint demonstrates an osteochondral lesion of the medial talar dome (*arrow*); however, the detailed morphology of the lesion is unclear. (B) Straight coronal fast spin-echo MR image of the ankle in the same patient (FOV 140 mm, 2.0-mm slice thickness) obtained at a plane directly parallel to the ankle joint more clearly depicts the morphology of the lesion with a partially loose in situ necrotic fragment (*arrow*).

body and perpendicular to the sole of the foot. Imaging of the foot is often optimized by focusing on a specific portion of the foot, that is, the ankle/hindfoot, midfoot, or forefoot (see **Tables 1–3**). This facilitates smaller fields of view and high spatial resolution imaging of the area of interest. In addition, it provides the opportunity to tailor imaging planes to anatomy of interest.[19] For example, images in the hindfoot can be oriented to the subtalar joint; images in the midfoot can be oriented to the tarsometatarsal joints and metatarsal bones, and images of the forefoot can be oriented to the metatarsal heads or metatarsophalangeal joints. When necessary, oblique sagittal images can be oriented along a specific ray of interest. Techniques for imaging for Morton neuroma, with the patient in the prone position, have also been described.[20]

Nowadays, most imaging centers have a choice of 1.5-T and 3.0-T magnets. MR imaging at 3.0 T results in nearly twice the signal-to-noise ratio (SNR) compared with 1.5 T, usually accompanied by concomitant advantages of improved gradient performance and wider bandwidths.[21] Overall, imaging at 3.0 T results in higher spatial resolution and increased contrast-to-noise ratios, usually with significant decreases in scanning time when combined with software that results in higher acceleration factors (parallel acquisition techniques).[21,22] Slight modifications of imaging parameters are required, however, when translating protocols from 1.5 T to 3.0 T, as T1- and T2-relaxation times are slightly different at the differing field strengths.

Additional MR sequences can be tailored to the specific clinical question. Gradient echo imaging, for example can be of use in certain specific diagnostic considerations. In children, 3-dimensional spoiled gradient echo imaging with fat suppression (3D-SPGR) has been shown to depict the morphology of the regional physes accurately and should be used (ideally in 2 planes, usually sagittal and coronal) to evaluate the integrity of the physes (physeal bars) in the setting of pediatric ankle fractures.[23–25] In addition, T2*W multiplanar gradient echo imaging (MPGR) demonstrates significant "blooming" artifact in the setting of pigmented villonodular synovitis (PVNS), thus contributing to making this diagnosis[26,27] (**Fig. 3**).

MAGNETIC RESONANCE ANGIOGRAPHY

Vascular mapping of the foot and ankle is often required, commonly in presurgical tumor removal planning or possibly if limb salvage is being considered in the setting of a traumatically

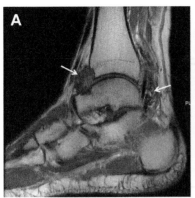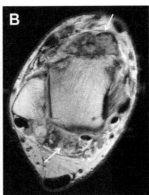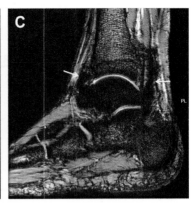

Fig. 3. Sagittal (*A*) (FOV, 160 mm, 3.5-mm slice thickness) and axial (*B*) (FOV, 140 mm, 3.5-mm slice thickness) fast spin-echo proton density–weighted images demonstrate heterogeneous nodular mass lesions in both the anterior and the posterior ankle joint recesses (*arrows*). Sagittal T2*-weighted MPGR image (*C*) (FOV, 160 mm, 3.0-mm slice thickness) demonstrates significant regional "blooming" artifact (*arrows*) corresponding to the areas identified on the fast spin-echo images, consistent with deposits of PVNS.

mangled limb. The location of the foot, away from the isocenter of the bore of the magnet, combined with its location at the periphery of the body, can make obtaining diagnostic MR angiographic images difficult. Some of the earliest developed MR angiographic sequences were non-contrast-enhanced techniques that relied on flow-related parameters such as systolic/diastolic phase differences and inflow and outflow phenomena.[28–31] Later, contrast-enhanced MR angiographic imaging was developed, with enhancement of T1 contrast parameters, largely relying on bolus timing.[32–34] There was a need, however, to improve both spatial and temporal resolution while maintaining SNR.[35] The advent of parallel imaging with high acceleration factors contributed to faster and more reliable MR angiographic techniques.[36] In the late 1990s, rapid imaging sequences based on keyhole techniques, wherein the central portion of *k*-space is sampled more frequently than the peripheral regions and the timeframes are interleaved, were developed.[37] These techniques (with proprietary names such as time resolved imaging of contrast kinetics or TRICKS, TWIST, TRAQ, 4DTRAK, and Freeze) can produce fast, high-resolution images that have greatly facilitated diagnostic MR angiography of the foot and ankle. Most original applications were implemented on standard 1.5-T units; however, advanced MR contrast-enhanced angiographic techniques can be applied to higher magnetic field strengths. The increased spatial and temporal resolution at 3.0 T as well as the increased contrast-to-noise ratio resulting from the accentuated T1 shortening effects of gadolinium contrast material at 3.0 T has resulted in improved diagnostic contrast-enhanced vascular imaging at higher field strengths with shortened imaging acquisition time.[21,22]

IMAGING THE POSTOPERATIVE FOOT AND ANKLE

The postoperative setting provides additional and different challenges for MR imaging of the foot and ankle. The presence of metal, whether from an open reduction internal fixation of an ankle fracture, realignment of adult acquired flatfoot deformity, or a total ankle arthroplasty, presents a serious challenge to the radiologist in obtaining diagnostic images.

Artifact caused by metal, such as that associated with orthopedic hardware, is based on differences in magnetic susceptibilities of the metal and the surrounding tissues. These differences in susceptibilities cause distortion of the local static magnetic field surrounding the metal, which varies with type of metal and its size, shape, and orientation in the magnetic field. Because the precessional frequency of protons depends on the magnetic field they experience, local variations in the field will cause localized variations in the protons' precessional frequencies. This results in accelerated T2* dephasing with resultant loss of signal, and, because precessional frequency serves as a surrogate for spatial localization in MR imaging, it also causes mismapping of the measured MR signal. The resultant metallic susceptibility artifact distorts the appearance of the surrounding soft tissues, with focal signal voids and also with focal areas of high signal attributed to "piling up" of mismapped signal. These same frequency variations interfere with effective frequency-selective fat saturation, making inversion recovery-based fat

Table 4
Suggested protocol for imaging the ankle with instrumentation

	Sagittal MAVRIC IR	Sagittal PD	Coronal PD	Axial PD
TR	4900	4100	5300	6900
TE	6	23	19	24
ST	3.0	3.0	4.0	3.3
ETL	24	18	18	21
FOV	260	200	150	160
Matrix	256 × 192	512 × 52	512 × 352	512 × 224
NEX	0.5	3	2	3

saturation (eg, STIR) a more robust option in this setting.[38,39]

Many of the same principles used in the preoperative setting also apply to postoperative imaging (a suggested imaging protocol can be found in **Table 4**). The STIR sequence remains the key "water-sensitive" pulse sequence to evaluate for areas of bone marrow edema pattern (fractures and so forth), because it is less susceptible to magnetic field inhomogeneities. For more detailed anatomic and morphologic analysis, fast spin-echo proton density–weighted sequences with long echo train lengths and shortened interecho spacing, should be used.[40,41] Short interecho spacing results in less time for dephasing to occur; this, combined with increasing echo train length, results in decreased frequency of mismapping and less image distortion[42–44] (**Fig. 4**). Last, increasing the frequency of the readout bandwidth can help to decrease overall artifact by increasing the strength of the readout gradient.[45,46]

Main magnetic field strength also will have an effect on the degree of artifact encountered: although many think that "bigger is better," in the postoperative setting, metal artifact is accentuated at higher field strengths (eg, 3.0 T), compared with conventional 1.5 T.

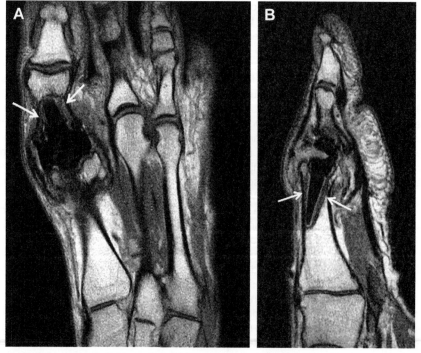

Fig. 4. Coronal (*A*) (FOV, 120 mm, 2.0-mm slice thickness) and sagittal (*B*) (FOV, 150 mm, 1.2-mm slice thickness) proton density fast spin-echo MR images optimized for metal demonstrates significant implant reaction and synovitis (*arrows*) surrounding a first metatarsophalangeal joint prosthesis placed 2 years before.

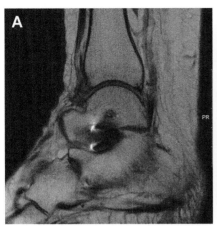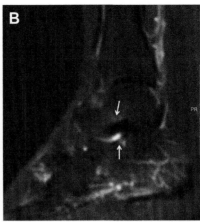

Fig. 5. (*A*) Sagittal proton density–weighted MR image in a patient with a subtalar arthrodesis implant (FOV, 170 mm, 3.0-mm slice thickness) demonstrates moderate flare artifact surrounding the implant obscuring the immediate surrounding tissues. (*B*) Sagittal composite MAVRIC inversion recovery image (FOV, 210 mm, 3.5-mm slice thickness) demonstrates reduced flare artifact about the subtalar arthrodesis implant with clearer visualization of its surrounding bone marrow edema pattern and fluid in the subtalar joint (*arrows*).

In addition to STIR and fast spin-echo proton density–weighted sequences, specific metal artifact reduction sequences are now available on most vendor platforms to aid in reducing the flare artifact around metal thus providing better image quality. These include techniques such as view angle tilting (VAT), multiacquisition variable-resonance image combination (MAVRIC), and slice encoding metal artifact correction (SEMAC).[47] Lu and colleagues[48] described the use of the slice encoding for SEMAC technique, which corrects artifacts by enhanced encoding of individual excited slices by using a VAT spin-echo sequence with additional z-phase encoding; the latter ensures improved visualization through decreased in-plane distortion. The MAVRIC technique has been validated largely in the setting of hip and knee arthroplasty to improve evaluation of the metal-bone interface, specifically in the setting of osteolysis, and can be applied to routine clinical MR imaging hardware.[49–51] MAVRIC works to decrease image artifacts by combining multiple individually acquired data sets at frequencies slightly offset from the dominant proton frequency.[52–55] A complementary technique to routine fast spin-echo imaging, MAVRIC can be useful when imaging around total ankle arthroplasty (**Fig. 5**).

ADDITIONAL CONSIDERATIONS

Additional specialized cartilage sequences can be applied to evaluate the foot and ankle, often in a research setting. T2 mapping takes advantage of differential T2 values of free water and collagen orientation to provide a semiquantitative evaluation of the status of the articular cartilage, often in the setting of evaluating the reparative cartilage scaffold after a cartilage restorative procedure, such as microfracture or osteochondral autograft transfer system.[56–59] T1 rho relaxation time measurements can be used in conjunction with routine spin-echo or fast spin-echo imaging and can help quantify areas of cartilage softening, with values increasing with loss of proteoglycan (glycosaminoglycan) content from the cartilaginous extracellular matrix.[60,61] Last, ultrashort TE sequences can be applied to evaluate the status of the articular cartilage, inclusive of its short T2* components, specifically, the calcified layer, for subclinical evaluation of cartilage degeneration.[62–64]

SUMMARY

In conclusion, MR imaging of the foot and ankle produces a unique set of technical challenges related to imaging small, curved structures located at the periphery of the body and offset from the isocenter of the magnet. Using high-resolution fast spin-echo proton-density imaging in 3 planes with at least one plane of STIR imaging to evaluate for bone marrow edema pattern should be satisfactory and produces diagnostic images in most cases. The postoperative setting is more complicated, however, using fast spin-echo proton density–weighted images with shortened interecho spacing, and using STIR imaging with inversion recovery fat suppression, as opposed to frequency selective fat suppression, which is more susceptible to local field inhomogeneities, will help to reduce the characteristic flare artifact, which can limit diagnostic interpretation. Additional sequences, such as MPGR, 3D-SPGR with fat suppression, and MR angiographic techniques, can also be used, tailored to answering specific clinical questions.

REFERENCES

1. Gusmer PB, Potter HG, Schatz J, et al. Labral injuries: accuracy of detection with unenhanced MR imaging of the shoulder. Radiology 1996;200:519–24.

2. Connell DA, Potter HG, Wickiewicz TL, et al. High resolution magnetic resonance imaging of superior labral pathology: 102 surgically-confirmed cases. Am J Sports Med 1999;27(2):208–13.

3. Magee TH, Williams D. Sensitivity and specificity in detection of labral tears with 3.0-T MRI of the shoulder. AJR Am J Roentgenol 2006;187:1448–52.

4. Mintz DN, Hooper TR, Connell DA, et al. Magnetic resonance imaging of the hip: detection of labral and chondral abnormalities using non-contrast imaging. Arthroscopy 2005;21(4):385–93.

5. Koff MF, Potter HG. Noncontrast MR techniques and imaging of cartilage. Radiol Clin North Am 2009;47: 495–504.

6. Rivera M, Vaquero JJ, Santos A, et al. MRI visualization of small structures using improved surface coils. Magn Reson Imaging 1998;16(2):157–66.

7. Russell JA, Shave RM, Yoshioka H, et al. Magnetic resonance imaging of the ankle in female ballet dancers en pointe. Acta Radiol 2010;6:655–61.

8. Tokuda O, Awaya H, Taguchi K, et al. Kinematic MRI of the normal ankle ligaments using a specially designed passive positioning device. Foot Ankle Int 2006;27(11):935–42.

9. Erickson SJ, Prost RW, Timins ME. The magic angle effect—background physics and clinical relevance. Radiology 1993;188(1):23–5.

10. Fullerton GD, Rahal A. Collagen structure: the molecular source of the tendon magic angle effect. J Magn Reson Imaging 2007;25(2):345–61.

11. Mengiardi B, Pfirmann CWA, Schöttle PB, et al. Magic angle effect in MR imaging of ankle tendons: influence of foot positioning on prevalence and site in asymptomatic subjects and cadaveric tendons. Eur Radiol 2006;16(10):2197–209.

12. Erickson SJ, Cox IH, Hyde JS, et al. Effect of tendon orientation on MR imaging signal intensity—a manifestation of the magic angle phenomenon. Radiology 1991;181(2):389–92.

13. Peh WCG, Chan JHM. The magic angle phenomenon in tendons: effect of varying the MR echo time. Br J Radiol 1998;71(841):31–6.

14. Fullerton GD, Cameron IL, Ord VA. Orientation of tendons in the magnetic field and its effect on T2 relaxation times. Radiology 1985;155(2):433–5.

15. Li T. Manifestation of magic angle phenomenon: comparative study on effects of varying echo time and tendon orientation among various MR sequences. Magn Reson Imaging 2003;21(7):741–4.

16. Bydder M, Rahal A, Fullerton GD, et al. The magic angle effect: a source of artifact, determinant of image contrast, and technique for imaging. J Magn Reson Imaging 2007;25(2):290–300.

17. Othman MI, Chew KM, Peh WC. Variants and pitfalls in MR imaging of foot and ankle injuries. Semin Musculoskelet Radiol 2014;18:54–62.

18. Srikhum W, Nardo L, Karampinos DC, et al. Magnetic resonance imaging of ankle tendon pathology: benefits of additional axial short-tau inversion recovery imaging to reduce magic angle effects. Skeletal Radiol 2013;42:499–510.

19. Rubin DA, Towers JD, Britton CA. MR imaging of the foot: utility of complex oblique imaging planes. AJR Am J Roentgenol 1996;166:1079–84.

20. Weishaupt D, Treiber K, Kundert HP, et al. Morton neuroma: MR imaging in prone, supine and upright weight-bearing body positions. Radiology 2003; 226(3):849–56.

21. Chhabra A, Soldatos T, Chalian M, et al. Current concepts review: 3T magnetic resonance imaging of the ankle and foot. Foot Ankle Int 2012;33(2): 164–71.

22. Chang KJ, Kamel IR, Macura KJ, et al. 3.0T MR imaging of the abdomen: comparison with 1.5T. Radiographics 2008;28(7):1983–98.

23. Lurie B, Koff MF, Shah P, et al. Three-dimensional magnetic resonance imaging of physeal injury: reliability and clinical utility. J Pediatr Orthop 2014;34: 239–45.

24. Ecklund K, Jaramillo D. Patterns of premature physeal arrest: MR imaging of 111 children. AJR Am J Roentgenol 2002;178:967–72.

25. Sailhan FDR, Chotel F, Guibal A-L, et al. Three-dimensional MR imaging in the assessment of physeal growth arrest. Eur Radiol 2004;14:1600–8.

26. Murphey MD, Rhee JH, Lewis RB, et al. Pigmented villonodular synovitis: radiologic-pathologic correlation. Radiographics 2008;28(5):1493–518.

27. Eckhardt BP, Hernandez RJ. Pigmented villonodular synovitis: MR imaging in pediatric patients. Pediatr Radiol 2004;34(12):943–7.

28. Wedeen VJ, Meuli RA, Edelman RR, et al. Projective imaging of pulsatile flow with magnetic resonance. Science 1985;230:946–8.

29. Gullberg GT, Wehrli FW, Shimikawa A, et al. MR vasculature imaging with a fast gradient focusing pulse sequence and reformatted images from transaxial sections. Radiology 1987;165:241–6.

30. Keller PJ, Drayer BP, Fram EK, et al. MR angiography with two dimensional acquisition and three dimensional display. Radiology 1989;173:527–32.

31. Laub GA, Kaiser WA. MR angiography with gradient motion refocusing. J Comput Assist Tomogr 1988; 12:377–82.

32. Prince MR, Yucel EK, Kaufman JA, et al. Dynamic gadolinium-enhanced three dimensional abdominal

MR arteriography. J Magn Reson Imaging 1993;3:877–81.

33. Foo TK, Saranathan M, Prince MR, et al. Automated detection of bolus arrival and initiation of data acquisition in fast, three-dimensional, gadolinium-enhanced MR angiography. Radiology 1997;203:275–80.

34. Lee VS, Martin DJ, Krinsky GA, et al. Gadolinium-enhanced MR angiography, artifacts and pitfalls. AJR Am J Roentgenol 2000;175:197–205.

35. Grist TM, Mistretta CA, Strother CM, et al. Time-resolved angiography: past, present, and future. J Magn Reson Imaging 2012;36:1273–86.

36. Haider CR, Glockner J, Stanson AW, et al. Peripheral vasculature: high temporal- and spatial-resolution three-dimensional contrast-enhanced MR angiography. Radiology 2009;253:831–43.

37. Korosec FR, Frayne R, Grist TM, et al. Time-resolved contrast-enhanced 3D MR angiography. Magn Reson Med 1996;36:345–51.

38. Hargreaves BA, Worters PW, Pauly KB, et al. Metal induced artifacts in MRI. AJR Am J Roentgenol 2011;197(3):547–55.

39. Lee MJ, Kim S, Lee SA, et al. Overcoming artifacts from metallic orthopedic implants at high-field strength MR imaging and multi-detector CT. Radiographics 2007;27(3):791–803.

40. Zanetti M, Saupe N, Espinosa N. Postoperative MR imaging of the foot and ankle: tendon repair, ligament repair, and Morton's neuroma resection. Semin Musculoskelet Radiol 2010;14(3):357–64.

41. Hilfiker P, Zanetti M, Debatin JF, et al. Fast spin-echo inversion-recovery imaging versus fast T2-weighted spin-echo imaging in bone marrow abnormalities. Invest Radiol 1995;30(2):110–4.

42. Bergin D, Morrison WB. Postoperative imaging of the ankle and foot. Radiol Clin North Am 2006;44:391–406.

43. Sofka C. Post operative magnetic resonance imaging of the foot and ankle. J Magn Reson Imaging 2013;37:556–65.

44. White LM, Kim JK, Mehta M, et al. Complications of total hip arthroplasty: MR imaging—initial experience. Radiology 2000;215:254–62.

45. Harris CA, White LM. Metal artifact reduction in musculoskeletal magnetic resonance imaging. Orthop Clin North Am 2006;37:349–59.

46. Potter HG, Nestor BJ, Sofka CM, et al. Magnetic resonance imaging after total hip arthroplasty: evaluation of periprosthetic soft tissue. J Bone Joint Surg Am 2004;86-A:1947–54.

47. Dillensegar JP, Moliere S, Choquet P, et al. An illustrative review to understand and manage metal-induced artifacts in musculoskeletal MRI: a primer and updates. Skeletal Radiol 2016;45(5):677–88.

48. Lu W, Pauly KB, Gold GE, et al. SEMAC: Slice encoding for metal artifact correction in MRI. Magn Reson Med 2009;62:66–76.

49. Sofka CM, Potter HG. MR imaging of joint arthroplasty. Semin Musculoskelet Radiol 2002;6:79–85.

50. Suh JS, Jeong EK, Shin KH, et al. Minimizing artifacts caused by metallic implants at MR imaging: experimental and clinical studies. AJR Am J Roentgenol 1998;171:1207–13.

51. Hayter C, Koff M, Shah P, et al. MRI after arthroplasty: comparison of MAVRIC and conventional fast spin-echo techniques. AJR Am J Roentgenol 2011;197:W405–11.

52. Koff M, Koch K, Potter HG. Magnetic resonance imaging of periprosthetic tissues in the presence of joint arthroplasty. Stockholm (Sweden): ISMRM; 2010.

53. Koff MF, Shah P, Koch KM, et al. Quantifying image distortion of orthopedic materials in magnetic resonance imaging. J Magn Reson Imaging 2013;38(3):610–8.

54. Koch KM, Lorbiecki JE, Hinks RS, et al. A multispectral three-dimensional acquisition technique for imaging near metal implants. Magn Reson Med 2009;61:381–90.

55. Koch KM, Brau AC, Chen W, et al. Imaging near metal with a MAVRIC-SEMAC hybrid. Magn Reson Med 2011;65:71–82.

56. Apprich S, Trattnig S, Welsch GH, et al. Assessment of articular cartilage repair tissue after matrix-associated autologous chondrocyte-transplantation or the microfracture technique in the ankle joint using diffusion-weighted imaging at 3 Tesla. Osteoarthritis Cartilage 2012;20:703–11.

57. Becher C, Zühlke D, Plaas C, et al. T2-mapping at 3T after microfracture in the treatment of osteochondral defects of the talus at an average follow up of 8 years. Knee Surg Sports Traumatol Arthrosc 2015;23:2406–12.

58. Domayer SE, Apprich S, Stelzeneder D, et al. Cartilage repair of the ankle: first results of T2 mapping at 7.0T after microfracture and matrix associated autologous cartilage transplantation. Osteoarthritis Cartilage 2012;20:829–36.

59. Tao H, Shang X, Lu R, et al. Quantitative magnetic resonance imaging (MRI) evaluation of cartilage repair after microfracture (MF) treatment for adult unstable osteochondritis dissecans (OCD) in the ankle: correlations with clinical outcome. Eur Radiol 2014;24:1758–67.

60. Jungmann PM, Baum T, Bauer JS, et al. Cartilage repair surgery: outcome evaluation by using noninvasive cartilage biomarkers based on quantitative MRI techniques? Biomed Res Int 2014;2014:840170.

61. Li X, Han ET, Ma CB, et al. In vivo 3T spiral imaging based multi-slice T(1rho) mapping of knee cartilage in osteoarthritis. Magn Reson Med 2005;54:929–36.

62. Chang EY, Du J, Chung CB. UTE imaging in the musculoskeletal system. J Magn Reson Imaging 2015;41:870–83.

63. Boyde A, Riggs CM, Bushby AJ, et al. Cartilage damage involving extrusion of mineralisable matrix from the articular calcified cartilage and subchondral bone. Eur Cell Mater 2011;21:470–8.

64. Bae WC, Dwek JR, Znamirowski R, et al. Ultrashort echo time MR imaging of osteochondral junction of the knee at 3T: identification of anatomic structures contributing to signal intensity. Radiology 2010;254:837–45.

Normal Variants
Accessory Muscles About the Ankle

Yvonne Cheung, MD, MS

KEYWORDS

- Accessory muscles • Ankle • Peroneus quartus • Accessory soleus
- Flexor digitorum accessorius longus • Peroneocalcaneus internus • Tibiocalcaneus internus

KEY POINTS

- Accessory muscles are commonly presented as incidental findings on cross-sectional imaging.
- Although most often asymptomatic, accessory muscles sometimes mimic mass lesions, and have been implicated as the cause of tarsal tunnel syndrome, impingement of surrounding structures, and pain related to muscle ischemia. Unless specifically injured, accessory muscles appear isointense to other muscles on all imaging sequences.
- Based on the location of the accessory muscles, including their origins, insertions, and relationships to the aponeurosis of the lower leg, an imaging algorithm is proposed to aid in their identification.

INTRODUCTION

Anatomic variations of muscles around the ankle consist predominantly of extra or accessory muscles. Generally asymptomatic, these supernumerary muscles are discovered incidentally on imaging studies. Accurate diagnosis of the infrequent symptomatic cases, presenting as mass lesions, tarsal tunnel syndromes, chronic ankle pain, or impingement, is important for management. However, distinguishing between these muscles can be challenging, because some travel along a similar path, and others have either similar origins or similar insertions. This article reviews each accessory muscle in detail, including those located lateral and posteromedial to the ankle. Each muscle's origin, insertion, imaging features, and clinical presentations, along with its relationship with the aponeurosis of the lower leg, are described (**Table 1**). In an effort to improve diagnostic accuracy, an imaging algorithm that can be readily applied in daily practice is proposed.

IMAGING OF ACCESSORY MUSCLES

Although the accessory muscles of the ankle can be detected on all cross-sectional imaging modalities, most published reports are of magnetic resonance (MR) imaging studies because of its superior soft tissue contrast. However, MR imaging does have limitations. First, the origins of these muscles may not be included in the field of view of a routine ankle examination. Second, if insertions are small, they can be difficult to separate from surrounding soft tissues. Lateral radiography captures only the accessory soleus and is therefore of limited use.

ACCESSORY MUSCLES IN THE LATERAL ANKLE
Peroneus Quartus

The peroneus quartus (PQ) (**Fig. 1**) refers to the fourth peroneal muscle, after peroneus longus, peroneus brevis, and peroneus tertius. It represents a group of accessory peroneal muscles

Disclosure: The author has nothing to disclose.
Department of Radiology, Dartmouth-Hitchcock Medical Center, One Medical Center Drive, Lebanon, NH 03756, USA
E-mail address: Yvonne.Y.Cheung@hitchcock.org

Magn Reson Imaging Clin N Am 25 (2017) 11–26
http://dx.doi.org/10.1016/j.mric.2016.08.002
1064-9689/17/© 2016 Elsevier Inc. All rights reserved.

Table 1
Summary of accessory muscles around the ankle

	Origin	Course	Insertion	Alternative Name	Relative to Deep Aponeurosis	Notes
Lateral Accessory Muscle						
			Alternative Name of PQ Based on Insertion			
PQ	Posterior surface of the fibula or peroneus longus or peroneus brevis	Travels medial and posterior to the peroneal tendons	Retrotrochlear eminence (most common insertion) Cuboid Peroneus longus Inferior retinaculum	Peroneocalcaneus externum Peroneocuboideus Peroneoperoneolongus		The insertion site is highly variable, which gives rise to subtypes and confusing terminology
Posteromedial Accessory Muscles						
Accessory soleus	Fibula, or soleal line of the tibia, or the anterior surface of the soleus muscle	Descends posterior to the neurovascular bundle	Upper or medial, calcaneal surface		Superficial	
FDAL	Variable origin, can arise from any structures of the posterior compartment	Descends with the posterior tibial neurovascular bundle in the tarsal tunnel	Quadratus plantae, or the FDL before its division	Long accessory of the quadratus plantae Long accessory of the long flexors Accessorius of the accessorius of Turner Second accessorius of Humphrey	Deep	Compare with other accessory muscles in or near the tarsal tunnel, such as the TCI or PCI; the FDAL does not insert onto the calcaneus
PCI	Lower third of the fibula	Travels parallel to but remains lateral to the FHL	Base of the sustentaculum		Deep	Not directly related to the neurovascular bundle, because it travels lateral to the FHL
TCI	Medial crest of the tibia	Travels posterior to the FHL, within the tarsal tunnel and superficial to the neurovascular bundle	Medial calcaneus		Deep	Has features of both the FDAL and the accessory soleus

Abbreviations: FDAL, flexor digitorum accessorius longus; FDL, flexor digitorum longus; FHL, flexor hallucis longus; PCI, peroneocalcaneus internus; PQ, peroneus quartus; TCI, tibiocalcaneus internus.

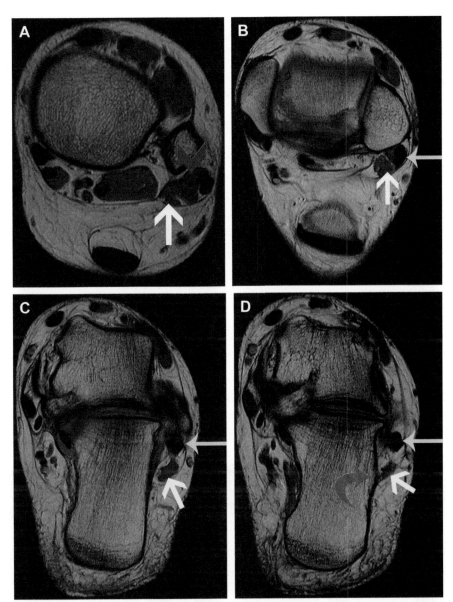

Fig. 1. PQ. Axial intermediate-weighted image of a 16-year-old girl with medial pain and instability following remote trauma, from above the ankle joint (*A*), at ankle joint (*B*), distal to ankle joint line (*C*) and beyond malleolar tips (*D*). In the lower leg, the PQ (*yellow arrow*) arises from the peroneus brevis muscle (*blue arrowhead*). The PQ descends with the peroneal tendons (*light blue arrow*). At the tip of the lateral malleolus, the PQ is posterior to the peroneal tendons. It then inserts onto the retrotrochlear eminence (*pink curved arrow* in *D*).

found only in humans. Its absence in other species and its function in stabilizing hind foot pronation led Hecker[1] to postulate that these muscles are evolutionary developments to accommodate the bipedal posture.

The reported prevalence of the PQ ranges from 5.2% to 22%.[1–6] A systematic review pooling 46 studies reported 16% prevalence.[7] The most common subtype is the peroneocalcaneus externum, found in 79%[5] and 91%[6] of all PQ.

Origin

The origin is variable and includes the posterior surface of the fibula or an origin from the peroneus longus or peroneus brevis muscle. Origin from the peroneus brevis origin is the most common based on both cadaveric studies[3,8] and imaging.[5,6]

Insertion

The insertion site is highly variable, which gives rise to subtypes and confusing terminology (**Fig. 2**). Hecker's[1] classification, based on the various insertions, is listed in **Table 2**.

The most common insertion of the PQ is at the retrotrochlear eminence,[1,5,6] one of 2 bony protuberances arising from the lateral cortex of the calcaneus (see **Fig. 1**). The retrotrochlear eminence lies posterior to the peroneal tubercle, which separates the 2 peroneal tendons.

Imaging Features

The tendon is described mostly in MR and infrequently in ultrasonography (US)[9] studies. The accessory muscle is seen as a separate structure traveling medial and posterior to the peroneal tendons (see **Fig. 2**). Its origin may be difficult to separate from the peroneal muscles. It becomes tendinous with variable insertions (see **Fig. 2** and **Table 2**).

Clinical Features

Although generally asymptomatic, the PQ muscles may contribute to crowding in the peroneal tunnel

Table 2 Insertion sites of PQ	
Insertion Site	**Alternative Name of PQ Based on Insertion**
Retrotrochlear eminence[a]	Peroneocalcaneus externum
Cuboid	Peroneocuboideus
Peroneus longus	Peroneoperoneolongus
Inferior retinaculum	

[a] Most common insertion site.

(**Fig. 3**), thereby predisposing patients to peroneal tendinopathy, peroneal brevis dislocation,[10] synovitis, pain, and snapping.[2,4] The use of PQ for repair of the superior peroneal retinaculum has also been reported.[11]

ACCESSORY MUSCLES IN THE POSTEROMEDIAL ANKLE

Despite traveling in a similar course in the posterior and medial ankle, the 4 accessory muscles of the posteromedial ankle (accessory soleus, flexor digitorum accessorius longus [FDAL], peroneocalcaneus internus [PCI], and tibiocalcaneus internus [TCI]) have distinct origins and insertions.

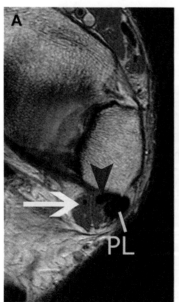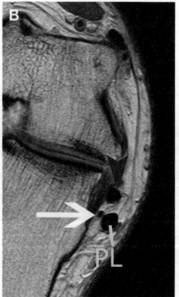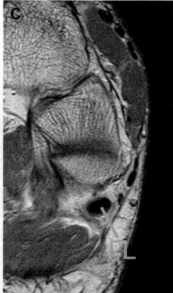

Fig. 2. Peroneoperoneolongus, a peroneus quartus variant that inserts onto the peroneus longus tendon. Axial intermediate-weighted image of a 47-year-old man with chronic ankle pain following injury, from ankle joint line (A) to cuboid fossa (C). At the lateral malleolus (A), the peroneoperoneolongus muscle (*yellow arrow*) travels medial and posterior to the peroneal tendons. It becomes tendinous (*yellow arrow* in B) before inserting onto the peroneus longus (PL). At the cuboid fossa (C), the tiny tendinous slip is no longer seen. Blue arrowhead in (A) and (B) indicates the peroneus brevis. Yellow arrow indicates peroneoperoneolongus muscle and tendon.

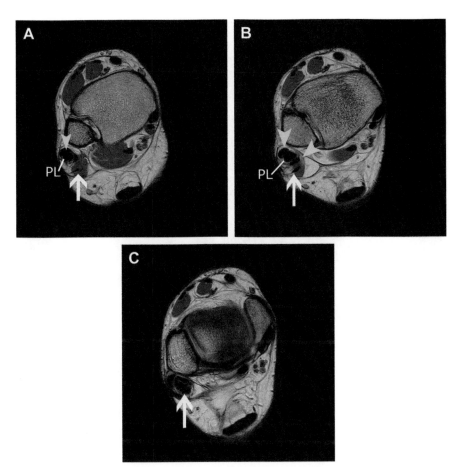

Fig. 3. Crowding at retromalleolar groove. Axial intermediate-weighted images of a 29-year-old woman with chronic lateral ankle pain, at lower leg (*A*), proximal to plafon (*B*) and at joint line (*C*). The PQ (*yellow arrow*) travels posterior to the PL and peroneus brevis (*arrowheads*) (*A*). At the retromalleolar groove, the fleshy muscle can cause crowding, leading to a split of the peroneus brevis (*B*) and tears of the PL. The PQ is difficult to separate from the split and torn peroneal tendons (*C*).

Moreover, their unique relations to the aponeurosis of the lower leg and the neurovascular bundle help to set them apart. **Figs. 4** and **5** described the aponeurosis of the lower leg, the flexor retinaculum, and the fibro-osseous tunnels in detail.

Accessory Soleus

The prevalence of accessory soleus in the general population is 0.7% to 5.5%,[12,13] but its prevalence is higher in athletes.[14] This muscle, bilateral in approximately 15% of cases,[12] is found most commonly in men. The posterior tibial artery provides the blood supply and the posterior tibial nerve innervates the accessory soleus.

Origin

The muscle may arise from the fibula, soleal line of the tibia, or the anterior surface of the soleus muscle[12,15,16] (**Fig. 6**).

Insertion

The accessory soleus inserts on the calcaneus at either the upper surface or the medial cortex. The insertion can be fleshy or tendinous (**Fig. 7**). There are 5 permutations of insertions: (1) into the Achilles tendon distally, (2) fleshy insertion into the upper surface of the calcaneus, (3) fleshy insertion into the medial cortex of the calcaneus, (4) tendinous insertion into the upper calcaneal surface, and (5) tendinous insertion into the medial surface of the calcaneus by way of a long tendon.[16,17]

Imaging Features

The accessory soleus can be detected using multiple modalities, including lateral radiographs,[16] computed tomography (CT),[18] US,[19] and MR imaging.[12–17,20–23] However, MR imaging allows the most specific diagnosis.

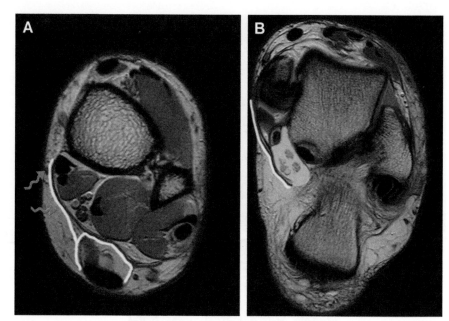

Fig. 4. Superficial and deep aponeurosis and flexor retinaculum. Axial intermediate-weighted MR images of the distal leg (*A*) and ankle (*B*). In the distal leg (*A*), the superficial aponeurosis (*yellow line*) splits and encircles the Achilles tendon. The deep aponeurosis (*blue line*) forms the boundary for the deep compartment as it blankets the 3 medial tendons and the posterior tibial neurovascular bundle. Distally, new fascial layers appear. They encircle individual tendons and the neurovascular bundle, creating 4 fibrous tunnels (*B*), housing the posterior tibial tendon (*blue tunnel*), the flexor digitorum longus (FDL) tendon (*red tunnel*), the flexor hallucis longus (FHL) tendon (*orange tunnel*), and the posterior tibial neurovascular bundle (*green tunnel*). The flexor retinaculum (*wavy orange arrows*), also known as the laciniate ligament, is formed by the fusion of the superficial and deep aponeurosis. The yellow and blue line represent the superficial and deep aponeurosis respectively in (*A*) and (*B*).

On lateral radiographs, the accessory soleus is seen as a tubular soft tissue density partially obscuring the Kager fat (**Fig. 8**). It travels anterior to the Achilles tendon, superficial to the deep aponeurosis, and is surrounded by its own fascial sheath. On US, the accessory soleus is isoechoic with muscle, located in between the flexor halluces longus (FHL) and the Achilles tendon. CT imaging, similar to MR imaging, reveals a well-defined soft tissue mass in Kager fat. The accessory soleus descends posterior to the tarsal tunnel, which contains the posterior tibial neurovascular bundle and its branches. In symptomatic cases, the MR signal of the accessory soleus may be altered by trauma, ischemia, or atrophy (see **Fig. 7**B).

Clinical Features

Symptoms generally arise from mass effect of the accessory muscle and are present predominantly in young men in the second and third decades of life.[12,16] The mass can be either painless or painful. For painless posterior masses, CT and MR imaging allow diagnosis without biopsy. Painful masses typically occur with exertion. Several hypotheses attempt to explain the cause of this pain. One theory suggests that exercise-induced hypertrophy of the accessory soleus leads to increased intrafascial pressure, subsequent development of a compartment syndrome, and pain.[12,15] Another theory suggests that increased activity may lead to inadequate blood supply, resulting in claudication. An alternative explanation is that the accessory soleus may compress on the adjacent posterior tibial nerve, resulting in pain. There are case reports of resolution of tarsal tunnel syndrome following excision of the accessory muscle, despite the accessory soleus being outside the tarsal tunnel.[23,24] Symptomatic cases have been successfully treated with fasciotomy, tendon release, and/or excision.[12,15] The accessory soleus has also been associated with clubfoot deformity[25] and Achilles tendinopathy (69.2%).[13]

FLEXOR DIGITORUM ACCESSORIUS LONGUS

Sometimes considered to be a variant of the quadratus plantae muscle,[26] the FDAL is one of the most common accessory muscles of the ankle,

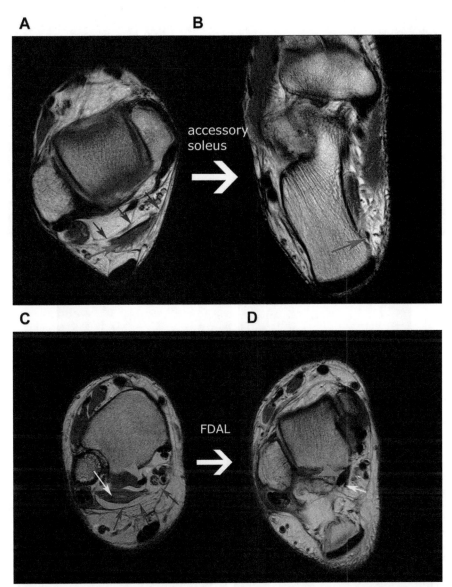

Fig. 5. Comparison of accessory muscle locations relative to the deep aponeurosis. Axial intermediate-weighted MR images of the ankle from 2 different patients: one with accessory soleus (*A*, *B*), and the other with FDAL (*C*, *D*). The images on the left (*A*, *C*) are more proximal, showing the muscle bellies. The images on the right (*B*, *D*) are more distal, near the accessory muscle insertions. The accessory soleus (*red arrow*) is superficial to the deep aponeurosis of the lower leg (*blue arrows*), whereas the FDAL (*yellow arrow*) is deep to the deep aponeurosis (*C*) and in the deep compartment. Both the PCI and the TCI (not shown) also travel in the deep compartment (FHL, *orange arrowhead*).

with a reported prevalence ranging from 6% to 8%. It is also most common in men.[27,28]

Origin

The origin of the FDAL is variable; it can arise from any structure in the posterior compartment, such as the FHL,[28] fascia of the deep posterior

compartment,[28] and medial and lateral margins of the fibula[29] (**Fig. 9**).

Insertion

The distal muscle tapers near its insertion, which can remain muscular or can become tendinous or aponeurotic.[26] Two sites of insertions have

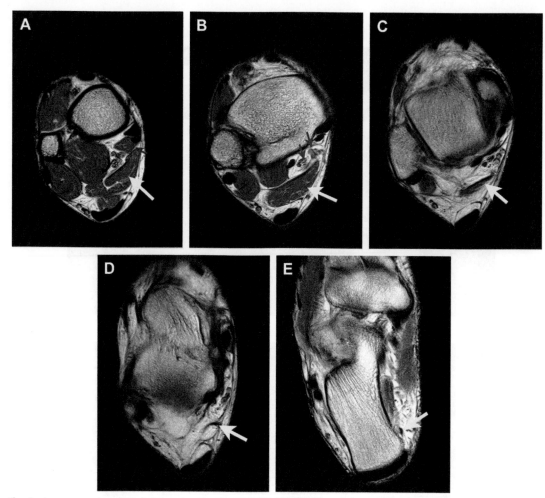

Fig. 6. Accessory soleus (AS). Axial proton density-weighted MR images of the ankle at distal tibia (*A*), proximal to plafond (*B*), tip of the medial malleolus (*C*), tip of the lateral malleolus (*D*) and body of calcaneus (*E*) in a 37-year-old man with ankle pain. The AS (*yellow arrow*) muscle belly is superficial to the deep aponeurosis (*blue arrows*) covering the posterior tibial, flexor digitorum longus and flexor hallucis longus, and the posterior tibial neurovascular bundle (*purple arrows*) (*A*, *B*). The AS descends posterior to the tarsal tunnel containing the neurovascular bundle (*purple arrows*) and inserts onto the medial cortex of the posterior calcaneus (*E*).

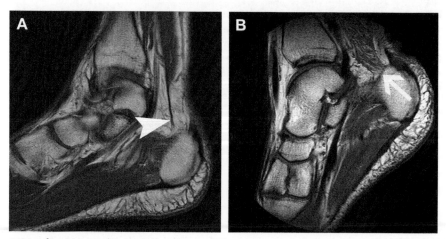

Fig. 7. Two types of accessory soleus insertion. Sagittal T1-weighted MR images of the ankle from 2 different patients showing tendinous insertion (*arrowhead*) in (*A*) and fleshy insertion (*arrow*) in (*B*). The accessory soleus in (*B*) is also mildly atrophic, infiltrated by fat.

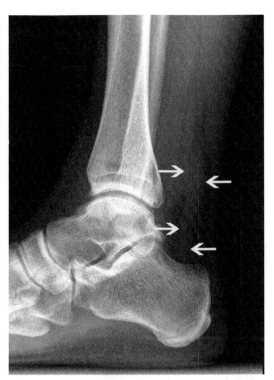

Fig. 8. Radiography of the accessory soleus. Lateral radiograph shows an accessory soleus (*yellow arrows*) with a tendinous insertion onto the calcaneus.

been described: the quadratus plantae, and the flexor digitorum longus (FDL) before its division[27,30] (**Fig. 10**).

Imaging Features

The FDAL is readily detected on axial MR images. In the lower leg, the FDAL is seen deep to the deep aponeurosis (see **Fig. 9**), within the common compartment that houses both the FHL and the posterior tibial neurovascular bundle. This feature differentiates the FDAL from the accessory soleus (see **Fig. 5**). It descends with the posterior tibial neurovascular bundle in the tarsal tunnel and can remain fleshy in the tight fibro-osseous tunnel (see **Fig. 9C**).[28] Its alternative insertion to the FDL before its division can sometimes be difficult to show because the small FDAL distal tendinous slip may be obscured by the surrounding muscles and soft tissues.[28] These sites of FDAL insertions distinguish it from other accessory muscles around the tarsal tunnel, such as PCI and TCI muscles, both of which insert onto the calcaneus.

Clinical Features

The presence of FDAL within the tight fibro-osseous tarsal tunnel increases the risk of

compression or impingement of the posterior tibial neurovascular bundle (**Fig. 11A**). One surgical report found that 12% of cases of tarsal tunnel syndrome were caused by an FDAL. Moreover, these cases were successfully treated by excision of the accessory muscle.[23] In another report, the mass effect created by the accessory muscle caused tethering of the flexor tendons at the fibro-osseous canal of the FHL. In this case, the acute pain with limited dorsiflexion of the foot and toes, which resembled flexor hallucis syndrome, was relieved following excision of the FDAL muscle.[29] Like any muscle, this accessory muscle can be injured after trauma or twisting. A strained FDAL, represented by bright T2 signal in the muscle, was reported in a case of ankle pain after twisting injury.[31]

PERONEOCALCANEUS INTERNUS

The PCI, a less frequently encountered accessory muscle first described by in 1817 in an anatomy dissection report,[32] has since been reported in cadaveric/anatomic, orthopedic, and MR imaging studies, most of which consisted of case reports of fewer than 5 cases.[33–36] It is also known as the fibulocalcaneus internus.[34] The reported prevalence of the PCI is 1%, based on a single MR imaging study of 100 asymptomatic patients.[35]

Origin

The PCI muscle arises from the lower third of the fibula and is located lateral to the FHL muscle (**Fig. 12A–C**).

Insertion

The PCI passes below the sustentaculum tali and inserts onto the medial aspect of the calcaneus, at the base of the sustentaculum (**Fig. 12D–F**).

Imaging Features

On ankle MR imaging, the muscle belly can be seen deep to the deep aponeurosis (see **Fig. 12C**) and interdigitates with the FHL muscle (see **Fig. 12A**). The PCI muscle belly not only runs parallel to but remains lateral to the FHL in the distal leg. It is not directly related to the neurovascular bundle and typically becomes tendinous 2 to 3 cm above the tibiotalar joint.[35] This tendon is slender, travels with the FHL tendon, and enters the calcaneal groove of the talus posterior to the FHL tendon (see **Fig. 12E, F**). Both travel under the sustentaculum, where the PCI inserts into a small tubercle on the medial aspect of the sustentaculum (**Fig. 13**).[35] This calcaneal insertion may be better seen on coronal images (see **Fig. 13B**).

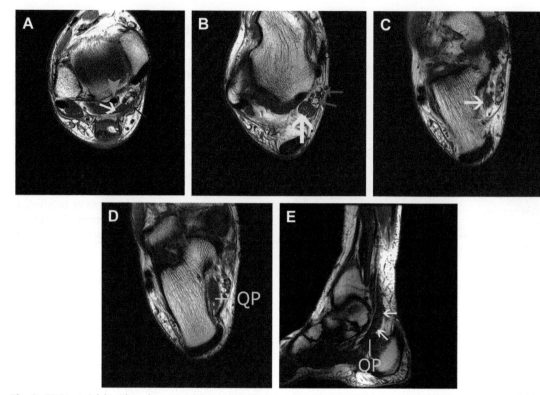

Fig. 9. FDAL. Axial (*A–D*) and sagittal (*E*) images of a 36-year-old man with suspected Achilles rupture. Axial images are intermediate weighted; (*A*) is more proximal than (*D*). The sagittal image (*E*) is medial and T1 weighted. In the lower leg (*A*), the FDAL is seen deep to the deep aponeurosis (*small blue arrows*), within the common compartment that houses both the FHL (*orange arrowhead*) and the posterior tibial neurovascular bundle (*pink arrow*). In this case, the FDAL remains fleshy as it descends with the posterior tibial neurovascular bundle in the tarsal tunnel (*B, C*). Its insertion to the quadratus plantae (QP) is muscular in this case. The sagittal image (*E*) best shows the merging of the FDAL with the QP. Yellow arrow indicates FDAL.

The PCI can be confused with the FDAL, because both the PCI and FDAL travel in a similar course. However, differentiation can be important because the FDAL is more closely applied to the posterior tibial neurovascular bundle and therefore more likely associated with nerve impingement. A major difference between the two is the site of insertion. The PCI inserts onto the calcaneus, whereas the FDAL inserts on the FDL tendon or the quadratus plantae. Another difference is the relationship of the accessory muscles relative to the neurovascular bundle. The PCI is typically not near the neurovascular bundle because the FHL is interposed between them (see **Fig. 12C**). In contrast, the FDAL stays immediately adjacent to the neurovascular bundle (see **Fig. 11**). In addition, unlike the PCI, a fat plane between the FDAL and the quadratus plantae may be absent.[35]

The PCI is similar to the accessory soleus in that both insert onto the medial calcaneal cortex. The PCI can be distinguished from the accessory soleus in that the latter is located superficial to the deep aponeurosis (blue arrow in **Fig. 5A, D**).

Occasionally, an FHL muscle with 2 tendinous slips may also be mistaken for a PCI tendon.[35]

Clinical Features

The PCI is generally asymptomatic but has been implicated as a cause of ankle pain, limitation of movement,[33,35,36] posterior ankle impingement, and FHL tenosynovitis.[33,37] Complications during hind foot arthroscopic surgery may arise when the PCI is misidentified as the FHL. During arthroscopy, the FHL commonly serves as an important landmark that denotes the medial margin of safety (ie, an area with low risk of neurovascular injury).[38] When the PCI is mistaken for the FHL during arthroscopic surgery, it is referred to as the false FHL. Failure to recognize the PCI (or false FHL) may lead to an altered surgical approach and

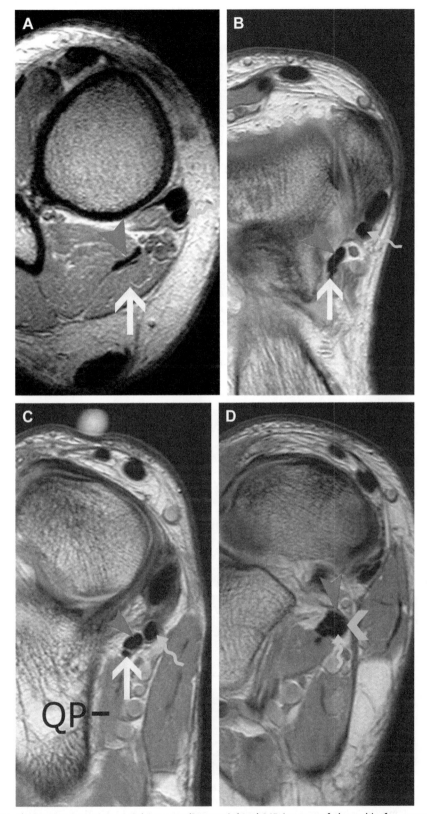

Fig. 10. FDAL alternative insertion. Axial intermediate-weighted MR images of the ankle from proximal (*A*) to distal (*D*) of the ankle joint. Two sites of FDAL (*yellow arrow*) have been described, the QP and the FDL (*curved arrow*) before its division near the knot of Henry (*green arrowhead*). This FDAL arises from the deep aponeurosis (*A*), becomes tendinous (*B*) and passes the QP (*C*). It follows the FHL (*orange arrowhead*) and disappears around the knot of Henry where the FHL and FDL cross over (*D*). The exact insertion site is frequently difficult to see because of overlapping structures (*D*).

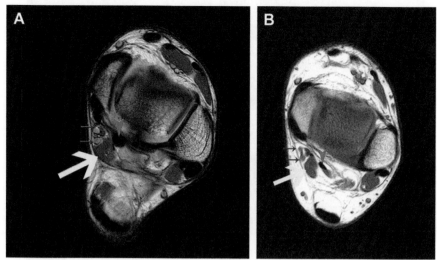

Fig. 11. FDAL and the neurovascular bundle. Axial intermediate-weighted MR images of the ankle from 2 male patients, 33 years old (*A*) and 50 years old (*B*). Both reported ankle pain. Compared with the smaller FDAL in (*B*), the FDAL in (*A*) has a fleshy belly resulting in a tight fibro-osseous tarsal tunnel, thus is at risk for tarsal tunnel syndrome. In one surgical report 12% of cases of tarsal tunnel syndrome were caused by an FDAL.[23] Purple arrows indicate posterior tibial neurovascular bundle. Yellow arrow indicates FDAL. Orange arrowhead indicates FHL.

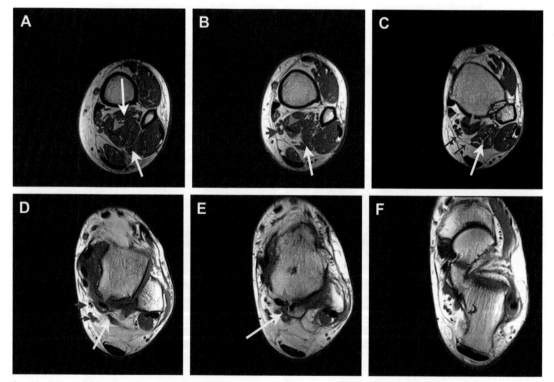

Fig. 12. PCI. Axial intermediate-weighted MR images of a 33-year-old man with ankle instability, from proximal (*A*) to distal (*F*). The PCI (*yellow arrow*) muscle belly is deep to the deep aponeurosis (*blue small arrows*) and lateral to the FHL muscle (*white arrow*) and tendon (*orange arrowhead*) (*A–C*). These 2 muscles interdigitate (*A*). The PCI then descends posterior to the FHL tendon (*arrowhead*) (*D–F*). Passing through the tarsal tunnel, the PCI then inserts onto the medial cortex of the calcaneus, at the base of the sustentaculum (*curved arrow*) (*F*). The PCI tendon is slender and does not encroach on the neurovascular bundle in the tarsal tunnel (*purple arrows*). Yellow arrow indicates PCI in **Fig. 12.**

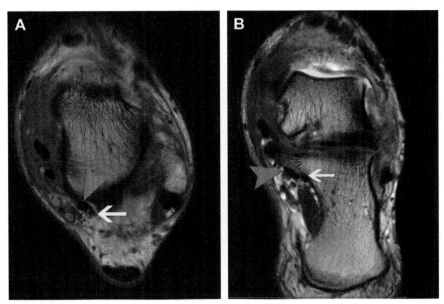

Fig. 13. PCI insertion beneath the sustentaculum tali. Axial (*A*) and coronal (*B*) images from a 19-year-old male athlete with persistent medial pain weeks after ankle sprain. The PCI (*yellow arrow* in *A*) travels with the FHL (*orange arrowhead*) (*A* and *B*). It passes below the sustentaculum tali (*purple asterisk* in *B*) and inserts onto the medial aspect of the calcaneus, at the base of the sustentaculum (*yellow arrow* in *B*). The insertion is best see on coronal images (*B*).

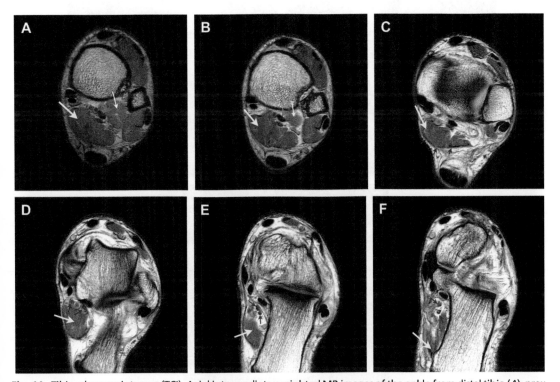

Fig. 14. Tibiocalcaneus internus (TCI). Axial intermediate-weighted MR images of the ankle from distal tibia (*A*), proximal to plafond (*B*), at tibiotalar joint line (*C*), at tip of medial malleolus (*D*), distal to lateral malleolus (*E*) and slightly beyond the posterior subtalar joint (*F*) to the ankle joint in a middle-aged recreational athlete with medial pain after 85-km (53-mile) Nordic race. The TCI (*yellow arrow*) is bounded by the deep aponeurosis of the lower leg (*blue arrows*) in (*C*) and lies medial to the FHL muscle (*white arrow* in *A* and *B*) and tendon (*arrowhead* in all images). The TCI travels posterior to the neurovascular bundle (*purple arrows*). It inserts on the medial cortex of the calcaneus (*F*). The deep location of the TCI relative to the deep aponeurosis (*blue arrows* in (*C*) distinguishes the TCI from the accessory soleus.

increased risk of neurovascular injury. Although the PCI does not travel with the neurovascular bundle, tarsal tunnel has been reported in some cases of PCI. One explanation is that the PCI muscle belly displaces the FHL medially in some patients,[35] leading to indirect encroachment of the neurovascular bundle. Although this creates a potential risk for nerve entrapment, the causal relationship between the PCI and the ankle symptoms remains unclear.

TIBIOCALCANEUS INTERNUS

There are no imaging reports on the TCI accessory muscle. The few reports on the TCI[1,39] are anatomic studies from dissections.

Origin

The TCI arises from the medial crest of the tibia.

Insertion

The TCI inserts onto the medial surface of the calcaneus approximately 1 to 2 cm anterior to the Achilles tendon (**Figs. 14 and 15**).[1,39]

Imaging Features

The TCI muscle travels deep to the deep aponeurosis, posterior to the FHL. It is located within the tarsal tunnel and superficial to the neurovascular bundle. It has features of both the FDAL and the accessory soleus. Similar to the FDAL but different from the accessory soleus, the TCI stays deep to the aponeurosis, whereas the accessory soleus stays superficial to the aponeurosis. Its course within the tarsal tunnel is also similar to that of FDAL. In contrast, its insertion onto the medial cortex of the calcaneus more closely resembles the accessory soleus than the FDAL.

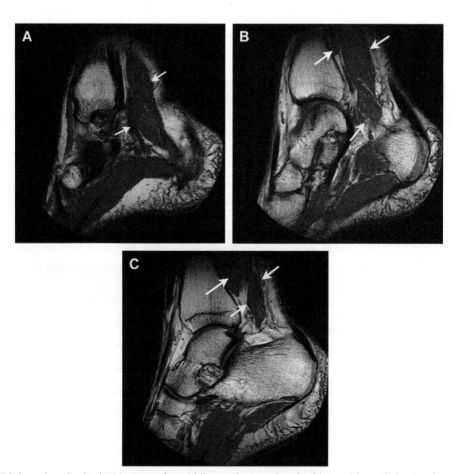

Fig. 15. TCI insertion. Sagittal T1 images of a middle-aged recreational athlete with medial pain after an 85-km (53-mile) Nordic race, from the medial malleolus (*A*), medial tibia (*B*), and midline (*C*). An anomalous muscle, TCI (*yellow arrows*), is noted medial to the FHL tendon (*white arrow*). The TCI inserts on the medial calcaneus (*A*), similar to an accessory soleus. In contrast with the accessory soleus, the TCI is located deep to the deep aponeurosis and the tarsal tunnel, best seen on axial images (*C*).

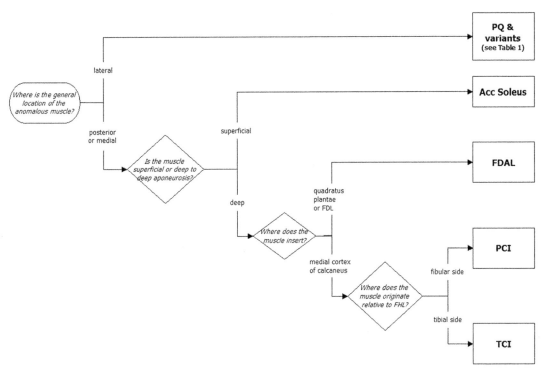

Fig. 16. Diagnostics algorithm for identification of accessory muscles of the ankle. Acc Soleus, accessory soleus.

The latter inserts onto either the quadratus plantae muscle or the FDL.

Clinical Features

It is likely that the lack of reported complications associated with TCI is related to its infrequent occurrence. However, with its close proximity to the neurovascular bundle in the tarsal tunnel, and similarity to FDAL, it may be associated with tarsal tunnel syndrome.

DIAGNOSTIC ALGORITHM TO IDENTIFY ACCESSORY MUSCLES OF THE ANKLE

Distinguishing one accessory muscle from another within the same region can be challenging because they can share similar origins, paths, insertions, and compartments. An algorithmic approach based on image analysis of the anatomy can help narrow the possibilities (**Fig. 16**).

First, for accessory muscles located in the lateral ankle, the possibilities are limited to PQ and its variants (see **Table 2**). Second, only the accessory soleus, located in the posterior ankle, resides superficial to the deep aponeurosis of the leg. In addition, the remaining muscles can be identified first by their insertion and then by their origin.

SUMMARY

Accessory muscles discovered incidentally in cross-sectional imaging of the ankle are generally asymptomatic. For the few symptomatic cases, the accessory muscle may mimic a mass lesion, and/or be implicated as a cause of tarsal tunnel syndrome, chronic pain, and impingement. Accurate diagnosis is therefore important for guiding patient care. Using an algorithm approach based on knowledge of the anatomy allows radiologists to accurately identify the muscle, resulting in appropriate management.

REFERENCES

1. Hecker P. Study on the peroneus of the tarsus. Anat Rec 1923;26(1):79–82.
2. Bilgili MG, Kaynak G, Botanlio H, et al. Peroneus quartus: prevalance and clinical importance. Arch Orthop Trauma Surg 2014;134(4):481–7.
3. Sobel M, Levy ME, Bohne WHO. Congenital variations of the peroneus quartus muscle: an anatomic study. Foot Ankle Int 1990;11(2):81–9.
4. Zammit J, Singh D. The peroneus quartus muscle. Anatomy and clinical relevance. J Bone Joint Surg Br 2003;85(8):1134–7.
5. Cheung YY, Rosenberg ZS, Ramsinghani R, et al. Peroneus quartus muscle: MR imaging features. Radiology 1997;202(3):745–50.

6. Saupe N, Mengiardi B, Pfirrmann CW, et al. Anatomic variants associated with peroneal tendon disorders: MR imaging findings in volunteers with asymptomatic ankles. Radiology 2007;242(2): 509–17.

7. Yammine K. The accessory peroneal (fibular) muscles: peroneus quartus and peroneus digiti quinti. A systematic review and meta-analysis. Surg Radiol Anat 2015;37(6):617–27.

8. Athavale SA, Gupta V, Kotgirwar S, et al. The peroneus quartus muscle: clinical correlation with evolutionary importance. Anat Sci Int 2012;87(2):106–10.

9. Chepuri NB, Jacobson JA, Fessell DP, et al. Sonographic appearance of the peroneus quartus muscle: correlation with MR imaging appearance in seven patients. Radiology 2001;218(2):415–9.

10. Rosenberg ZS, Bencardino J, Astion D, et al. MRI features of chronic injuries of the superior peroneal retinaculum. Am J Roentgenol 2003;181(6):1551–7.

11. Mick C, Lynch F. Reconstruction of the peroneal retinaculum using the peroneus quartus: a case report. J Bone Joint Surg Am 1987;69-A(2):296–7.

12. Brodie JT, Dormans JP, Gregg JR, et al. Accessory soleus muscle. A report of 4 cases and review of literature. Clin Orthop Relat Res 1997;4(337):180–6.

13. Luck MD, Gordon AG, Blebea JS, et al. High association between accessory soleus muscle and Achilles tendonopathy. Skeletal Radiol 2008;37(12): 1129–33.

14. Rossi R, Bonasia DE, Tron A, et al. Accessory soleus in the athletes: literature review and case report of a massive muscle in a soccer player. Knee Surg Sports Traumatol Arthrosc 2009;17(8):990–5.

15. Kendi TK, Erakar A, Oktay O, et al. Accessory soleus muscle. J Am Podiatr Med Assoc 2004;94(6):587–9.

16. Lorentzon R, Wirell S. Anatomic variations of the accessory soleus muscle. Acta Radiol 1987;28(5):627–9.

17. Yu JS, Resnick D. MR imaging of the accessory soleus muscle appearance in six patients and a review of the literature. Skeletal Radiol 1994;23(7):525–8.

18. Assoun J, Railhac J, Richardi G, et al. CT and MR of accessory soleus muscle. J Comput Assist Tomogr 1995;19(2):333.

19. Bianchi S, Abdelwahab IF, Oliveri M, et al. Sonographic diagnosis of accessory soleus muscle mimicking a soft tissue tumor. J Ultrasound Med 1995;14(9):707–9.

20. Del Nero FB, Ruiz CR, Aliaga Júnior R. The presence of accessory soleus muscle in humans. Einstein (São Paulo, Brazil) 2012;10(1):79–81.

21. Buschmann WR, Cheung Y, Jahss MH. Magnetic resonance imaging of anomalous leg muscles: accessory soleus, peroneus quartus and the flexor digitorum longus accessorius. Foot Ankle 1991;12(2):109–16.

22. Rossi F, Dragoni S. Symptomatic accessory soleus muscle: report of 18 cases in athletes. J Sports Med Phys Fitness 2005;45(1):93–7.

23. Kinoshita M, Okuda R, Morikawa J, et al. Tarsal tunnel syndrome associated with an accessory muscle. Foot Ankle Int 2003;24(2):132–6.

24. Sookur PA, Naraghi AM, Bleakney RR, et al. Accessory muscles: anatomy, symptoms, and radiologic evaluation. Radiographics 2008;28(2):481–99.

25. Danielsson LG, El-Haddad I, Sabri T. Clubfoot with supernumerary soleus muscle. Report of 2 cases. Acta Orthop Scand 1990;61(4):371–3.

26. Athavale SA, Geetha GN, Swathi. Morphology of flexor digitorum accessorius muscle. Surg Radiol Anat 2012;34(4):367–72.

27. Peterson DA, Stinson W, Lairmore JR. The long accessory flexor muscle: an anatomical study. Foot Ankle Int 1995;16(10):637–40.

28. Cheung YY, Rosenberg ZS, Colon E, et al. MR imaging of flexor digitorum accessorius longus. Skeletal Radiol 1999;28(3):130–7.

29. Eberle CF, Moran B, Gleason T. The accessory flexor digitorum longus as a cause of flexor hallucis syndrome. Foot Ankle Int 2002;23(1):51–5.

30. Gümüşalan Y, Kalaycioglu A. Bilateral accessory flexor digitorum longus muscle in man. Ann Anat 2000;182(6):573–6.

31. Ho VW, Peterfy C, Helms CA. Tarsal tunnel syndrome caused by strain of an anomalous muscle: an MRI-specific diagnosis. J Comput Assist Tomogr 1993;17(5):822–3.

32. Macalister A. Additional observations on muscular anomalies in human anatomy. Trans R Irish Acad 1871;25:1–134.

33. Seipel R, Linklater J, Pitsis G, et al. The peroneocalcaneus internus muscle: an unusual cause of posterior ankle impingement. Foot Ankle Int 2005;26(10): 890–3.

34. Lambert HW, Atsas S, Fox JN. The fibulocalcaneus (peroneocalcaneus) internus muscle of Macalister: clinical and surgical implications. Clin Anat 2011; 24(8):1000–4.

35. Mellado JM, Rosenberg ZS, Beltran J, et al. The peroneocalcaneus internus muscle: MR imaging features. AJR Am J Roentgenol 1997;169(2): 585–8.

36. Howe BM, Murthy NS. An accessory peroneocalcaneus internus muscle with MRI and US correlation. J Radiol Case Rep 2012;6(10):20–5.

37. Best A, Giza E, Linklater J, et al. Posterior impingement of the ankle caused by anomalous muscles. A report of four cases. J Bone Joint Surg Am 2005; 87(9):2075–9.

38. Phisitkul P, Amendola A. False FHL: a normal variant posing risks in posterior hindfoot endoscopy. Arthroscopy 2010;26(5):714–8.

39. Kelikian A, Sarrafian S. Sarrafian's anatomy of the foot and ankle: descriptive, topographic, functional. 3rd edition. Philadelphia: Lippincott Williams & Wilkins; 2011.

MR Imaging of the Pediatric Foot and Ankle
What Does Normal Look Like?

Grace Mang Yuet Ma, MD[a], Kirsten Ecklund, MD[b],*

KEYWORDS

• Pediatric • Ankle • Normal • MR Imaging • Children • Physis

KEY POINTS

- The MR appearance of the pediatric foot and ankle depends on the predictable pattern of chondral, osseous, and marrow maturation.
- An understanding of normal age-related development is essential to differentiating normal findings from common pathologies.
- The distal tibial and fibular physes have undulating, trilaminar appearances with consistent width until skeletal maturity; physeal widening or bridging indicates disrupted endochondral ossification.
- Epiphyseal and tarsal ossification centers are surrounded by secondary physes, identical to primary physes. Osteochondral abnormalities often result from injury/insult to the secondary physis.
- Residual hematopoietic marrow has a characteristic appearance in the foot and ankle and may persist into young adulthood.

INTRODUCTION

The MR imaging appearance of the pediatric ankle reflects the dynamic process of skeletal growth and maturation. An understanding of the normal age-related development within the chondroosseous structures is essential to an appreciation of the common pathologic conditions affecting the ankle in children. This article focuses on the MR imaging appearance of the maturing ankle and the disorders that can impact this appearance. The imaging manifestations of trauma, developmental disorders, infection, avascular necrosis, and tumors depend on the developmental maturation of the physis, epiphysis/apophysis, and marrow.

In the neonate, the epiphyses at the distal ends of the tibia and fibula are composed entirely of hyaline cartilage, and the physes separating the epiphyses from the metaphyses are transversely oriented. The ultimate shape and growth of the ends of these long bones depends on a balance between endochondral ossification and intramembranous ossification. Endochondral ossification is the highly organized process converting cartilage to bone. The primary physis provides for linear growth of the long bones and centrifugal growth of the tarsal bones, whereas the secondary physis that surrounds the secondary center of ossification is responsible for spherical growth of the epiphyses. The periosteum contributes to transverse growth (diameter increase) of the long bones through intramembranous ossification with direct mineralization of the vascular connective tissue without a cartilaginous mold.[1] This dynamic ossification process dictates the age-related appearance of the ankle on MR images. In the newborn

Disclosure: The authors have nothing to disclose.
[a] Department of Radiology, Ohio State University Wexner Medical Center, 410 West 10th Avenue, Columbus, OH 43210, USA; [b] Department of Radiology, Harvard Medical School, Boston Children's Hospital, 300 Longwood Avenue, Boston, MA 02115, USA
* Corresponding author.
E-mail address: Kirsten.Ecklund@childrens.harvard.edu

Magn Reson Imaging Clin N Am 25 (2017) 27–43
http://dx.doi.org/10.1016/j.mric.2016.08.010
1064-9689/17/© 2016 Elsevier Inc. All rights reserved.

period, epiphyseal cartilage is homogeneously intermediate signal intensity on T1-weighted images (T1WI) and low signal intensity on water-sensitive sequences.[2] The high water concentration of marrow in the newborn period leads to homogeneous low signal intensity on T1WI and high signal intensity on water-sensitive sequences. As the secondary ossification centers appear and the marrow converts from hematopoietic to fatty, the adult MR imaging features develop with a predictable pattern[2,3] (**Fig. 1**).

The vascularity of the growing bones predisposes to pathology and its associated appearance. Transphyseal vascular canals in infants and toddlers allow infection and tumor to pass between the metaphysis and epiphysis. These channels disappear by 18 months of age and do not normally recur until skeletal maturity.[2] If these transphyseal vascular communications are reestablished owing to trauma, endochondral ossification along the vessels may ensue leading to physeal bone bridge formation. Embryologic vascular channels may persist within the epiphyses and epiphyseal equivalents and should not be confused for infection or tumor. This is most commonly seen in the mid portion of the calcaneus where vascular remnants near the insertion of the cervical and interosseous ligaments can create a moderately sized pseudolesion[4] (**Fig. 2**). These vascular remnants are more prevalent on MR imaging studies of children, but are also seen in adults. **Table 1** summarizes several normal developmental features that may be confused for pathology.

PHYSEAL DEVELOPMENT

The distal tibial and fibular physes are highly organized cartilaginous structures responsible for linear growth of the ankle. T2-weighted fat-suppressed MR images are best suited for evaluation of the physis, which has a trilaminar appearance, with high signal intensity in the physeal resting and hypertrophic zones adjacent to the epiphysis, low signal intensity in the zone of provisional calcification, and high signal intensity in the metaphyseal vascular primary spongiosa[2,5,6] (see **Fig. 1**). Physeal cartilage has a higher signal intensity than the adjacent epiphyseal cartilage on long repetition time sequences owing to the greater amount of free water in the physeal hyaline cartilage.[2] By 2 years of age, the distal tibial physis is normally undulating with a focal anteromedial upward deviation often called Kump's bump or Poland's hump.[7] This represents the site of initial physiologic physeal closure, which is completed in girls from 12 to 15 years and boys from 15 to 18 years[7] (**Fig. 3**). This asymmetric early physeal fusion tethers the growth plate and predisposes to Tillaux (Salter Harris type III) and triplane physeal fractures in this age group. Distal tibial physeal fractures have a high rate of growth arrest because

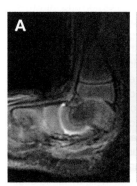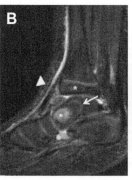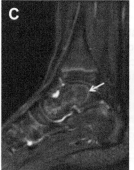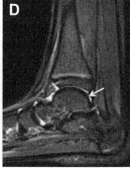

Fig. 1. Normal skeletal maturation of the ankle. Sagittal short T1 inversion recovery images in different children at 23 days old (*A*), 15 months old (*B*), 5 years old, (*C*) and 12 years old (*D*) demonstrating progressive ossification of the distal tibia and talus. At 23 days (*A*), the distal tibial physis is concave and the entirely cartilaginous epiphysis has intermediate signal intensity. At 15 months (*B*), the tibial epiphyseal and anterior talar preossification centers (*asterisk*) have increased signal owing to normal increased water content in the developing ossification centers. The posterior talus remains cartilaginous. Note the high signal intensity spherical physis of the talus posteriorly (*arrow*) similar to the primary physis of the distal tibia, which is now straighter than in the newborn. The tibial epiphysis has become more rectangular and is diffusely low signal owing to fatty marrow. Dorsal inflammatory changes in this toddler are related to spondyloarthropathy (*solid arrow head*). By age 5 years (*C*), the tibial physis has an undulating contour and the talar ossification center and physis are well developed (*arrow*). The posterior talus is increasingly ossified. Patchy high signal in the talar ossification center is normal red marrow. At 12 years of age (*D*), the ankle has a mature appearance. The physis is narrow and the epiphysis is completely ossified. The talus is completely ossified and maintains the adult configuration (*arrow*).

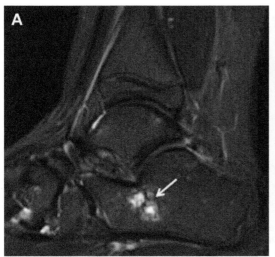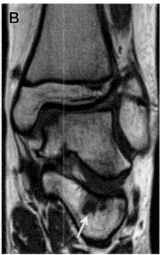

Fig. 2. Calcaneal vascular remnant. Sagittal short T1 inversion recovery (STIR; *A*) and coronal T1 (*B*) images demonstrate the characteristic T1 hypointense and STIR hyperintense multilocular focus (*arrow*) within the calcaneus in the typical subtalar location. Notice the fine streaks of lower T1 signal intensity residual red marrow within the tibial metaphysis of this 10-year-old girl.

the undulating physis predisposes to the creation of transphyseal vascular connections and subsequent physeal bone bridge formation at the fracture site. Large bone bridges lead to limb length discrepancy, whereas small, eccentric bridges lead to angular deformity. Growth recovery lines tethered to the physis, best seen on T1WI, indicate asymmetric physeal growth (**Fig. 4**). The distal

Table 1
Normal skeletal developmental features and their potential pathologic mimics

Normal Development	Distinguishing Feature(s)	Pathologic Mimic
Calcaneal vascular remnant: persistent embryologic vascular channels	Characteristic location in the mid portion of the calcaneus, extending from the sinus tarsi	Tumor or infection
Kump's bump or Poland's hump: Site of initial distal tibial physeal closure	Characteristic location in the anteromedial distal tibial physis	Fracture with osseous bridging of physis
Focal periphyseal edema: diminished bone flexibility at the site of transphyseal osseous fusion	Centered in the closing physis of adolescents	Physeal stress injury or infection
Calcaneal apophyseal fragmentation: normal developmental ossification	Absence of marrow edema or surrounding soft tissue edema, especially at the Achilles tendon insertion	Sever's apophysitis
Epiphyseal ossification center irregularity, especially of the tarsal bones and malleoli: normal ossification center development	Absence of subjacent marrow edema. Intact adjacent trilaminar physis of the ossification center and articular cartilage	Osteochondritis dissecans or malleolar fracture.
Normal residual hematopoietic marrow	T1 signal greater than that of the adjacent muscle. Characteristic speckled appearance in the tarsal bones and geometric shape tethered to physis in long bones.	Stress-related edema. Perivascular foci of red marrow often magnified by osteoporosis from disuse

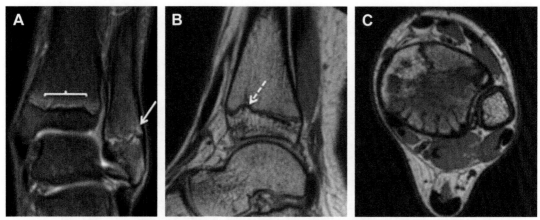

Fig. 3. A 12-year-old ballet dancer with normal distal tibial and fibular physis. Coronal proton density (PD) with fat suppression (*A*), sagittal PD (*B*), and axial PD (*C*) demonstrate the development of normal spiculations within the trilaminar physis indicating impending fusion (*curly braces*). Notice the normal laterally undulating distal fibular physis (*solid arrow*). Kump's bump (*dashed arrow*) anteriorly in the tibia reflects the location of earliest physiologic fusion. Axial image at the level of the fusing physis (*C*) reveals spoke wheel low signal spiculations radiating from the periphery. The physis has a heterogeneous signal intensity when viewed axially owing to its undulating orientation in the longitudinal axis.

fibular physis is highly undulating, especially laterally where the peripheral margins can be spiculated and should not be mistaken for fracture.

The distal tibiofibular physeal relationship is dynamic early in growth. In infancy, the distal fibular physis is at the level of the midpoint of the tibial epiphysis. By 5 years of age, the distal fibular physis has migrated to the level of the distal tibial articular surface. Disruption of this relationship indicates growth disturbance. Additionally, the physis should be uniform in thickness throughout growth up until skeletal maturity.[2,8] Physeal widening, either diffuse or focal owing to unossified physeal cartilage extending into the metaphysis, indicates physeal injury and disruption of endochondral ossification (**Fig. 5**). This growth

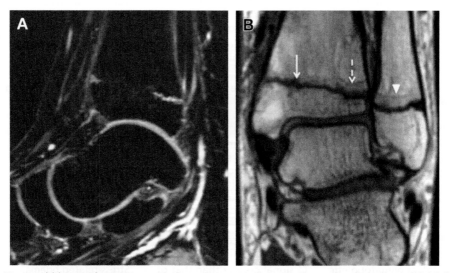

Fig. 4. A 12-year-old boy with posttraumatic premature growth arrest 7 months after distal tibial Salter Harris type II fracture. A large anteromedial bone bridge is seen on the gradient echo fat-suppressed sagittal image (*A*) as a low signal intensity fatty marrow interrupting the high signal intensity cartilaginous physis. This bone bridge or physeal arrest would appear as high signal intensity marrow fat on T1-weighted imaging (not shown). Coronal PD image (*B*) shows a growth recovery line, which is tethered to the physis medially (*solid arrow*) and separated laterally (*dashed arrow*), indicating asymmetric growth and angular deformity. The fibular growth recovery line (*arrow head*) is parallel to the physis indicating normal symmetric growth.

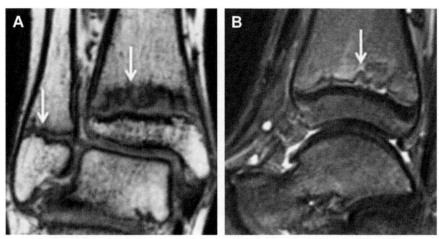

Fig. 5. Physeal stress injury in a 10-year-old gymnast with chronic ankle pain and recurrent inversion injuries. Coronal T1 (*A*) and sagittal short T1 inversion recovery (*B*) images demonstrate focal "tonguelike" extensions of the physeal cartilage into the metaphysis (*arrows*). These indicate disruption of endochondral ossification and typically resolve with rest.

disturbance is typically the result of chronic overuse stress in young athletes.

As the distal tibial and fibular physes begin to fuse normally with growth, at age 12 to 16 years in girls and age 15 to 18 years in boys, localized marrow edema can be seen in the epiphysis and metaphysis surrounding the closing physis, termed focal periphyseal edema zone[9] (**Fig. 6**). This normal phenomenon is commonly seen in the adolescent knee and ankle and may be a cause of joint pain. The etiology of the marrow edema may relate to relatively diminished bone flexibility at the sites of earliest transphyseal osseous fusion. The edema resolves with

progressive physeal closure and no treatment or imaging follow-up is necessary.[9]

EPIPHYSEAL/APOPHYSEAL CHONDRAL DEVELOPMENT

The cartilaginous epiphyses, spherical in the fetus, become increasingly hemispherical and concave postnatally. The distal tibial epiphyseal ossification center appears between 3 and 10 months of age with the distal fibular center appearing slightly later at 9 to 22 months of age.[10] The ossification begins centrally and extends peripherally but typically in an asymmetric fashion (**Fig. 7**). The medial and

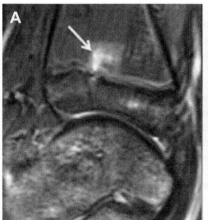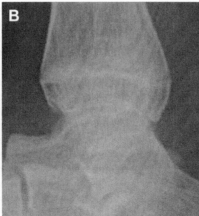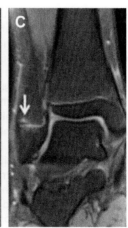

Fig. 6. Focal periphyseal edema. Sagittal short T1 inversion recovery (*A*) and lateral radiograph (*B*) of a 14-year-old boy with ankle pain. Focal increased fluid signal is centered at the distal tibial physis extending into the metaphysis (*solid arrow*) and the epiphysis to a lesser degree. Corresponding lateral radiograph confirms impending physeal fusion. A similar lesion in the distal fibula (*solid arrow*) is seen on the coronal proton density fat-suppressed image of another adolescent (*C*).

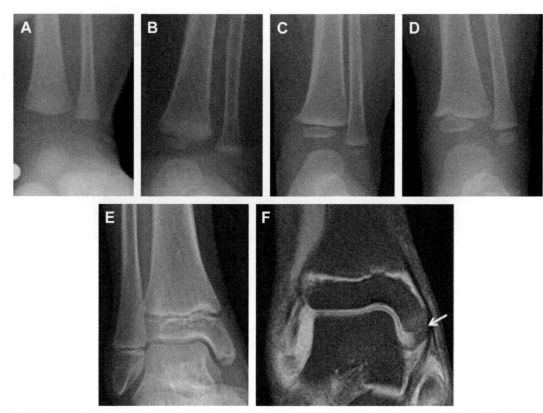

Fig. 7. Series of anteroposterior ankle radiographs in normal children at advancing ages: 52 days (*A*), 6 months (*B*), 11 months (*C*), 18 months (*D*), and 11 years (*E*). Note the appearance and development of the distal tibial and fibular epiphyses over time. They evolve from spherical to hemispherical and assume their terminal configurations by the second decade of life. The radiographically fragmented medial malleolus (*E*) should not be confused for a fracture. Coronal fat-suppressed proton density MR imaging (*F*) confirms cartilaginous continuity with the distal tibial ephiphysis (*arrow*). The distal fibular physis is at the level of the distal tibial physis at birth. Owing to asymmetric growth of these 2 physes, the distal fibular physis migrates distally to the level of the ankle mortise by age 5 (*E*).

lateral malleolar ossification centers appear later and are commonly separated from the dominant ossification center radiographically, but MR imaging shows the continuous surrounding cartilaginous anlage (see **Fig. 7**). The tarsal bones develop in a process similar to the long bone epiphyses. Single or multiple ossification centers appear, often eccentrically, within the epiphyseal cartilage and subsequently coalesce.[2,11] Unossified epiphyseal cartilage is intermediate signal on T1 and low signal intensity on water sensitive sequences owing to the strong binding of water by macromolecules within the cartilage.[6] These macromolecules are broken down at the onset of ossification, freeing the previously bound water molecules and resulting in increased signal intensity on water sensitive sequences.[2] These high signal intensity "preossification centers" should not be mistaken for cartilaginous injury or inflammation[12,13] (see **Fig. 1**). The epiphyseal and tarsal ossification centers are surrounded by secondary physes, which are thinner but otherwise identical to the primary long bone physeal trilaminar appearance on T2-weighted MR images.

Articular cartilage can be differentiated from the less well-organized hyaline cartilage of the developing epiphysis/epiphyseal equivalents on MR imaging. The articular cartilage appears as a thin hyperintense rim along the articular surfaces of hypointense unossified tarsal cartilage on fluid sensitive sequences.[2,12,13]

The calcaneal apophysis typically develops with multiple secondary ossification centers beginning in the plantar third of the cartilaginous apophysis at approximately age 5 to 7 years.[11] These ossification centers often have an irregular fragmented appearance as they elongate and coalesce to form a cap like structure.[11] Fusion of the calcaneal apophysis begins at around 12 years old and is completed by the end of the second decade of life.[11] High signal intensity within the calcaneal apophysis on fluid sensitive sequences may reflect normal red marrow within the ossification center. Surrounding soft tissue edema and fluid at the Achilles tendon insertion are helpful indicators of Sever's calcaneal apophysitis[11,14,15] (**Fig. 8**).

Osteochondral Lesions

Osteochondritis dissecans (OCD) is an acquired lesion of subchondral bone characterized by osseous resorption and collapse, sequestrum formation, and variable involvement of the overlying articular cartilage. There is no consensus about the etiology of this condition, although repetitive minor trauma is suggested by many.[16] In young children, disruption of the spherical physeal trilaminar signal characteristics suggests that OCD may be related to secondary physeal injury[17]

(**Fig. 9**). The talus and navicular are frequent sites of foot and ankle OCD in children and adolescents. MR imaging is helpful to stage the lesions and to differentiate them from epiphyseal ossification center irregularity associated with normal developmental ossification in children. Disruption of the overlying articular cartilage and undercutting fluid indicate instability. Marrow edema within the fragment and subjacent bone as well as disruption of the spherical physis favor OCD over developmental ossification. This is especially helpful in the tarsal bones and malleoli, which characteristically develop with multifocal or fragmented ossification centers. OCD-associated intraarticular chondral fragments are also well demonstrated by MR imaging.

Another cause of apparent intraarticular osteochondral lesions of the ankle is dysplasia

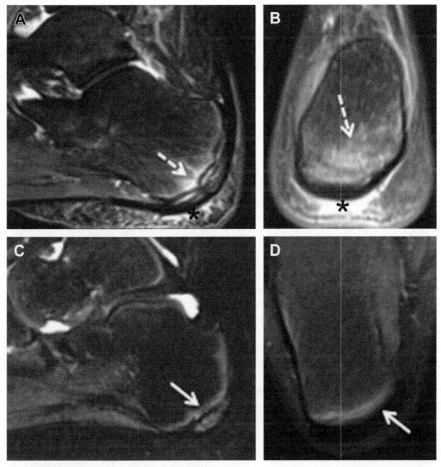

Fig. 8. Calcaneal apophysitis (Sever's disease). (*A, B*) Sagittal short T1 inversion recovery (STIR) and coronal proton density (PD) images of a 14-year-old girl with heel pain. There is marrow edema within the calcaneal apophysis extending into the calcaneal metaphyseal equivalent (*dashed arrow*) as well as adjacent soft tissue edema (*asterisk*). (*C, D*) Sagittal STIR and coronal PD images of a normal calcaneal apophysis for comparison. High signal intensity along the chondroosseous margin represents normal physis (*solid arrow*) and should not be mistaken for calcaneal apophysitis. Note that there is no adjacent soft tissue edema.

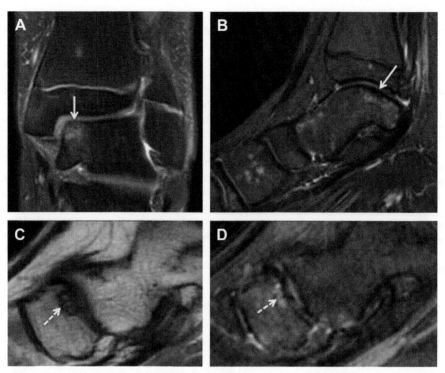

Fig. 9. Osteochondritis dissecans lesions. Coronal T1 and sagittal short T1 inversion recovery (STIR) images (*A, B*) of a 10-year-old girl show a medial talar dome osteochondral lesion (*solid arrow*) with subjacent marrow edema. There is irregularity of the overlying cartilage but no signs of instability. (*C, D*) Sagittal T1-weighted and fat-saturated T2-weighted images of a 14-year-old girl show a similar lesion within the navicular bone at the talonavicular joint (*dashed arrow*). Both lesions show typical peripheral sclerosis. The sagittal STIR image (*B*) demonstrates normal hematopoietic marrow within the anterior talus and navicular.

epiphysealis hemimelica or Trevor disease, which is the osteocartilaginous overgrowth of 1 or more epiphyses, typically involving the ankle or knee. Trevor disease is classified into 3 forms: (1) classic with involvement of one or more epiphyses of the same limb, (2) localized with involvement of only one epiphysis, and (3) diffuse with involvement of the entire lower limb (pelvis to foot).[18] Radiographically, multicentric calcifications are seen in the region of an epiphysis or apophysis. MR imaging differentiates this condition from other paraarticular calcifications including synovial chondromatosis, vascular malformation, and tumoral calcinosis. MR imaging will demonstrate the extent of epiphyseal involvement and the unossified chondral component, necessary for surgical planning.[19,20] The osteocartilaginous overgrowths in dysplasia epiphysealis hemimelica have similar signal intensities as the normal epiphyseal cartilage[21] (**Fig. 10**).

Osteochondroses

Osteochondroses are benign lesions of the immature epiphyses or epiphyseal equivalents that are likely the result of repetitive mechanical stress leading to vascular compromise, collapse, and fragmentation of the involved bone.[22] Osteochondroses of the tarsal navicular and metatarsal head are known as Kohler disease and Freiberg infraction, respectively. Kohler disease has a male predilection and typically affects younger patients between the of ages 4 and 6 years.[22,23] The condition is self-limited and most resolve with no significant deformity.[24] In contrast, Freiberg infraction has a female predilection and typically affects adolescents between 12 and 18 years of age, often involving the second or third metatarsal heads.[24] MR imaging is helpful when radiographs demonstrate navicular ossification center irregularity and fragmentation, which may be developmental. On MR imaging, the involved bone will be hypointense on T1 and demonstrate edema (early) or sclerosis (late) on fluid sensitive sequences[24] (**Fig. 11**). Surrounding soft tissue edema with cortical irregularity, flattening, and fragmentation may be present.[24] Freiberg infraction can result in deformity of the affected bone but complete healing may be seen even after several years.[25]

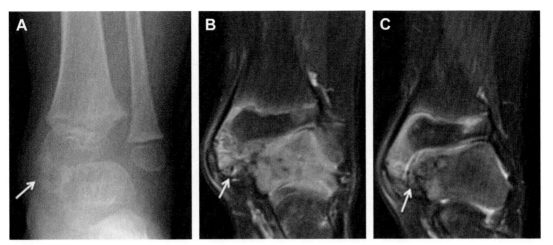

Fig. 10. Dysplasia epiphysealis hemimelica (Trevor disease) in a 3-year-old girl with a medial ankle mass. Anteroposterior radiograph (*A*) shows the calcified mass adjacent to the medial talus (*arrow*). Consecutive coronal fat-suppressed proton density images (*B, C*) show that the complex mass is composed of chondral and osseous signal and arises from the medial malleolar epiphyseal cartilage (*arrow in B*). The more anterior image (*C*) shows an additional, similar masslike enlargement of the medial talus (*solid arrow*) owing to classical dysplasia epiphysealis hemimelica.

PERIOSTEUM

The periosteum in children is loosely attached to the cortex along the shaft of the tibia and fibula, but becomes tightly adherent at the physis.[2] This configuration allows tumor, hematoma, or pus to extend under the periosteum leading to periosteal elevation and subperiosteal collections (**Fig. 12**). Normally, a fibrovascular layer of tissue separates the periosteum from the cortex of the metaphysis.[2]

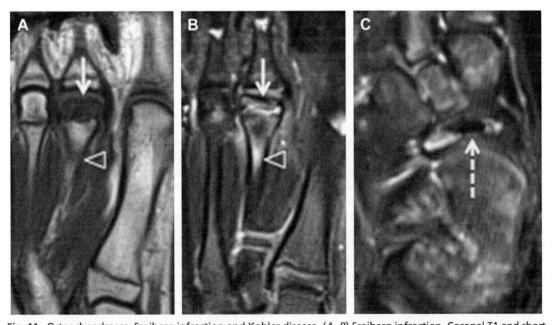

Fig. 11. Osteochondroses. Freiberg infraction and Kohler disease. (*A, B*) Freiberg infraction. Coronal T1 and short T1 inversion recovery (STIR) images of a 12-year-old girl with foot pain. Heterogenous hypointense T1 and increased STIR signal and flattening of the articular surface of the second metatarsal epiphysis (*solid arrow*) are related to ischemia. Stress-induced marrow edema is present in the second metatarsal shaft (*arrow head*). (*C*) Kohler disease. Coronal STIR image of a 7-year-old boy shows a small navicular ossification center with central hypointense signal surrounded by peripheral increased signal intensity compatible with late changes of Kohler disease (*dashed arrow*).

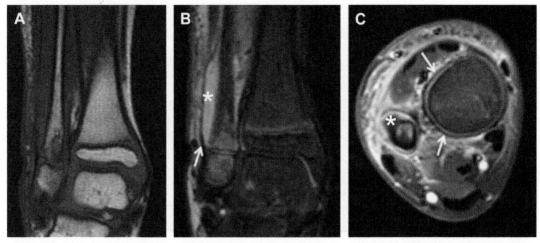

Fig. 12. Osteomyelitis with subperiosteal abscesses. Coronal T1 (*A*), coronal inversion recovery (*B*) and axial fat-saturated T1 postcontrast (*C*) images of a 4-year-old girl with distal fibular osteomyelitis. The distal fibular metaphyseal marrow signal is lower than muscle on T1 and high signal intensity on the inversion recovery sequence. There is circumferential periosteal elevation with a large subperiosteal fluid collection (*asterisk*), surrounding soft tissue edema, and a nonenhancing intraosseous collection. Note that the periosteum is attached at the physis, preventing the subperiosteal abscess from extending distally (*arrow in B*). Coronal inversion recovery image (*B*) shows marrow edema within the distal fibular epiphysis and periphyseal metaphysis. The axial image also demonstrates the normal tibial metaphyseal collar related to highly vascular spongiosum (*arrows in C*). This should not be mistaken for periosteal reaction or subperiosteal collection.

On MR images, this normal structure is often seen as a metaphyseal stripe (long axis images) or collar (axial images) of fluid signal intensity or enhancement underlying the distal tibial and fibular periosteum[2] (see **Fig. 12**). The metaphyseal stripe disappears at skeletal maturity.[2]

MARROW DEVELOPMENT

Distinguishing normal age-appropriate marrow from pathology can be a source of concern on MR imaging of the pediatric skeleton. The neonatal marrow is completely red/hematopoietic and converts to adult yellow/fatty marrow in a predictable pattern. Within the long bones, the conversion occurs first within the epiphyses and then proceeds from central to peripheral or diaphysis to metaphysis. Within the skeleton as a whole, the conversion is peripheral to central or distal to proximal.[3,26] The epiphysis undergoes conversion to fatty marrow within 6 months of the appearance of the secondary ossification center, which begins to form between 6 months and 2 years of age in the distal tibia.[27]

Isolated foci of residual red marrow may remain in the metaphyses into early adulthood and can mimic pathology. Typically, retained hematopoietic marrow in the long bones is flame-shaped or vertically striated with a base that extends to the physis.[28,29] The T1 signal intensity of these regions should be greater than that of the adjacent

muscle.[2] Residual red marrow in the ankle and foot, especially in the talus, calcaneus, and tarsal bones, often appears as speckled hyperintense foci on fluid sensitive sequences and as hypointense foci on T1WI[29,30] (**Fig. 13**). Hematopoietic marrow is hyperenhancing after contrast administration (**Fig. 14**). These areas of signal change are often attributed to stress-related edema in athletes, but they more likely to represent normal perivascular foci of red marrow, which are magnified by the osteoporosis associated with immobilization.[14]

Marrow signal intensity that is lower than adjacent muscle on T1WI should be viewed with concern at any age. Localized marrow edema in the ankle and hindfoot of young children is commonly owing to osteomyelitis. Many of these children have a history of minor trauma and their symptoms may be attributed to radiographically occult fracture. MR imaging evaluation should be considered in any child with a limp, ankle pain and fever. MR imaging of chondroosteomyelitis of the tarsal bones in infants and toddlers reveals increased fluid signal intensity within the ossification centers and surrounding cartilaginous anlage (**Fig. 15**). Marrow edema owing to trauma, infection, or inflammation typically has indistinct, irregular margins with the adjacent normal fatty marrow (see **Fig. 12**). Sharp, well-defined borders between abnormal and normal marrow raise suspicion for neoplasm (**Fig. 16**).

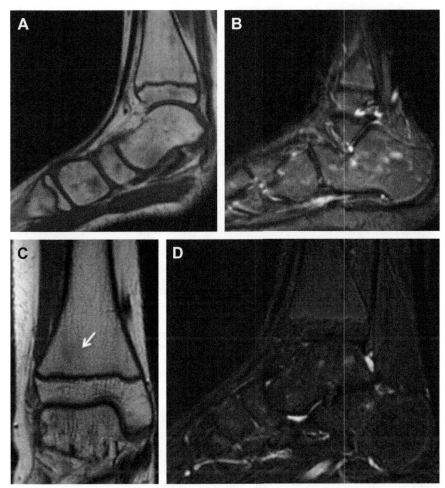

Fig. 13. Physiologic residual red marrow, changes with age. A 9-year-old active soccer player with lateral ankle pain. Sagittal T1 (*A*) and inversion recovery (*B*) images show speckled residual red marrow normally present in the distal tibia and tarsal bones. The T1 signal intensity of the red marrow foci is higher than the plantar muscles. Coronal T1 (*C*) and sagittal inversion recovery (*D*) images of the same child 4 years later shows decreasing red marrow with mild residual in the talus, navicular, and distal tibial metaphysis where it is striated and extends from the physis (*arrow*).

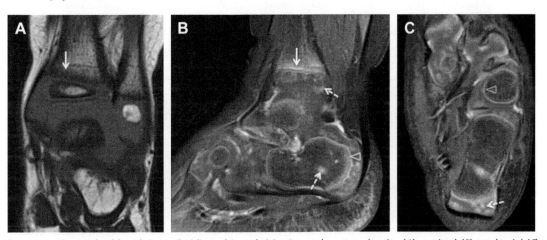

Fig. 14. A 22-month-old with juvenile idiopathic arthritis. Coronal proton density (*A*), sagittal (*B*), and axial (*C*) fat-suppressed postcontrast images show minimal synovitis and hyperenhancement of normal vascular structures including the primary and secondary physes (*open arrowheads*) and residual red marrow within the distal tibial metaphysis (*solid arrows*), epiphysis, and tarsal cartilaginous anlage (*dashed arrows*).

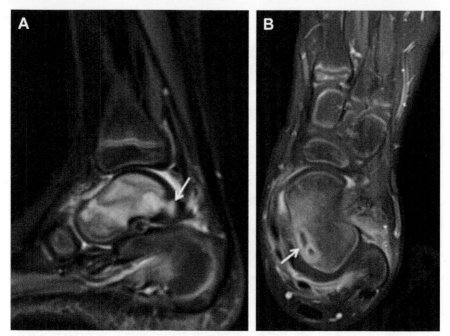

Fig. 15. A 4-year-old girl with talar chondroosteomyelitis. The patient fell from a chair and had been immobilized for presumed distal fibular physeal fracture. When the cast was removed 3 weeks later, she refused to bear weight on the extremity. Sagittal T2 fat-suppressed image (*A*) shows extensive edema throughout the talar ossification center with a more focal fluid collection extending through the physis into the posterior talar epiphyseal cartilage (*arrow*). Effusion and soft tissue edema surround the bone. The postcontrast image (*B*) confirms the peripherally enhancing multilocular abscess within the talar ossification center (*arrow*). Note the normal appearing trilaminar distal tibial physis and enhancing tarsal physes.

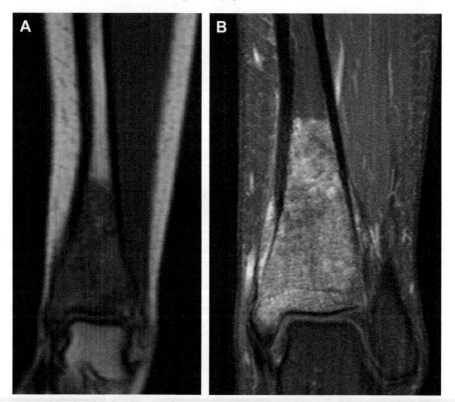

Fig. 16. A 14-year-old girl with left ankle pain for several months secondary to distal tibial osteosarcoma. Coronal T1-weighted MR image without fat suppression (*A*), low resolution owing to magnification of the large field of view image for the entire tibia, and coronal T1 fat-suppressed postcontrast image (*B*) show sharp demarcation between the medullary tumor and the adjacent normal marrow. Well-defined margins between normal and abnormal marrow should raise suspicion for neoplasm. This is in contrast with ill-defined margins, which suggest inflammatory conditions.

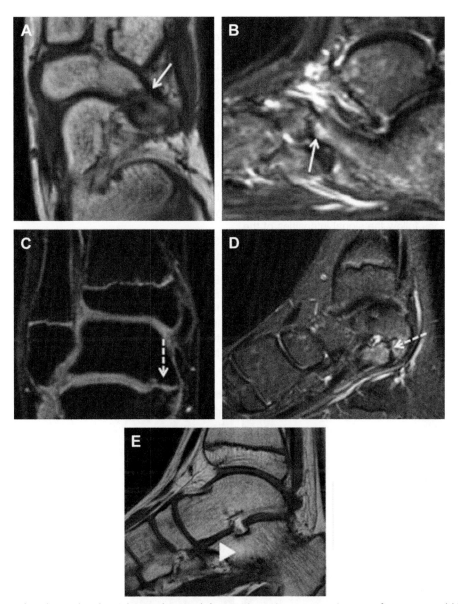

Fig. 17. Tarsal coalition. (*A, B*) Axial T1 and sagittal short T1 inversion recovery images of an 11-year-old boy with soft tissue and marrow edema along the elongated calcaneal anterior process, related to stress changes at the calcaneonavicular fibrous coalition (*solid arrow*). (*C–E*) Coronal fat-suppressed gradient echo, sagittal fat-suppressed T2, and sagittal proton density images of another patient with foot pain demonstrate the variant ta-localcaneal posteromedial facet coalition with marrow edema on either side of the coalition (*dashed arrow*). The middle facet (*arrow head* in *E*) is normal in this variant condition, which represents one-quarter of all subtalar coalitions. The majority of subtalar coalitions, in contrast, involve the middle facet.

DEVELOPMENTAL ABNORMALITIES
Tarsal Coalition

Tarsal coalition refers to congenital osseous, cartilaginous, or fibrous fusion of 2 or more adjacent bones in the mid and hind foot. Calcaneonavicular and talocalcaneal coalitions represent nearly 90% of all tarsal coalitions and are bilateral in approximately 50% of affected individuals.[31–35] Children

and adolescents often present with vague foot pain, fatigability, and peroneal spasms, owing to the heel valgus and altered mechanics associated with the coalition.[35,36] Calcaneonavicular coalitions are easily identified on well-positioned oblique radiographs of the foot as an elongated anterior process of the calcaneus, which represents fusion or narrowed articulation to the lateral aspect of the navicular.[36] Radiographs are less definitive in talocalcaneal coalitions. Computed tomography and MR imaging reveal osseous or nonosseous fusion between the talus, most commonly the middle facet, and the sustantaculum tali of the calcaneus.[36] A recent study found that more than 25% of subtalar (talocalcaneal) coalitions involve a variant posteromedial facet of the talus, associated with a short middle facet and elongated sustentaculum tali.[37] All of the posteromedial coalitions were nonosseous. In addition to the osseous changes elegantly shown by computed tomography, MR imaging reveals associated marrow and soft tissue edema. Cartilaginous coalitions follow the signal intensities of the articular cartilage, hypointense on T1 and hyperintense on fluid sensitive sequences, whereas fibrous and osseous coalitions are typically low signal intensity on all sequences[24,35] (**Fig. 17**).

Clubfoot Deformity

Clubfoot or talipes equinovarus occurs in 1 to 4 in 1000 live births and preferentially affects boys. It is congenital and may be isolated or associated with other abnormalities including myelomeningocele, arthrogryposis, and dysplasias. Radiographically, the hallmarks are fixed calcaneal plantarflexion (equinus) with tibiocalcaneal angle of greater than 90°, hindfoot varus with talocalcaneal angle of less than 30°, and forefoot varus.[38] The navicular bone is medially subluxed relative to the talus but not evident radiographically because the navicular ossification center is eccentric and does not appear until 2 to 5 years of age. Ultrasound and MR imaging may be used to evaluate the unossified cartilaginous tarsal bones in these young children (**Fig. 18**).

SOFT TISSUE TUMORS AND TUMORLIKE LESIONS

Benign soft tissue tumors and tumorlike lesions far outnumber malignant lesions in the pediatric foot and ankle. Small, superficial lesions should initially be evaluated on ultrasound examination to determine whether the mass is solid or cystic. MR imaging is the modality of choice for

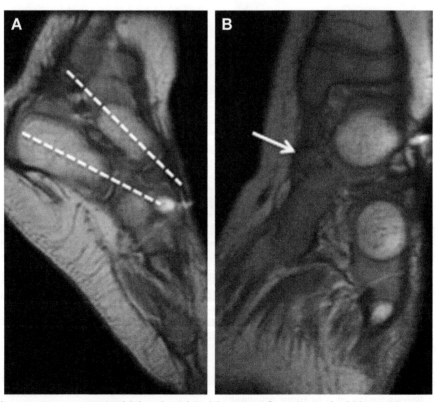

Fig. 18. Talipes equinovarus. Sagittal (*A*) and axial T1 (*B*) images of an 18-month-old boy with neurogenic clubfoot. The talocalcaneal angle, formed by lines drawn along the axes of the talus and calcaneus, is decreased (18° compared with normal >30°). There is mild medial subluxation of the unossified navicular relative to the talus (*arrow*). Varus deformity of the forefoot with adduction of the metatarsals is partially visualized. There is suggestion of an elevated plantar arch on sagittal view.

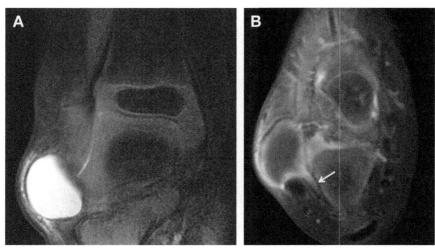

Fig. 19. Ganglion cyst. Coronal proton density (*A*) and axial postcontrast fat-suppressed T1-weighted (*B*) images in this 23-month-old with a painless mass on the lateral aspect of the right ankle. The cyst is just anterior to the peroneal tendon and a thin tail insinuates between the tendon and the adjacent calcaneus (*arrow*). Peripheral enhancement is present on the postcontrast images.

evaluation of complex cystic and solid masses.[39] Fluid-filled lesions are most commonly benign ganglion or synovial cysts or vascular malformations. Both can be seen in early childhood through adulthood. Ganglion cysts are unilocular or multilocular lobular fluid signal intensity masses adjacent to a joint or tendon sheath[22] (**Fig. 19**). Both benign lesions may occasionally demonstrate heterogeneous internal signal owing to hemorrhage or proteineous contents within the cyst. Postcontrast imaging may be required to exclude solid components and differentiate them from neoplastic processes, such as synovial sarcoma.

Synovial sarcomas are the most common soft tissue malignancy of the adult and pediatric foot.[40,41] These are most commonly periarticular multiloculated masses with multiple internal septations, heterogeneous enhancement, and mixed low T1 and high signal intensity on water-sensitive sequences.[39,41] Small lesions in the feet, however, may have a nonaggressive, well-defined, unilocular appearance with heavy T2 weighting similar to that of a ganglion cyst on precontrast images[39,41] (**Fig. 20**). Comparison between precontrast and postcontrast T1WI with fat suppression will document enhancement of these tumors. Synovial sarcoma may also have indolent growth with

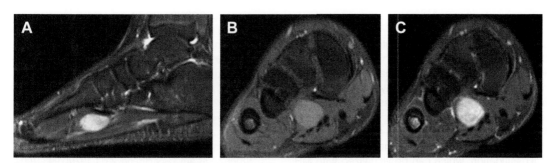

Fig. 20. Synovial sarcoma in a typical location in this 11-year-old girl with a plantar arch bump for more than 2 years. Sagittal short T1 inversion recovery imaging (*A*) shows a heterogeneously hyperintense, well-circumscribed lesion deep to the extensor tendons of the midfoot. The diffuse enhancement documented by comparison of the axial T1 fat-suppressed images before (*B*) and after (*C*) distinguishes this lesion from ganglion/synovial cysts, which should only show peripheral enhancement. Even though it is malignant, this synovial sarcoma displayed all of the imaging features typically thought of as nonaggressive, including sharp margins, little surrounding edema, and slow growth.

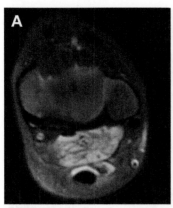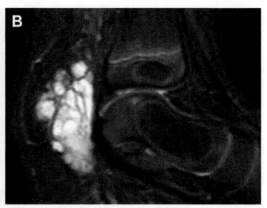

Fig. 21. A 2-year-old with venous malformation of the heel. Axial (*A*) and sagittal short T1 inversion recovery (*B*) images show a multilocular, hyperintense lesion in the posterior soft tissues of the ankle, involving the Achilles' and flexor hallucis longus tendons. This slow flow lesion contains characteristic fluid–fluid levels and low signal intensity phleboliths.

apparent stability on consecutive imaging studies, further complicating their diagnosis.[41]

The most common vascular lesion in the pediatric foot and ankle is the venous malformation, composed of an abnormal network of thin-walled dysplastic venous spaces with slow flow.[42,43] These venous channels are present at birth with gradual expansion, but may not become symptomatic until later in childhood when they present with a painful mass that often fluctuates in size and may have overlying cutaneous bluish discoloration.[42,43] Venous malformations have characteristic MR imaging appearances with T2 hyperintense tubular or cystic spaces often with fluid–fluid levels owing to hemorrhage or high protein content, as well as small phleboliths, which are low signal intensity on all sequences.[43] Generally, diffuse enhancement of the lesion is seen on delayed images after administration of an intravenous contrast agent[43] (**Fig. 21**).

SUMMARY

Accurate diagnosis of abnormalities of the pediatric ankle and foot requires an understanding of normal development and the changing MR imaging appearances that accompany growth. Maturation of the cartilaginous structures and the marrow occurs in a predictable pattern. Abnormalities of the physis and epiphysis owing to trauma, infection, or disease lead to disturbances in endochondral ossification, which can be visualized with MR imaging. Physiologic bone marrow conversion from neonatal hematopoietic marrow to adult fatty marrow also occurs in a predictable pattern. Recognition of the characteristic appearances of persistent red marrow can help to distinguish normal pediatric marrow from disease.

REFERENCES

1. Scheuwer L, Black S. The juvenile skeleton. 2nd edition. London: Elsevier; 2004. p. 23–45, 341–466.
2. Laor T, Jaramillo D. MR imaging insights into skeletal maturation: what is normal? Radiology 2009;250(1): 28–38.
3. Jaramillo D, Laor T, Hoffer F, et al. Epiphyseal marrow in infancy: MR imaging. Radiology 1991; 180(3):809–12.
4. Fleming J, Dodd L, Helms C. Prominent vascular remnants in the calcaneus simulating a lesion on MRI of the ankle: findings in 67 patients with cadaveric correlation. AJR Am J Roentgenol 2005;185(6): 1449–52.
5. Jaramillo D, Shapiro F. Growth cartilage: normal appearance, variants and abnormalities. Magn Reson Imaging Clin N Am 1998;6(3):455–71.
6. Menezes NM, Olear EA, Li X, et al. Gadolinium-enhanced MR images of the growing piglet skeleton: ionic versus nonionic contrast agent. Radiology 2006;239(2):406–14.
7. Love S, Ganey T, Ogden J. Postnatal epiphyseal development: the distal tibia and fibula. J Pediatr Orthop 1990;10(3):298–305.
8. Ecklund K, Jaramillo D. Imaging of growth disturbance in children. Radiol Clin North Am 2001; 39(4):823–41.
9. Zbojniewicz AM, Laor T. Focal periphyseal edema (FOPE) zone on MRI of the adolescent knee: a potentially painful manifestation of physiologic physeal fusion? AJR Am J Roentgenol 2011;197(4):998–1004.
10. Bedoya MA, Chauvin NA, Jaramillo D, et al. Common patterns of congenital lower extremity shortening: diagnosis, classification, and follow-up. Radiographics 2015;35(4):1191–207.
11. Rossi I, Rosenberg Z, Zember J. Normal skeletal development and imaging pitfalls of the calcaneal

apophysis: MRI features. Skeletal Radiol 2016;45(4): 483–93.

12. Rivas R, Shapiro F. Structural stages in the development of the long bones and epiphyses: a study in the New Zealand white rabbit. J Bone Joint Surg Am 2002;84-A(1):85–100.

13. Varich LJ, Laor T, Jaramillo D. Normal maturation of the distal femoral epiphyseal cartilage: age-related changes at MR imaging. Radiology 2000;214(3): 705–9.

14. Shabshin N, Schweitzer ME, Morrison WB, et al. High-signal T2 changes of the bone marrow of the foot and ankle in children: red marrow or traumatic changes? Pediatr Radiol 2006;36(7):670–6.

15. Ogden JA, Ganey TM, Hill JD, et al. Sever's injury: a stress fracture of the immature calcaneal metaphysis. J Pediatr Orthop 2004;24(5):488–92.

16. Edmonds EW, Polousky J. A review of knowledge in osteochondritis dissecans: 123 years of minimal evolution from Konig to the ROCK study group. Clin Orthop Relat Res 2013;471(4):1118–26.

17. Laor T, Zbojniewicz A, Eismann E, et al. Juvenile osteochondritis dissecans: is it a growth disturbance of the secondary physis of the epiphysis? AJR Am J Roentgenol 2012;199(5):1121–8.

18. Azouz EM. MRI of dysplasia epiphysealis hemimelica. Pediatr Radiol 1996;26(12):904.

19. Merzoug V, Wicard P, Dubousset J, et al. Bilateral dysplasia epiphysealis hemimelica: report of two cases. Pediatr Radiol 2002;32(6):431–4.

20. Lang I, Azouz E. MRI appearances of dysplasia epiphysealis hemimelica of the knee. Skeletal Radiol 1997;26(4):226–9.

21. Iwasawa T, Aida N, Kobayashi N, et al. MRI findings of dysplasia epiphysealis hemimelica. Pediatr Radiol 1996;26(1):65–7.

22. Rosenberg ZS, Beltran J, Bencardino JT. MR imaging of the ankle and foot. Radiographics 2000;20(suppl_1):S153–79.

23. Stanton BK, Karlin JM, Scurran BL. Kohler's disease. J Am Podiatr Med Assoc 1992;82(12):625–9.

24. Iyer RS, Thapa MM. MR imaging of the paediatric foot and ankle. Pediatr Radiol 2013;43(Suppl 1): S107–19.

25. Baert A, editor. Encyclopedia of diagnostic imaging, vol. 2. New York: Springer-Verlag Verlin Heidelberg; 2008.

26. Vogler JB, Murphy WA. Bone marrow imaging. Radiology 1988;168(3):679–93.

27. Ogden J, Phillips S. Radiology of postnatal skeletal development. VII. The scapula. Skeletal Radiol 1983;9(3):157–69.

28. Foster K, Chapman S, Johnson K. MRI of the marrow in the paediatric skeleton. Clin Radiol 2004;59(8): 651–73.

29. Babyn PS, Ranson M, McCarville ME. Normal bone marrow: signal characteristics and fatty conversion. Magn Reson Imaging Clin N Am 1998;6(3):473–95.

30. Dwek JR, Shapiro F, Laor T, et al. Normal gadolinium-enhanced MR images of the developing appendicular skeleton: Part 2. Epiphyseal and metaphyseal marrow. AJR Am J Roentgenol 1997;169(1): 191–6.

31. Gessner AJ, Kumar SJ, Gross GW. Tarsal coalition in pediatric patients. Semin Musculoskelet Radiol 1999;3(3):239–46.

32. Bohne WH. Tarsal coalition. Curr Opin Pediatr 2001; 13(1):29–35.

33. Schoenberg NY, Lehman WB. Magnetic resonance imaging of pediatric disorders of the ankle and foot. Magn Reson Imaging Clin N Am 1994;2(1):109–22.

34. Newman JS, Newberg AH. Congenital tarsal coalition: multimodality evaluation with emphasis on CT and MR imaging. Radiographics 2000;20(2):321–32.

35. Patel CV. The foot and ankle: MR imaging of uniquely pediatric disorders. Magn Reson Imaging Clin N Am 2009;17(3):539–47, vii.

36. Murphy JS, Mubarak SJ. Talocalcaneal Coalitions. Foot Ankle Clin 2015;20(4):681–91.

37. Bixby SD, Jarrett DY, Johnston P, et al. Posteromedial subtalar coalitions: prevalence and associated morphological alterations of the sustentaculum tali. Pediatr Radiol 2016;46(8):1142–9.

38. Kamegaya M, Shinohara Y, Kuniyoshi K, et al. MRI study of talonavicular alignment in clubfoot. J Bone Joint Surg Br 2001;83(B):726–30.

39. Waldt S, Rechl H, Rummeny E, et al. Imaging of benign and malignant soft tissue masses of the foot. Eur Radiol 2003;13(5):1125–36.

40. Kransdorf M. Malignant soft-tissue tumors in a large referral population: distribution of diagnoses by age, sex, and location. AJR Am J Roentgenol 1995; 164(1):129–34.

41. Morton M, Berquist T, McLeod R, et al. MR imaging of synovial sarcoma. AJR Am J Roentgenol 1991; 156(2):337–40.

42. Fayad LM, Hazirolan T, Bluemke D, et al. Vascular malformations in the extremities: emphasis on MR imaging features that guide treatment options. Skeletal Radiol 2006;35(3):127–37.

43. Flors L, Leiva-Salinas C, Maged IM, et al. MR imaging of soft-tissue vascular malformations: diagnosis, classification, and therapy follow-up. Radiographics 2011;31(5):1321–40.

Aftermath of Ankle Inversion Injuries
Spectrum of MR Imaging Findings

Timothy M. Meehan, MD,
Edgar Leonardo Martinez-Salazar, MD,
Martin Torriani, MD, MMSc*

KEYWORDS

• Ankle • Injuries • Sprain • MR imaging • Ligaments

KEY POINTS

• MRI is the method of choice to characterize soft tissue and osseous injuries, which can involve both the lateral and medial ankle after inversion injuries.
• Injury to anterior talofibular ligament is the most common sequela of ankle inversion injury, however additional ligamentous and bony lesions may be present.
• MRI can detect occult injuries that are not apparent during radiographic or clinical workup, which may affect functional outcome.

INTRODUCTION

Acute ankle injuries rank among the most common musculoskeletal injuries, affecting both elite athletes and the general population, resulting in up to 10% of emergency room visits.[1,2] Approximately 80% to 90% of injuries involve the lateral ankle ligaments, being more common in sports that require running and jumping, which account for up to 25% of total injuries.[3] Importantly, long-term residual symptoms after an acute injury are increasingly reported. In prior studies, 74% of patients had recurrent or residual symptoms up to 4 years after an acute inversion injury,[4] and 32% of patients had recurrent complaints up to 7 years following the initial injury.[5]

Traditional assessment with clinical examination and radiographs is usually performed for inversion injuries. However, clinical examination alone can be unreliable in the acute setting because of pain,[6] with standard and stress-view radiographs being limited by ankle orientation, amount of force applied, and the patient's ability to cooperate with the examination. In contrast, MR imaging grading of ligamentous injury can predict clinical outcomes and correlates with return to sporting activity.[2] MR arthrography may also be useful in patients with chronic lateral ankle instability compared with stress radiographs and conventional MR imaging when assessing for full-thickness tears.[7] Importantly, the accurate delineation of soft tissue and osseous anatomy and the characterization of ankle ligamentous injury by MR imaging have been well documented.[2]

Although anterior talofibular ligament injury is by far the most common occurrence in ankle inversion injuries, additional findings that go underdiagnosed by usual radiographic or clinical work-up may affect the clinical course and outcome in both acute and chronic cases. Osteochondral injuries and occult fractures, complex lateral ankle ligament tears, syndesmotic injury, sinus tarsi syndrome, countercoup and deltoid ligament injury, as well as tendon and retinacular injury occur in

Disclosure: The authors have nothing to disclose.
Division of Musculoskeletal Imaging and Intervention, Department of Radiology, Massachusetts General Hospital, Harvard Medical School, 55 Fruit Street, Boston, MA 02114, USA
* Corresponding author. Division of Musculoskeletal Imaging and Intervention, Department of Radiology, Massachusetts General Hospital, 55 Fruit Street, YAW 6048, Boston, MA 02114.
E-mail address: mtorriani@mgh.harvard.edu

Magn Reson Imaging Clin N Am 25 (2017) 45–61
http://dx.doi.org/10.1016/j.mric.2016.08.012
1064-9689/17/© 2016 Elsevier Inc. All rights reserved.

inversion injuries and can be diagnosed by MR imaging. Therefore, familiarity with features of ankle inversion injury by MR imaging is important to comprehensively characterize the consequences of this type of skeletal trauma.

MR IMAGING PROTOCOL

A detailed description of MR imaging technique for foot and ankle is beyond the scope of this article and is covered elsewhere (see Won C. Bae, Thumanoon Ruangchaijatuporn, Christine B. Chung's article, "New Techniques in MR Imaging of the Ankle and Foot," in this issue).

However, brief general comments on technique are worth emphasizing in the context of lateral ankle ligamentous injury. MR imaging of the ankle is challenging because of a combination ankle spatial configuration, anatomic complexity, and inherent small size of ankle ligaments. Accurate diagnosis of disorder after an inversion injury hinges on the ability to assess the integrity of ligaments and articular cartilage, as well as identify subtle areas of bone marrow or soft tissue edema. Hallmarks of high-quality ankle MR imaging include uniform fat suppression, high signal-to-noise ratio (SNR), and elimination/minimization of artifacts. Although 3.0-T MR imaging systems allow higher spatial resolution and/or shorter imaging times, MR imaging at 1.5 T has proved effective for almost all musculoskeletal imaging applications, including the ankle.[8] Nonetheless, the benefit of obtaining ankle MR imaging at higher field strengths is apparent when assessing subtle ligamentous injury that may require higher spatial resolution, or when attempting to grade the severity of ligamentous injury, which may benefit from higher SNR.

Fat-suppressed images are necessary to detect subtle soft tissue or bone marrow edema, which are critical to fully characterize an injury. Although frequency-selective suppression of fat signal on fast spin-echo imaging is accepted practice, alternative techniques are emerging to improve fat suppression, increase SNR, and optimize image quality. One such technique uses multiecho Dixon techniques for fat and water separation to produce more uniform fat suppression with high SNR. This technique is less sensitive to magnetic field inhomogeneities and eliminates the need for selective fat suppression,[9] which frequently is uneven adjacent to curved surfaces of the ankle. This characteristic may be especially problematic adjacent to the malleoli and in the setting of prior metallic hardware placement, and can be exacerbated when using higher field strengths.

In order to adequately evaluate the lateral ankle ligaments and adjacent soft tissues, it is necessary to optimize the imaging planes and coverage during MR imaging examination. Coronal and axial images are most appropriate for ankle ligament assessment.[9] Axial coverage should extend from above the distal tibiofibular syndesmosis to the plantar soft tissues to ensure visualization of all lateral ligamentous structures. The coronal plane should be optimally placed along a line connecting both malleoli, which provides the best depiction of medial and lateral ligaments. If more detailed assessment is required, multiplanar reconstruction from two-dimensional or three-dimensional image data sets may be useful to provide nonstandard planes to visualize medial and lateral ankle ligaments.[10]

The optimal positioning of the foot and ankle before imaging is debated, with evidence showing no significant difference in ligament assessment between dorsiflexion and usual position of the ankle (20° of plantar flexion) in the supine position.[11] Further, strict positioning of the ankle during MR imaging examination may not be reproducible depending on foot size, coil configuration, and discomfort during scanning. Therefore, a balance between optimal positioning and comfort to avoid motion should be considered. Although no uniform standard exists for appropriate coil selection in ankle imaging, dedicated MR imaging coils with multichannel phase-array elements provide best results. However, excellent images can also be obtained with surface or extremity coils, as long as adequate coverage and contact are achieved.

DISORDERS
Lateral Ligamentous Injuries

Anterior talofibular ligament, calcaneofibular ligament, posterior talofibular ligament
Biomechanical studies have shown that the anterior talofibular ligament (ATFL) is the weakest of the lateral ankle ligaments, followed by the calcaneofibular ligament (CFL) and posterior talofibular ligament (PTFL).[12] As such, the ATFL is most susceptible to injury, with the remaining ligaments being involved sequentially based on their biomechanical properties.[13] The PTFL is rarely torn, except in cases of complete ankle dislocation and/or severe tibiofibular syndesmotic injury, and is consistently associated with injury of ATFL and CFL.[14] The most common mechanisms for lateral ankle ligamentous injury are inversion and plantar flexion.[15]

The ATFL originates at the anterior margin of the lateral malleolus and attaches to the talar body, anterior to the articular surface. Although variation does occur, the normal thickness of the ATFL on MR imaging has been described to be approximately 2 mm.[16] The ATFL is generally divided into 2 bands by perforating branches of the peroneal artery, which occasionally can be appreciated on MR imaging. The number of ATFL bands varies between 1 and 3, with different descriptions found in the literature.[15] Although these bands are inconsistently visualized on MR imaging, the increasing use of high field strength imaging has made such identification more common.[17] Functionally, the ATFL is important during plantar flexion, preventing anterior displacement of the talus. As such, the ATFL is vulnerable to injury especially under plantar flexion and inversion, placing the ligament under maximal strain.[18]

The CFL originates from the anterior aspect of the lateral malleolus, often with a partial connection to the ATFL at the fibula, and runs caudally and posteriorly to its attachment site on the lateral calcaneus. It is the second most commonly injured ligament of the lateral ankle. The CFL can be injured even in the absence of dorsiflexion or plantar flexion if stressed under varus foot positioning.[18] The CFL is an important lateral stabilizer and helps restrain calcaneal inversion,[15] elongating mostly during dorsiflexion and pronation. The peroneal retinaculum is in close proximity to the CFL and should not be confused with the ligament, because the retinaculum courses superficial, whereas the CFL runs deep to the peroneal tendons. The normal thickness of the CFL on MR imaging has been described to be approximately 3 mm.[16] When evaluating the CFL by MR imaging, note that the peroneal tendons travel superficial to the ligament, often resulting in an indentation.

The PTFL is the strongest of the lateral ankle ligaments and is rarely injured. It spans from the lateral malleolar fossa to the posterolateral talus, with a horizontal trajectory. It is usually interconnected with fibers from the posterior intermalleolar ligament and contains numerous fascicles that yield a normal striated appearance on MR imaging, which should not be confused with abnormality. Dorsiflexion increases tensile stress to the PTFL[18] and the ligament limits anterior and posterior displacement of the talus in relation to the tibia and fibula.[15]

During an acute ankle sprain, an acute inflammatory response occurs during the first 3 days and a hematoma can form at the margins of a complete ligamentous tear.[19] Defects within the ligament can generally be seen within the first 2 weeks of injury, and by 7 weeks reparative remodeling has occurred to the point that the defect is no longer visualized, and the injured ligament is either attenuated or thickened, findings that are seen with subacute and chronic injuries.[20] However, the reparative process may fail to reconstitute the ligament, in which case it will not be visualized on MR imaging.[20] Bony proliferative changes can occur at attachment sites or within

the substance of the ligament with chronic injuries.[19] Although MR imaging is excellent to assess the integrity and stage of healing of ligamentous injuries, false-positive results do occur. In one prospective study, approximately 30% of patients with asymptomatic lateral ankles had an abnormal-appearing ATFL on MR imaging, which should be considered when evaluating lateral ankle ligaments.[21] Correlation with physical examination and clinical history are important components of accurate image interpretation.

As seen in other anatomic sites, MR imaging findings of acute ankle ligamentous injury include fiber discontinuity, thickening or attenuation of ligament, contour abnormalities, and intrasubstance signal changes. MR imaging grading of ligamentous injuries of the ankle follows the usual schema suggested for other ligaments based on T2-weighted MR imaging findings: grade 1, intrasubstance stretching without visible tears; grade 2, partial thickness tear; and grade 3, complete disruption of the ligament. As an important aside, MR imaging grading must be used with caution and in agreement with referring specialists, because it does not always reliably correlate with surgical findings.[2] Extra-articular joint fluid arising from a fluid-filled ligamentous defect, particularly with injury to the ATFL,[22] can be helpful to identify high-grade tears (**Figs. 1** and **2**). Other findings may include bone marrow edema/contusion, adjacent soft tissue edema, or associated avulsion fracture (**Fig. 3**). A common finding in chronic high-grade lateral ligament injuries is nonvisualization of a given ligament, with resulting prominent articular recess (**Figs. 4** and **5**). Acute CFL injury can result in thickening or discontinuity of fibers with surrounding soft tissue edema (**Fig. 6**). Associated thickening caused by sprain of the superior peroneal retinaculum and fluid in the peroneal tendon sheath are common secondary findings seen in lateral ankle ligament injuries.[23] The PTFL is rarely ruptured because of its intrinsic load capacity, therefore injury often results in intrasubstance loss of its normal fascicular appearance.

Injury to lateral ankle ligaments is linked to lateral ankle instability and functional ankle instability can result from unbalanced loading to the ankle joint. Studies evaluating cartilage T2 mapping and other advanced imaging techniques have shown peak cartilage strain as well as increased T2 relaxation time after lateral ligamentous injury,[24,25] suggesting that lateral ankle ligament injury can lead to acceleration of tibiotalar osteoarthritis in combination with chronic ankle instability.

Regarding evaluation of chronic lateral ankle ligament injuries, MR imaging has been proposed as an important component of patient work-up;

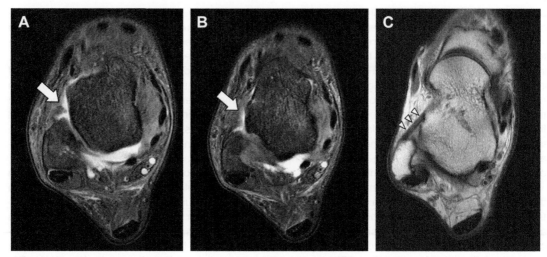

Fig. 1. A 21-year-old female patient presenting with ATFL full-thickness tear. (*A, B*) Ligamentous discontinuity at the talar attachment is seen (*arrow*) with fluid-filled ligamentous defect on axial T2-weighted fat-suppressed MR images. The normal appearance of the ATFL (*arrowheads*) in another patient is shown in a PD-weighted axial image (*C*).

however, a study by Park and colleagues[14] showed that the sensitivity of MR imaging to detect CFL chronic injuries was higher than for ATFL (44%–75% for ATFL, 50%–83% for CFL). In contrast, Kumar and colleagues[26] reported higher MR imaging sensitivity for detection of ATFL tears compared with CFL tears (87% for ATFL, 47% for CFL). Nonetheless, there is a high specificity and positive predictive value compared with arthroscopic findings in the diagnosis of chronic ankle pain and/or instability, showing up to 100% specificity for the diagnosis of ATFL and CFL tears and osteochondral lesions.[27] For these reasons, symptomatic patients with negative MR imaging findings may still require an arthroscopy for a definitive diagnosis.[27]

Tibiofibular syndesmosis

Injury to the distal tibiofibular syndesmosis, or high ankle sprain, is a well-recognized but often overlooked cause of chronic lateral ankle pain and instability. The incidence of tibiofibular syndesmosis injury ranges from 1% to 20%,[28] commonly with a protracted recovery time. Injury can be associated with other ligaments or ankle fractures[22]; however, isolated syndesmotic injury in

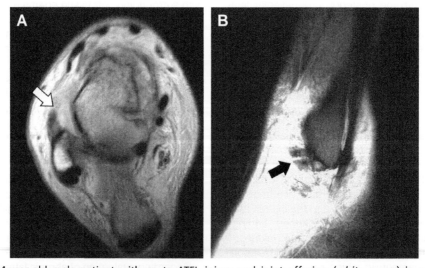

Fig. 2. A 24-year-old male patient with acute ATFL injury and joint effusion (*white arrow*) in axial (*A*) PD-weighted MR image. (*B*) T2 sagittal fat-suppressed MR image showing 2 distinct bands of the torn ATFL (*black arrow*), seen amid surrounding joint effusion and hematoma.

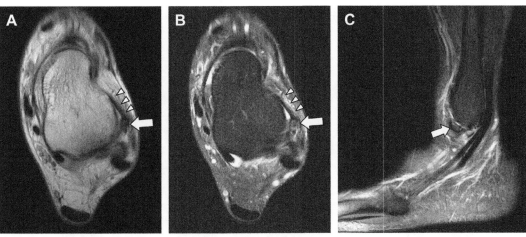

Fig. 3. A 29-year-old woman with an acute inversion injury. The ATFL (*arrowheads*) is attached to the avulsed lateral malleolar fracture fragment (*arrows*) seen in (*A*) axial T1-weighted, (*B*) axial, and (*C*) sagittal T2 fat-suppressed MR images. Note the bone marrow edema of the fracture fragment on T2 fat-suppressed images. The ATFL is otherwise continuous.

acute scenarios can occur in approximately 16% of athletes,[29] with the most common injury patterns being dorsiflexion and external rotation. Functionally, the syndesmotic ligament complex

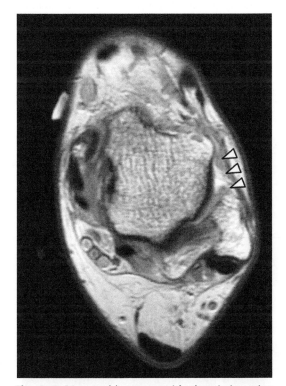

Fig. 4. A 34-year-old woman with chronic inversion injury. Axial PD-weighted MR image showing absent ATFL (*white arrowheads*) caused by prior full-thickness tear.

serves as a stabilizer of the distal tibia and fibula, resisting axial, rotational, and translational forces.

The distal tibiofibular syndesmosis is a complex structure composed of 4 syndesmotic ligaments: anterior inferior tibiofibular ligament (AITFL), posterior inferior tibiofibular ligament (PITFL), interosseous tibiofibular ligament (IOTFL), and inferior transverse tibiofibular ligament.[28] Although syndesmotic injury has traditionally been associated with high fibular fractures and certain types of Weber B fibular fractures, pure ligamentous injury without fracture is possible. In the acute traumatic setting, MR imaging has been shown to reliably identify syndesmotic injuries that were otherwise occult on radiographs and clinically.[30] MR imaging findings of acute syndesmotic injury consist of rupture or abnormal intrasubstance signal within the ligaments, occasionally with bony avulsion from either the tibial or fibular attachment sites,[30] which often result in widening of the syndesmosis. The reported sensitivity of MR imaging for syndesmotic injury ranges from 93% to 100%.[29]

The AITFL is the most commonly injured syndesmotic ligament and is almost always injured before other syndesmotic ligaments. Because of its oblique trajectory from the tibia to the fibula, it usually is seen in multiple consecutive axial images and requires careful assessment, because this off-axial orientation has been reported to affect diagnostic accuracy.[31] The origin of the AITFL is the anterolateral tibial tubercle and it extends laterally and distally to insert in the anterior margin of the fibula,[18,32] coursing in an oblique fashion. The MR imaging features of an acute

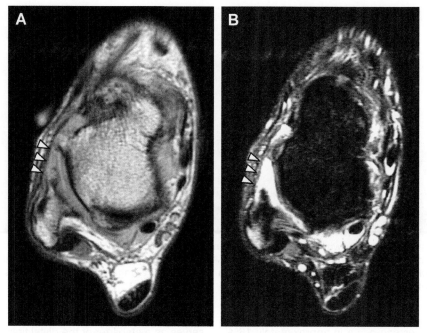

Fig. 5. A 31-year-old man with full-thickness chronic tear of the ATFL. Axial PD-weighted (*A*) and (*B*) fat-suppressed T2-weighted MR images show the high-grade chronic ATFL tear (*white arrowheads*). Note the enlarged articular recess in expected location of ATFL (*B*), typical of this type of chronic injury.

injury to the AITFL include discontinuity, laxity, or irregular configuration (**Fig. 7**). Although a small amount of fluid can be seen in a normal recess of distal tibiofibular syndesmosis, a recess height greater than 1 cm might prompt consideration of prior syndesmotic injury.[33] Chronic injury patterns span from complete disruption to a diminutive or thickened appearance, frequently with adjacent

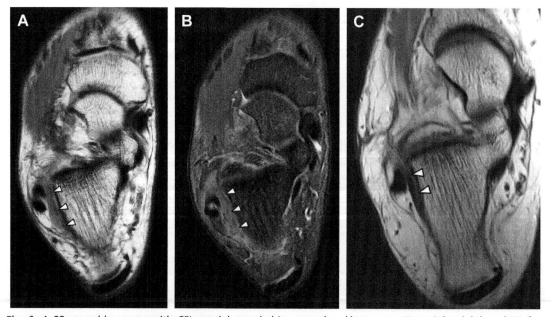

Fig. 6. A 22-year-old woman with CFL partial tear (*white arrowheads*) seen on PD-weighted (*A*) and T2 fat-suppressed (*B*) axial images. Note thickening and edema without evidence of full-thickness fluid-filled gap. The normal appearance of the CFL (*arrowheads*) in another patient is shown in a T1-weighted axial image (*C*).

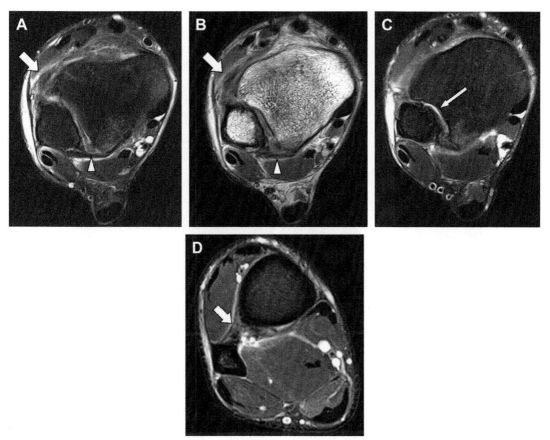

Fig. 7. A 33-year-old man with acute ankle injury showing high-grade AITFL partial tear (*arrow*) and PITFL partial tear (*arrowhead*) on (*A*) axial T2 fat-suppressed and (*B*) PD-weighted axial images. Axial T2 fat-suppressed images more proximally show excess fluid in the syndesmosis (*C, long arrow*) and involvement of the interosseous membrane (*D, arrow*).

small areas of mineralization (**Fig. 8**). Synovial hypertrophy is a commonly reported finding both at arthroscopy and MR imaging as a secondary finding. Thickening of an accessory AITFL can abut the talar dome and cause pain, resulting in anterolateral impingement. This accessory ligament resides inferior to the AITFL and is also known as the Basset ligament. Because of the high incidence of this variant (70%–92% incidence on MR imaging), many investigators believe it to be a normal anatomic structure and may refer to it as the distal fascicle of the AITFL[34] (**Fig. 9**).

The PITFL has a trapezoidal appearance and is divided into a superficial and deep component. It is the strongest syndesmotic ligament and isolated injury is rare.[35] The superficial component spans from the posterior margin of the distal fibula and inserts on the posterolateral tibial tubercle.[18,32] The deep component originates in the proximal area of the malleolar fossa and inserts on the posterior edge of the tibia.[18] The IOTFL

is an inferior continuation of the interosseous membrane and is composed of short fibers. Although there is no consensus regarding the biomechanical significance of the IOTFL,[18] injury usually occurs concurrently with other syndesmotic ligamentous injury or fracture. MR imaging findings include increased T2 signal, with or without disruption of ligamentous fibers (see **Fig. 7**). The inferior transverse tibiofibular ligament lies in close continuity to the PITFL and can be difficult to identify as a separate structure on MR imaging.[36]

Chronic symptoms related to syndesmotic injury may occur from either mechanical instability or impingement of hypertrophic soft tissue within the joint.[31] Sensitivity and specificity of chronic syndesmotic injuries are lower than those for acute injuries, ranging from 54% to 62%. Contrast enhancement on T1-weighted images has been described as a useful diagnostic indicator for chronic AITFL injury[37] and may improve sensitivity and specificity.

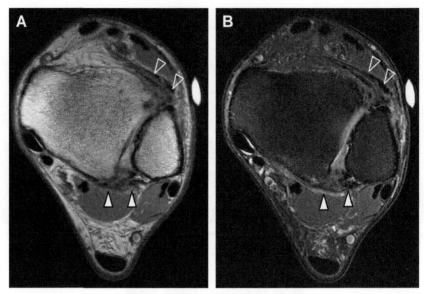

Fig. 8. A 29-year-old man with chronic tear of AITFL (*empty arrowheads*) and PITFL (*white arrowheads*) seen on axial PD-weighted (*A*) and T2 fat-suppressed (*B*) MR images. The ligaments are diffusely thickened and show heterogeneous signal intensity suggesting a chronic stage.

Sinus tarsi syndrome

The sinus tarsi is a conical anatomic space between the talus and calcaneus, which contains fatty tissue, nerve endings, arterial anastomoses, joint capsule, and ligaments (cervical ligament; interosseous talocalcaneal ligament; and the medial, intermediate, and lateral roots of inferior extensor retinaculum). The sinus tarsi spans between the anterior and posterior subtalar joints, occasionally communicating with the posterior subtalar joint. The ligaments of the sinus tarsi contribute to lateral stabilization of the ankle and hindfoot.[38] The cervical ligament is extracapsular and spans from the cervical tubercle of talar neck to the calcaneus, medial to the origin of the extensor digitorum brevis. The cervical ligament functions as a stabilizer that limits inversion of the hindfoot[39] and is therefore potentially affected in an inversion injury. The interosseous talocalcaneal ligament extends from the anterior margin of the posterior subtalar joint to the talus, functioning as a hindfoot stabilizer. The extensor retinaculum extends along the lateral margin of the sinus tarsi and, along with the cervical ligament, limits subtalar inversion.[39] The inferior extensor retinaculum has several components and appears as a Y-shaped connective tissue structure with medial, intermediate, and lateral roots with several attachment sites to both the calcaneus and the talus that provide stability to the hindfoot.

Sinus tarsi syndrome (STS) is a spectrum of abnormalities often clinically present with lateral or subtalar pain during weight bearing. Trauma often precedes STS, usually after an inversion ankle injury, therefore it is common for ligamentous injury of sinus tarsi to be present in up to 39% of patients with prior lateral ankle ligamentous tears.[38] The interosseous talocalcaneal ligament is the sinus tarsi ligament most commonly injured.

MR imaging findings of STS include diffuse low signal on T1-weighted images of the hyperintense sinus tarsi fat, with or without ligamentous injury (**Fig. 10**). The abnormal tissue is hyperintense on T2-weighted images and has been shown to reflect inflammation and fibrosis at histopathology.[40] Ligamentous injury is most commonly manifested as abnormal signal or disruption of the cervical and/or interosseous talocalcaneal ligaments. Association between several different types of ankle injuries and abnormal signal within the sinus tarsi has been reported, including posterior tibialis tendon injury, subtalar joint osteoarthritis, gout, tenosynovial giant cell tumor, and ganglion cyst formation.[39]

Deltoid ligament

The deltoid ligament is a strong multifascicle ligamentous medial stabilizer of the ankle, and consists of superficial and deep components. The deep deltoid ligament arises from the anterior colliculus of the tibia, inserting in the medial fovea of the talus, whereas the superficial deltoid ligament arises from the medial tibial periosteum, with insertions at sustentaculum tali, talar neck, spring

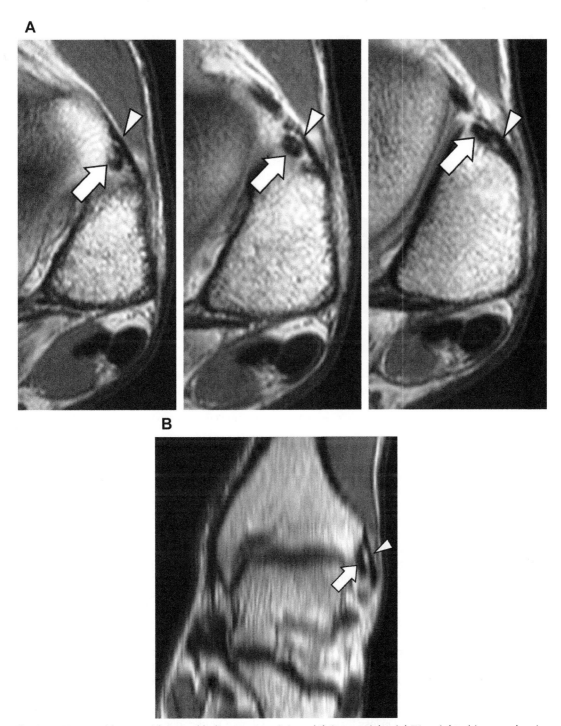

Fig. 9. A 50-year-old man without ankle ligamentous injury. (*A*) Sequential axial T1-weighted images showing accessory AITFL (Bassett ligament) (*arrows*) adjacent to the more caudal component of AITFL (*arrowheads*). (*B*) Oblique coronal reconstruction showing the anatomic relationship between both ligaments (Bassett ligament, *arrow*; AITFL, *arrowhead*).

ligament, navicular median eminence, and posterior talus.[41] The deep layers comprise the deep anterior and posterior tibiotalar ligaments, whereas the superficial layers include the tibionavicular ligament, tibiospring ligament, tibiocalcaneal ligament, and superficial posterior tibiotalar ligament. The tibiospring, tibionavicular, and the posterior tibiotalar ligament are the most

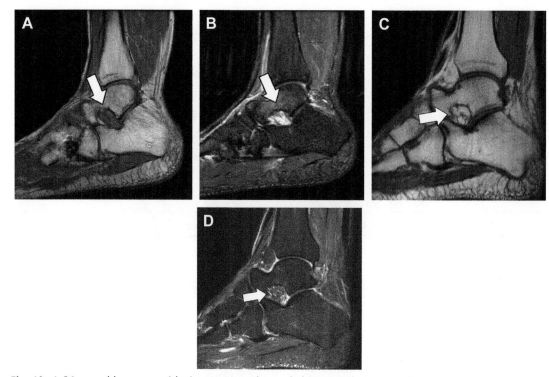

Fig. 10. A 34-year-old woman with sinus tarsi syndrome (*white arrow*) seen in (*A*) T1 and (*B*) fast multiplanar inversion recovery sagittal MR images. Note loss of normal fat signal in the sinus tarsi in (*A*) and edema in (*B*). The normal appearance of sinus tarsi (*white arrow*) in another patient is observed in (*C*) T1 and (*D*) T2 fat-suppressed sagittal MR images.

commonly visualized structures on MR imaging.[22] However, an important consideration is that variability in the presentation of superficial components should be expected and therefore most attention is usually directed to the deep components. Of these, the posterior tibiotalar ligament is the strongest ligament of the deltoid complex, which, in concert with the remaining medial ligaments, limits anterior, posterior, and lateral motion of the talus.[18]

Although injuries to the deltoid ligamentous complex are commonly linked to eversion (ie, pronation) injuries, inversion injuries can also affect the deltoid ligament. Common injury patterns include associated syndesmotic or lateral ankle ligamentous injury as well as in patients with chronic ankle instability, with isolated deltoid ligament injury being rare, reported in less than 3% of ankle injuries. Studies have shown 33% to 35% incidence of deltoid ligament injury after an acute inversion injury (see **Fig. 9**), whereas up to 68% of patients had medial ligament injury when undergoing lateral ligamentous surgery for chronic instability.[42] After an acute ankle sprain, superficial deltoid ligament injuries are more frequent than deep deltoid ligament injuries.[43] There is moderate

agreement between radiographic medial clear space widening and complete tear of deltoid ligament on MR imaging[43]; however, MR imaging is more sensitive for deltoid ligament injury.[41] Injury to deltoid ligament components follows similar MR imaging signal abnormalities seen in lateral ankle ligaments, being diffusely thickened and increased in signal intensity in lower-grade lesions and showing focal or full-thickness discontinuities in tears (**Fig. 11**).

Ankle impingement syndromes

Posttraumatic ankle soft tissue impingement is produced by entrapment of abnormal, hypertrophic tissue and is most commonly seen in the anterolateral recess (or anterolateral gutter). The anterolateral recess is triangular shaped, with anatomic boundaries including the tibia posteromedially, the fibula laterally, and the tibiotalar joint capsule. It is reinforced anteriorly by the anteroinferior tibiofibular and ATFLs, and laterally by the calcaneofibular ligament.[44] The anterolateral impingement syndrome occurs as a result of ankle inversion, commonly after lateral or syndesmotic injuries, with approximately 3% of ankle sprains potentially evolving to anterolateral impingement,

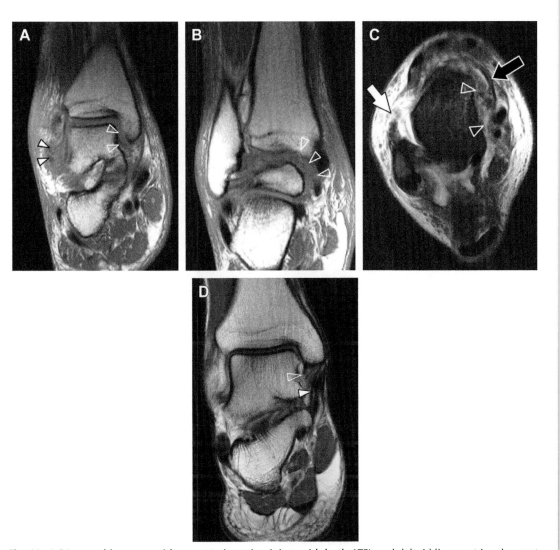

Fig. 11. A 24-year-old woman with an acute inversion injury with both ATFL and deltoid ligament involvement. (*A*, *B*) Coronal T1-weighted MR images showing rupture of the ATFL (*white arrowheads*). The deep fibers (*open arrowheads*) of the deltoid ligament are torn anteriorly (*A*) and posteriorly (*B*). (*C*) Axial T2-weighted MR image shows tear involving both the anterior and posterior tibiotalar ligaments (*open arrowheads*), which comprise the deep layer of the deltoid ligament. The superficial fibers (*black arrow*) are sprained. The full-thickness ATFL tear is also appreciated (*white arrow*). (*D*) The normal deep fibers of the deltoid ligament (*empty arrowhead*) and tibiospring ligament (*white arrowhead*) on coronal T1-weighted image in another patient.

leading to pain, synovitis, and mechanical blocking.[45]

MR imaging findings include the presence of intermediate signal intensity soft tissue thickening or fibrosis in the anterolateral recess (**Fig. 12**). Absence of normal recess fluid between the anterolateral soft tissues and the anterior surface of the fibula has been described as a pertinent MR arthrographic finding.[46,47] As the disease advances, synovitis may coalesce into a hyalinized meniscoid-type lesion.[46,48]

An additional cause of anterolateral impingement that is less common relates to the thickened accessory AITFL (Bassett's ligament) mentioned earlier, which can result in erosive injury to the anterolateral talar dome cartilage. The ligament is separated by a fibrofatty septum from the inferior margin of the anteroinferior tibiofibular ligament.[44] This accessory ligament is common, and can be clearly visualized with standard MR imaging protocols without contrast (see **Fig. 9**). The ligament has been reported to be present in up to 92% of cadaveric specimens.[49]

Anteromedial impingement is a less common form of ankle impingement and is also associated with lateral and medial ligamentous injury in the

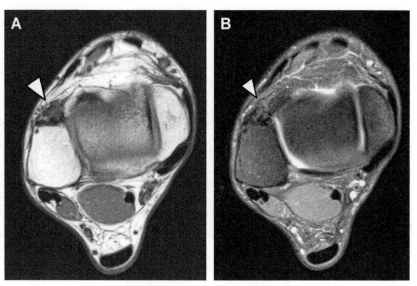

Fig. 12. A 42-year-old man with anterolateral impingement from prior lateral ankle inversion injury. Note the intermediate-signal/low-signal scar formation (*arrowheads*) in the anterolateral gutter observed on axial (*A*) T1 and (*B*) T2 fat-suppressed MR images.

context of inversion mechanism injury. It can be a result of anteromedial capsular thickening and, over time, osteophyte formation develops as the impinged tissues abut the anteromedial corner of the talus during ankle dorsiflexion.[44,50] Additional sites of impingement are less common after inversion injury, but include posteromedial, posterior, and extra-articular impingement.

OSSEOUS INJURIES

Fractures, bone contusions, and osteochondral lesions are associated with acute inversion injuries and can play an important role in treatment planning. Bone bruises or trabecular microcontusion occur in up to half of all acute inversion injuries and osteochondral lesions have been reported in up to 14% of patients.[6] MR imaging is a useful and sensitive tool to assess osseous injury, because these abnormalities can be occult on radiographs. The most common MR imaging findings are T2 subchondral hyperintensity with T1 hypointensity, representing hemorrhage, edema, and microfracture of the underlying trabecular bone.[51] In the pediatric population, it is important to differentiate the presence of T2 prolongation of the bone marrow signal intensity from presence of normal hematopoietic marrow.[52]

Bone Bruise

Although detection of fractures and osteochondral lesions may affect clinical outcome and recovery time, the significance of bone marrow edema is

unclear. One study found no change in clinical outcome, time to return to work, or mobility at 3 months compared with patients injured without bone marrow edema.[53] However, in another study, medial joint line bone bruises of the tibia, calcaneus, or talus were associated with longer delay in return to normal walking and sporting activity, as well as increased incidence of ATFL injuries.[54]

Osteochondral Lesions and Loose Bodies

Osteochondral lesions are most common in the talus after inversion injury and can accelerate the development of osteoarthritis (**Fig. 13**). MR imaging is sensitive for detecting osteochondral lesions and affords characterization of the underlying cartilage and fragment stability,[55] with T2-hyperintense signal undermining the osteochondral fragment, suggesting an unstable fragment (see **Fig. 13**C). Although it has been reported that the lateral talar dome is the most common location for osteochondral lesions after an acute inversion injury, the most common location is the medial talar dome when including all types of injuries.[55,56] Less common locations of osteochondral injuries include the tibial plafond, navicular, and cuboid. Intra-articular loose bodies occur after inversion injury as a result of osteochondral lesions with unstable fragments or chronic secondary osteoarthritis, being a chronic source of pain and morbidity. MR imaging is useful in this regard because it can detect both calcified and noncalcified loose bodies. MR arthrography improves

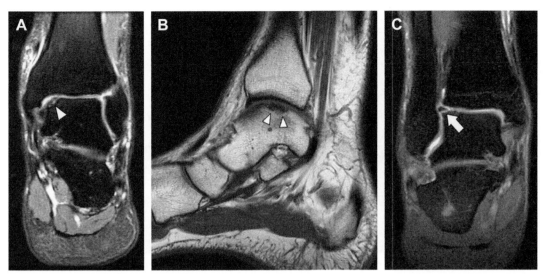

Fig. 13. A 34-year-old man after inversion injury. An osteochondral lesion of the medial talar dome is seen (*white arrowhead*) on (*A*) coronal T2 fat-suppressed and (*B*) sagittal T1-weighted images. In a different patient (*C*) a coronal T2 fat-suppressed image shows an unstable fragment, with high signal undercutting the lateral talar dome osteochondral lesion (*white arrow*).

detection of loose bodies with accuracy reported up to 92%.[55]

Fractures

Radiographic assessment remains the first line in fracture detection after inversion injury with well-codified malleolar fracture classifications that often constitute the basis for treatment. However, MR imaging is a useful method to uncover occult fractures in the setting of negative radiographs and persistent symptoms after inversion injury. Typical sites of occult fractures include medial and lateral malleoli, navicular, lateral process of the talus, proximal fifth metatarsal, and cuboid[1,6] (**Fig. 14**).

Fracture of the anterior process of the calcaneus (APC) is a unique injury that has been associated with acute inversion injuries.[57] The principal mechanism during an inversion injury is distraction of the bifurcate ligament leading to avulsion of variable size from the anterior calcaneal process.[58] The sudden ankle inversion with a plantar-flexed foot is the typical mechanism for fractures affecting the APC. MR imaging is useful for assessment of this type of fracture, because it

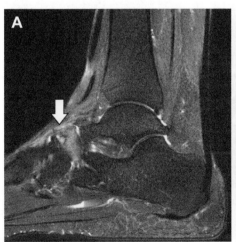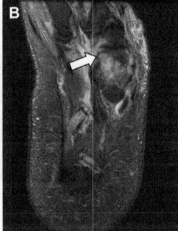

Fig. 14. In 2 different patients with inversion injury, sagittal (*A*) and axial (*B*) T2 fat-suppressed MR images show subchondral fractures of the navicular (*A*) and cuboid (*B*) (*arrows*) with surrounding marrow edema pattern.

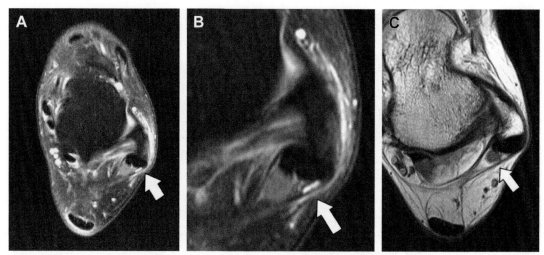

Fig. 15. A 26-year-old woman after inversion injury with abnormal SPR consistent with a low-grade SPR injury (*A*, *B*). Axial T2 fat-suppressed MR image showing edema surrounding the SPR and fibular periosteum (*arrow*). The peroneus brevis and longus tendons are intact. In another patient (*C*), the normal appearance of the SPR is shown (*arrow*).

can distinguish between a radiographic pitfall of an anatomic variant (os secondarium) in the acute setting. Calcaneonavicular coalitions have been reported to be a risk factor for this type of injury, seen in up to 60% of all APC fractures.[58]

Avulsion fractures at the superior and lateral calcaneus may also result from extensor digitorum brevis muscle avulsion from its origin caused by forceful inversion injury. Because these injuries may be difficult to diagnose radiographically, MR imaging may provide additional insight if there is clinical suspicion for injury.[59]

Superior Peroneal Retinaculum Injuries

The superior peroneal retinaculum (SPR) is a stabilizer of the peroneal complex at the level of

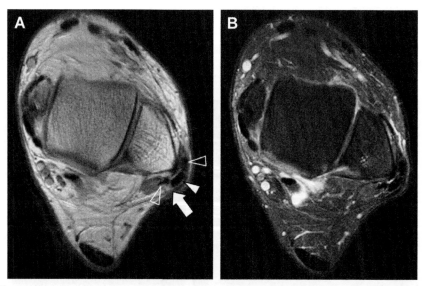

Fig. 16. A 65-year-old man with chronic SPR tear and stripping, peroneus brevis tendon split tear, and peroneal brevis and longus tendon subluxation. Axial T1 (*A*) and T2 fat-suppressed (*B*) MR images showing SPR tear and displacement of the SPR (*white arrow*), which is being stripped from fibular attachment, creating a pocket for peroneal tendon subluxation. The peroneus brevis tendon has a split tear (*open arrowheads*) with dislocation of the most anterior limb (*more anterior open arrowhead*). The peroneus longus tendon is also subluxed (*white arrowhead*).

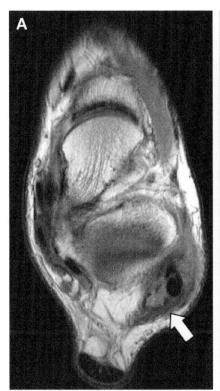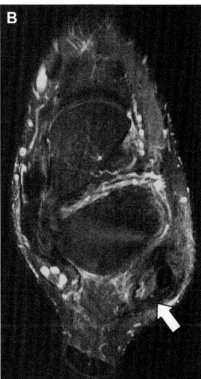

Fig. 17. A 41-year-old man with chronic injury to the SPR. (*A*) Axial T1-weighted images obtained below the level of the fibula show a markedly thickened SPR (*white arrow*) without substantial increased signal on axial T2 fat-suppressed image (*B*). These findings are consistent with chronic injury to the SPR.

retromalleolar groove that serves as an important restraint and that can be injured during an ankle inversion injury.[60] The SPR is a fibrous band of tissue that extends from the posterior ridge of the fibula at the retromalleolar groove and most commonly attaches distally at the lateral margin of the calcaneus. Medial fibers may also blend with the aponeurosis of the lateral Achilles tendon.[61] The SPR provides stability to peroneal tendons within the retromalleolar groove and prevents tendon subluxation. Because its trajectory is similar to that of the CFL, ankle inversion injuries that involve the CFL may also involve the SPR.[62] Although a detailed description of the classification of SPR injuries is beyond the scope of this article, such lesions can range from low-grade stripping of SPR from fibular attachment to full-thickness tears with bony avulsions.

At MR imaging, injuries to the SPR appear as thickening with increased T2 signal of the surrounding soft tissues (**Fig. 15**). In addition, SPR injury can show stripping from the periosteum allowing peroneal tendons to lodge within an adjacent pouch, whereas in higher-grade lesions an avulsed bony fragment may be identified. Subluxation or dislocation of peroneal tendons is typically

seen in higher-grade lesions of the SPR (**Fig. 16**). Injury of the SPR is underdiagnosed and can be a cause of chronic lateral ankle pain in the setting of a chronic injury[23] (**Fig. 17**).

SUMMARY

The aftermath of ankle inversion injuries covers a wide spectrum of abnormalities and patterns. MR imaging provides the most comprehensive assessment of osseous and soft tissue injuries, with the ability to uncover otherwise overlooked abnormalities. In the appropriate clinical setting, MR imaging is the imaging method of choice to characterize soft tissue and osseous injuries, which are common sources of pain and morbidity following ankle inversion injuries.

REFERENCES

1. Campbell SE, Warner M. MR imaging of ankle inversion injuries. Magn Reson Imaging Clin North Am 2008;16(1):1–18, v.
2. Langner I, Frank M, Kuehn JP, et al. Acute inversion injury of the ankle without radiological abnormalities: assessment with high-field MR imaging and

correlation of findings with clinical outcome. Skeletal Radiol 2011;40(4):423–30.

3. Mack RP. Ankle injuries in athletics. Clin Sports Med 1982;1(1):71–84.

4. Anandacoomarasamy A, Barnsley L. Long term outcomes of inversion ankle injuries. Br J Sports Med 2005;39(3):e14 [discussion: e14].

5. Konradsen L, Bech L, Ehrenbjerg M, et al. Seven years follow-up after ankle inversion trauma. Scand J Med Sci Sports 2002;12(3):129–35.

6. Khor YP, Tan KJ. The anatomic pattern of injuries in acute inversion ankle sprains: a magnetic resonance imaging study. Orthop J Sports Med 2013; 1(7):2325967113517078.

7. Chandnani VP, Harper MT, Ficke JR, et al. Chronic ankle instability: evaluation with MR arthrography, MR imaging, and stress radiography. Radiology 1994;192(1):189–94.

8. Bolog N, Nanz D, Weishaupt D. Muskuloskeletal MR imaging at 3.0 T: current status and future perspectives. Eur Radiol 2006;16(6):1298–307.

9. Fuller S, Reeder S, Shimakawa A, et al. Iterative decomposition of water and fat with echo asymmetry and least-squares estimation (IDEAL) fast spin-echo imaging of the ankle: initial clinical experience. AJR Am J Roentgenol 2006;187(6):1442–7.

10. Duc SR, Mengiardi B, Pfirrmann CWA, et al. Improved visualization of collateral ligaments of the ankle: multiplanar reconstructions based on standard 2D turbo spin-echo MR images. Eur Radiol 2007;17(5):1162–71.

11. Hua J, Xu JR, Gu HY, et al. Comparative study of the anatomy, CT and MR images of the lateral collateral ligaments of the ankle joint. Surg Radiol Anat 2008; 30(4):361–7.

12. Siegler S, Block J, Schneck CD. The mechanical characteristics of the collateral ligaments of the human ankle joint. Foot Ankle 1988;8(5):234–42.

13. Rosenberg ZS, Beltran J, Bencardino JT. From the RSNA refresher courses. Radiological Society of North America. MR imaging of the ankle and foot. Radiographics 2000;20 Spec No:S153–79.

14. Park H-J, Cha S-D, Kim SS, et al. Accuracy of MRI findings in chronic lateral ankle ligament injury: comparison with surgical findings. Clin Radiol 2012; 67(4):313–8.

15. Boonthathip M, Chen L, Trudell D, et al. Lateral ankle ligaments: MR arthrography with anatomic correlation in cadavers. Clin Imaging 2011;35(1):42–8.

16. Dimmick S, Kennedy D, Daunt N. Evaluation of thickness and appearance of anterior talofibular and calcaneofibular ligaments in normal versus abnormal ankles with MRI. J Med Imaging Radiat Oncol 2008;52(6):559–63.

17. Choo HJ, Lee SJ, Kim DW, et al. Multibanded anterior talofibular ligaments in normal ankles and sprained ankles using 3D isotropic proton density-weighted fast spin-echo MRI sequence. AJR Am J Roentgenol 2014;202(1):W87–94.

18. Golano P, Vega J, de Leeuw PAJ, et al. Anatomy of the ankle ligaments: a pictorial essay. Knee Surg Sports Traumatol Arthrosc 2016;24(4):944–56.

19. Dubin JC, Comeau D, McClelland RI, et al. Lateral and syndesmotic ankle sprain injuries: a narrative literature review. J Chiropr Med 2011;10(3):204–19.

20. Labovitz JM, Schweitzer ME, Larka UB, et al. Magnetic resonance imaging of ankle ligament injuries correlated with time. J Am Podiatr Med Assoc 1998;88(8):387–93.

21. Saxena A, Luhadiya A, Ewen B, et al. Magnetic resonance imaging and incidental findings of lateral ankle pathologic features with asymptomatic ankles. J Foot Ankle Surg 2011;50(4):413–5.

22. Perrich KD, Goodwin DW, Hecht PJ, et al. Ankle ligaments on MRI: appearance of normal and injured ligaments. AJR Am J Roentgenol 2009; 193(3):687–95.

23. Taljanovic MS, Alcala JN, Gimber LH, et al. High-resolution US and MR imaging of peroneal tendon injuries. Radiographics 2015;35(1):179–99.

24. Bischof JE, Spritzer CE, Caputo AM, et al. In vivo cartilage contact strains in patients with lateral ankle instability. J Biomech 2010;43(13):2561–6.

25. Golditz T, Steib S, Pfeifer K, et al. Functional ankle instability as a risk factor for osteoarthritis: using T2-mapping to analyze early cartilage degeneration in the ankle joint of young athletes. Osteoarthritis Cartilage 2014;22(10):1377–85.

26. Kumar V, Triantafyllopoulos I, Panagopoulos A, et al. Deficiencies of MRI in the diagnosis of chronic symptomatic lateral ankle ligament injuries. Foot Ankle Surg 2007;13(4):171–6.

27. Joshy S, Abdulkadir U, Chaganti S, et al. Accuracy of MRI scan in the diagnosis of ligamentous and chondral pathology in the ankle. Foot Ankle Surg 2010;16(2):78–80.

28. Kim S, Huh Y-M, Song H-T, et al. Chronic tibiofibular syndesmosis injury of ankle: evaluation with contrast-enhanced fat-suppressed 3D fast spoiled gradient-recalled acquisition in the steady state MR imaging. Radiology 2007;242(1):225–35.

29. Schoennagel BP, Karul M, Avanesov M, et al. Isolated syndesmotic injury in acute ankle trauma: comparison of plain film radiography with 3T MRI. Eur J Radiol 2014;83(10):1856–61.

30. Hermans JJ, Wentink N, Beumer A, et al. Correlation between radiological assessment of acute ankle fractures and syndesmotic injury on MRI. Skeletal Radiol 2012;41(7):787–801.

31. Han SH, Lee JW, Kim S, et al. Chronic tibiofibular syndesmosis injury: the diagnostic efficiency of magnetic resonance imaging and comparative analysis of operative treatment. Foot Ankle Int 2007; 28(3):336–42.

32. Williams BT, Ahrberg AB, Goldsmith MT, et al. Ankle syndesmosis: a qualitative and quantitative anatomic analysis. Am J Sports Med 2015;43(1):88–97.

33. Brown KW, Morrison WB, Schweitzer ME, et al. MRI findings associated with distal tibiofibular syndesmosis injury. AJR Am J Roentgenol 2004;182(1):131–6.

34. Nazarenko A, Beltran LS, Bencardino JT. Imaging evaluation of traumatic ligamentous injuries of the ankle and foot. Radiol Clin North Am 2013;51(3): 455–78.

35. Botchu R, Allen P, Rennie WJ. Isolated posterior high ankle sprain: a report of three cases. J Orthop Surg (Hong Kong) 2013;21(3):391–5.

36. Oae K, Takao M, Naito K, et al. Injury of the tibiofibular syndesmosis: value of MR imaging for diagnosis. Radiology 2003;227(1):155–61.

37. Vogl TJ, Hochmuth K, Diebold T, et al. Magnetic resonance imaging in the diagnosis of acute injured distal tibiofibular syndesmosis. Invest Radiol 1997; 32(7):401–9.

38. Thacker P, Mardis N. Ligaments of the tarsal sinus: improved detection, characterisation and significance in the paediatric ankle with 3-D proton density MR imaging. Pediatr Radiol 2013;43(2):196–201.

39. Lektrakul N, Chung CB, Ym L, et al. Tarsal sinus: arthrographic, MR imaging, MR arthrographic, and pathologic findings in cadavers and retrospective study data in patients with sinus tarsi syndrome. Radiology 2001;219(3):802–10.

40. Balen PF, Helms CA. Association of posterior tibial tendon injury with spring ligament injury, sinus tarsi abnormality, and plantar fasciitis on MR imaging. AJR Am J Roentgenol 2001;176(5):1137–43.

41. Crim J, Longenecker LG. MRI and surgical findings in deltoid ligament tears. AJR Am J Roentgenol 2015;204(1):W63–9.

42. Crim JR, Beals TC, Nickisch F, et al. Deltoid ligament abnormalities in chronic lateral ankle instability. Foot Ankle Int 2011;32(9):873–8.

43. Jeong MS, Choi YS, Kim YJ, et al. Deltoid ligament in acute ankle injury: MR imaging analysis. Skeletal Radiol 2014;43(5):655–63.

44. Donovan A, Rosenberg ZS. MRI of ankle and lateral hindfoot impingement syndromes. AJR Am J Roentgenol 2010;195(3):595–604.

45. Umans H. Ankle impingement syndromes. Semin Musculoskelet Radiol 2002;6(2):133–9.

46. Robinson P, White LM. Soft-tissue and osseous impingement syndromes of the ankle: role of imaging in diagnosis and management. Radiographics 2002;22(6):1451–7.

47. Robinson P, White LM, Salonen DC, et al. Anterolateral ankle impingement: MR arthrographic assessment of the anterolateral recess. Radiology 2001; 221(1):186–90.

48. Robinson P, White LM, Salonen D, et al. Anteromedial impingement of the ankle: using MR arthrography to assess the anteromedial recess. AJR Am J Roentgenol 2002;178(3):601–4.

49. Subhas N, Vinson EN, Cothran RL, et al. MRI appearance of surgically proven abnormal accessory anterior-inferior tibiofibular ligament (Bassett's ligament). Skeletal Radiol 2008;37(1):27–33.

50. Cerezal L, Abascal F, Canga A, et al. MR imaging of ankle impingement syndromes. AJR Am J Roentgenol 2003;181(2):551–9.

51. Boks SS, Vroegindeweij D, Koes BW, et al. Follow-up of occult bone lesions detected at MR imaging: systematic review. Radiology 2006;238(3):853–62.

52. Shabshin N, Schweitzer ME, Morrison WB, et al. High-signal T2 changes of the bone marrow of the foot and ankle in children: red marrow or traumatic changes? Pediatr Radiol 2006;36(7):670–6.

53. Alanen V, Taimela S, Kinnunen J, et al. Incidence and clinical significance of bone bruises after supination injury of the ankle. A double-blind, prospective study. J Bone Joint Surg Br 1998;80(3):513–5.

54. Chan VO, Moran DE, Shine S, et al. Medial joint line bone bruising at MRI complicating acute ankle inversion injury: what is its clinical significance? Clin Radiol 2013;68(10):e519–23.

55. Cerezal L, Llopis E, Canga A, et al. MR arthrography of the ankle: indications and technique. Radiol Clin North Am 2008;46(6):973–94, v.

56. Naran KN, Zoga AC. Osteochondral lesions about the ankle. Radiol Clin North Am 2008;46(6):995–1002, v.

57. Ouellette H, Salamipour H, Thomas BJ, et al. Incidence and MR imaging features of fractures of the anterior process of calcaneus in a consecutive patient population with ankle and foot symptoms. Skeletal Radiol 2006;35:833–7.

58. Petrover D, Schweitzer ME, Laredo JD. Anterior process calcaneal fractures: a systematic evaluation of associated conditions. Skeletal Radiol 2007;36(7): 627–32.

59. Norfray JF, Rogers LF, Adamo GP, et al. Common calcaneal avulsion fracture. AJR Am J Roentgenol 1980;134(1):119–23.

60. Geppert MJ, Sobel M, Bohne WH. Lateral ankle instability as a cause of superior peroneal retinacular laxity: an anatomic and biomechanical study of cadaveric feet. Foot Ankle 1993;14(6):330–4.

61. Wang X-T, Rosenberg ZS, Mechlin MB, et al. Normal variants and diseases of the peroneal tendons and superior peroneal retinaculum: MR imaging features. Radiographics 2005;25(3):587–602.

62. Rosenberg ZS, Bencardino J, Astion D, et al. MRI features of chronic injuries of the superior peroneal retinaculum. Am J Roentgenol 2003;181(6):1551–7.

Medial-sided Ankle Pain
Deltoid Ligament and Beyond

Julia Crim, MD

KEYWORDS

- Deltoid ligament • Ankle sprain • Spring ligament • Posterior tibial tendon • Flexor retinaculum
- Ankle impingement • Ankle instability

KEY POINTS

- Abnormalities of the medial ligaments and posterior tibial tendon can occur because of acute injury or chronic instability or malalignment.
- Medial ankle injuries may occur because of pronation or supination–external rotation injuries.
- Deltoid ligament injuries have a significant impact on lateral ankle instability but can be overlooked in patients with lateral ligament injuries.
- Posterior tibial tendon dysfunction is usually associated with spring ligament or flexor retinaculum injury.
- Tarsal tunnel syndrome, accessory flexor muscles, and subtalar coalition should be considered as well as ligament and tendon tears in differential diagnosis of chronic medial ankle pain.

INTRODUCTION

The medial soft tissue anatomy of the ankle is complex; the ligaments and posterior tibial tendon are closely interrelated both anatomically and functionally. The medial soft tissues may be acutely injured, or may undergo degeneration caused by hindfoot instability or malalignment. Abnormalities may be limited to the medial side of the foot, or occur in conjunction with lateral hindfoot abnormalities. Clinically, medial ankle abnormalities are often underestimated, or overshadowed by lateral injuries, and magnetic resonance (MR) imaging is useful in showing the full extent of injury and guiding surgical management.

A systematic analysis of medial soft tissue structures on MR imaging should begin with the deltoid ligament, followed by the flexor retinaculum, the spring ligament, and the posterior tibial tendon. The tarsal tunnel is examined next, and the intrinsic muscles of the foot. In addition, a search for tarsal coalition should be made because this diagnosis is often overlooked, especially in subtle cases. The medial findings should be analyzed in conjunction with lateral abnormalities, which may have precipitated the medial findings, or may have resulted from them. Integrating the entire MR imaging picture usually enables radiologists to diagnose the type of injury and to guide treatment.

IMAGING PROTOCOLS

Images obtained through the hindfoot should be aligned with the axis of the talus. The axial plane is the long axis of the talus, and the coronal plane is perpendicular to it. At least 1 T1-weighted sequence should be obtained to evaluate for bone marrow. Fluid-sensitive sequences should be acquired in all 3 planes. A second short echo time plane, either T1 or proton density, is recommended to improve identification of normal anatomy and variants. The field of view is generally 12 to 14 cm, and a dedicated ankle coil is preferred.

Disclosure: The author has nothing to disclose.
Department of Radiology, University of Missouri, 3801 Kinsey Court, Columbia, MO 65203, USA
E-mail address: crimj@health.missouri.edu

Magn Reson Imaging Clin N Am 25 (2017) 63–77
http://dx.doi.org/10.1016/j.mric.2016.08.003
1064-9689/17/© 2016 Elsevier Inc. All rights reserved.

ANATOMY

The medial ankle ligaments are closely associated anatomically and functionally. A robust understanding of their interconnections is necessary to evaluate medial ankle pain.

Deltoid Ligament Anatomy Overview

The constituent parts of deltoid ligament anatomy have been debated by numerous anatomists,

perhaps because cadaveric studies tend to be performed in an elderly population that has a high likelihood of prior ankle injury. The appearance of the ligament on MR imaging is fairly constant (**Figs. 1–3**).[1]

Deep Deltoid Ligament Anatomy

The deep deltoid ligament prevents lateral talar shift and external rotation of the talus. It has 2 bands. The posterior band of the deep ligament

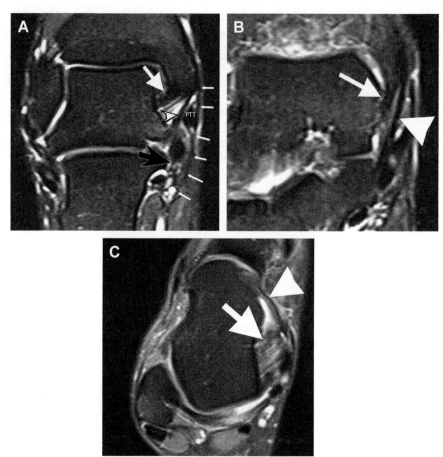

Fig. 1. Normal appearance of the deltoid ligament. (*A*) Coronal fast spin echo T2 weighted fat-suppressed (FSE T2FS) image through the midportion of the ankle joint shows the posterior band of the deep deltoid ligament (*white arrow*) coursing obliquely from the medial malleolus to the fovea at the medial margin of the talar body. Note that the ligament insertion does not entirely fill the fovea. The posterior band of the deep deltoid ligament has a striated appearance. A small portion of the tibiocalcaneal band of the superficial deltoid (*white arrowhead*) is also visible. Superficial to this, and separated from it by the soft tissue contents of the tarsal tunnel, is the vertically oriented portion of the flexor retinaculum (*small arrows*). Black arrow points to tibial nerve. (*B*) Coronal FSE T2FS image anterior to prior image shows the small anterior band of the deep deltoid ligament (*arrow*) inserting on the talar neck. The tibiocalcaneal band of the deltoid ligament, its strongest band, is seen coursing from the superficial margin of the medial malleolus to the sustentaculum tali (*arrowhead*). (*C*) Axial proton density weighted fat-suppressed (PDFS) image MR image at level of talar body fovea shows a portion of the deep deltoid ligament posterior band (*arrow*). Although the tibial attachment is not included on this slice, the tautness of the ligament fibers indicates an intact ligament, which should be confirmed by correlation with other slices. The tibionavicular band of the superficial deltoid ligament (*arrowhead*) is also included. The tibionavicular band merges distally with the superomedial band of the spring ligament. PTT, posterior tibial tendon.

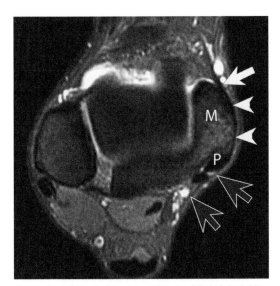

Fig. 2. Normal relationships of superficial deltoid ligament to flexor retinaculum. Axial PDFS image at the level of the talar dome shows the common origin of the superficial deltoid fibers from the anteromedial corner of the medial malleolus (M; *white arrow*). The fibers are continuous with the periosteum of the medial malleolus (*arrowheads*), which is continuous with the flexor retinaculum (*black arrows*). The flexor retinaculum stabilizes the flexor tendons and continues horizontally to insert on the deep flexor fascia. P, posterior tibial tendon.

(often called simply the deep deltoid) is the larger of the bands. It is a short, cone-shaped ligament that arises from the posterior margin of the anterior colliculus and from the posterior colliculus. It courses inferiorly, posteriorly, and laterally from the medial malleolus to insert on the fovea at the medial margin of the talar body. Because of its obliquity, it is not visualized in its entirety on a single axial image, and the talar attachment is seen on slices inferior to the tip of the medial malleolus. The ligament has a striated appearance similar to that of the anterior cruciate ligament of the knee, and it is normal to see a small amount of high signal intensity between the fibers. The individual fibers should always appear taut and sharply demarcated. The small anterior band of the deep ligament inserts on the medial talus at the junction of the talar neck and body, and is not always visible on MR imaging.

Superficial Deltoid Ligament Anatomy

The superficial deltoid ligament helps maintain rotational stability of the ankle. It has multiple bands that originate from the superficial surface of the medial malleolus and together make the fanlike shape that gives the ligament its name. The tibiocalcaneal band is the strongest band and inserts on the medial margin of the sustentaculum tali. Although cadaveric studies indicate that it may be absent, it is always visible on coronal MR

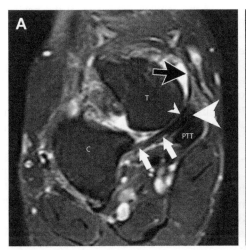
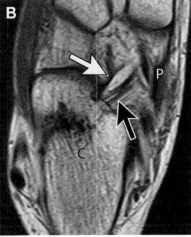

Fig. 3. Normal appearance of tibiospring, tibionavicular, and spring ligaments. (*A*) Coronal FSE T2FS image shows the tibiospring band of the superficial deltoid ligament (*black arrow*) merging with the superomedial (*small arrowhead*) and medioplantar oblique (*white arrows*) bands of the spring ligament. The tibionavicular band of the superficial deltoid ligament (*large arrowhead*) lies immediately deep to the posterior tibial tendon. (*B*) Axial T1 weighted image (T1WI) shows a portion of the plantar portions of the spring ligament arising from the sustentaculum tali and immediately anterior to it. The inferoplantar band (*white arrow*) is sagittally oriented and inserts on the beak of the navicular. The medioplantar oblique band (*black arrow*) has a diagonal orientation, inserting on the plantar aspect of the medial margin of navicular. C, calcaneus; T, talus.

imaging in patients who have not had a deltoid ligament injury. The tibiospring band merges with the superomedial band of the spring ligament, and is also best evaluated on coronal images. The tibionavicular band is deep to the posterior tibial tendon, and also merges with the superomedial band of the spring ligament. The anterior tibiotalar band is variably present, seen on axial or coronal images. The posterior tibiotalar band inserts on the body of the talus, posterior to the medial malleolus, and is best seen on axial images.

At their origin from the superficial margin of the medial malleolus, the superficial deltoid fibers merge with the periosteum of the malleolus, which in turn merges with the flexor retinaculum (see **Fig. 2**). This continuous sheet formed by the superficial deltoid, periosteum, and flexor retinaculum has been termed the medial malleolar fascial sleeve.[2] The fascial sleeve can be detached completely in twisting injuries, explaining the frequent association of superficial deltoid ligament injuries with injuries of the flexor retinaculum. This relationship should always be scrutinized on fluid-sensitive axial images.

Flexor Retinaculum Anatomy

The flexor retinaculum originates from the superficial margin of the medial malleolus, and extends both laterally and inferiorly.[3] Horizontally oriented fibers insert on the deep flexor fascia (see **Fig. 2**). They maintain the position of the flexor tendons posterior to the medial malleolus. Longitudinally oriented fibers extend inferiorly from the medial malleolus to form the roof to the tarsal tunnel, merging with the fascia of the abductor hallucis muscle and inserting on the calcaneus (see **Fig. 1A**). On MR imaging, the normal flexor retinaculum forms a thin, taut line that is low signal intensity on all sequences. Axial images are key to evaluate the insertion of the flexor retinaculum onto a pointed promontory at the posteromedial corner of the tibia.

Spring Ligament Anatomy

The spring ligament helps maintain the medial arch of the foot, although its importance has been debated. The spring ligament is composed of 3 bands.[4] The superomedial spring ligament forms a broad sling, arising from the surface of the sustentaculum tali and inserting on the superomedial surface of the navicular, dorsal to the insertion of the tibialis posterior tendon. It merges with the tibiospring band of the superficial deltoid ligament (see **Fig. 3A**). There are 2 deep plantar bands of the spring ligament (see **Fig. 3B**). The medioplantar oblique ligament is a narrow straplike ligament

that arises immediately anterior to the sustentaculum tali, and has a diagonal course, inserting on the median eminence of the navicular. The inferoplantar ligament is a short, broad ligament that arises from the calcaneus just lateral to the medioplantar oblique ligament and inserts on the lateral beak of the navicular. A joint recess of the talonavicular joint lies between the 2 plantar bands.[5] The plantar fascicles of the spring ligament are usually best seen on sequential axial images. The superomedial band is best seen on coronal images.

Tibiocalcaneonavicular Ligament

It is evident from the earlier descriptions that the tibionavicular, tibiospring, and superomedial spring ligament are closely linked, and they coalesce on MR imaging. In practice, they can be described together as the tibiocalcaneonavicular ligament[6] or the spring ligament complex.

Posterior Tibial Tendon Anatomy

The posterior tibial muscle is the most important dynamic stabilizer of the medial longitudinal arch of the foot.[7] It originates in the calf, and becomes tendinous in the distal one-third of the leg. At the ankle, the posterior tibial tendon is the most medial of the extrinsic flexor tendons and is held in place in a shallow groove behind the medial malleolus by the flexor retinaculum (see **Fig. 2**). It continues into the hindfoot within the tarsal tunnel, superficial to the deltoid ligament (see **Figs. 1A and 3A**), and has its primary insertion on the plantar aspect of the median eminence of the navicular. Small tendon slips continue anterior to the navicular to insert on the second and third cuneiforms, the bases of the second to fourth metatarsals, and the cuboid. A recurrent slip inserts on the sustentaculum tali.

On MR imaging, the normal tendon is twice the size of the adjacent flexor digitorum longus tendon. A small amount of fluid is often seen in its tendon sheath, and does not indicate tenosynovitis. The tendon normally shows slightly increased signal intensity as it inserts on the navicular. The anterior tendon slips to the cuneiforms, metatarsals, and cuboid are well seen on MR imaging and are rarely abnormal. A small recurrent tendon slip inserts on the anterior margin of the sustentaculum tali, and may be injured but is hard to distinguish from the spring ligament on imaging.

Accessory Navicular Bone

The accessory navicular bone (also called the os tibiale externum) is a normal variant that can be associated with posterior tibial tendon dysfunction.

A type 1 accessory navicular is a sesamoid in the distal tendon, and is not associated with tendon abnormalities. A type 2 accessory navicular is an accessory center of ossification, connected to the main portion of the navicular by a synchondrosis. The posterior tibial tendon attaches at least partly to the ossicle. This construct is vulnerable, and increases likelihood of acute or chronic posterior tibial tendon injury.

Tarsal Tunnel Anatomy

Students first learning the anatomy of the ankle are sometimes confused by 3 similar-sounding structures: the tarsal tunnel, the tarsal sinus (sinus tarsi), and the tarsal canal. It becomes easy to remember the location of the tarsal tunnel if you remember that it is analogous to the carpal tunnel: a space with a fibrous roof and bony floor, transited by nerves, vessels and tendons, within which the nerve is vulnerable to compression. In the case of the tarsal tunnel, the vulnerable nerves are the tibial nerve and its branches. The tarsal sinus is a lateral space between the calcaneus and talus, and the tarsal canal is the posteromedial continuation of the sinus.

The tibial nerve and its branches are most easily evaluated within the tarsal tunnel on fluid-sensitive coronal or axial MR imaging. The nerve is lower in signal intensity than the veins, but higher in signal intensity than the tendons (see **Fig. 1**A). Fascicles should be visible within it. The nerve branches in

the tarsal tunnel into a medial calcaneal nerve, and medial and lateral plantar nerves. The branching pattern may vary.[8]

DELTOID LIGAMENT INJURIES
Acute Deltoid Injuries

Deltoid ligament injuries were at one time thought to be uncommon, but are now known to be fairly common.[9,10] They are significantly less common than medial malleolar fractures. Injuries may occur either because of pronation or because of supination–external rotation injury.

Pronation injuries apply a direct abduction force to the deep deltoid ligament and may result in medial malleolar fracture or deltoid ligament tear (**Fig. 4**). The deltoid can be injured in isolation, but, in more severe injuries, there is a fibular fracture or a tear of the tibiofibular syndesmosis.

Both ankle sprain (injury to the lateral collateral ligament complex) and Weber B fractures are caused by supination–external rotation injuries. A supination–external rotation injury occurs when the foot is planted and inverted; the tibia rotates internally on the planted talus. By convention, ankle injuries are described by the force applied on the talus, hence the term supination–external rotation.

The twisting component of the supination–external injury mechanism may also result in deltoid ligament injury.[6,7,11] The risk of deltoid ligament injury increases with the severity of the

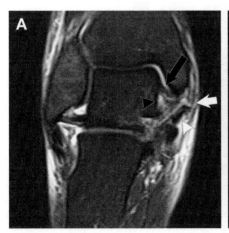
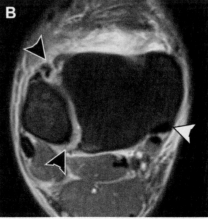

Fig. 4. Traumatic pronation injury of deltoid ligament. Twenty-year-old woman who incurred a pronation injury playing basketball, resulting in complete tears of deltoid ligament and tibiofibular syndesmotic ligaments. (*A*) Coronal FSE T2FS image through the midportion of the ankle joint shows the deep deltoid fibers (*black arrow*) flipped up in the medial ankle gutter. No fibers attach to their normal insertion on the fovea of the talus (*black arrowhead*). Superficial deltoid is stripped from the medial malleolus (*white arrow*). The posterior tibial tendon (*white arrowhead*) is small and irregular in shape, indicating partial tear. (*B*) Axial PDFS image immediately superior to the ankle joint shows the associated complete tears of the syndesmotic ligaments (*black arrowheads*). The horizontal portion of the flexor retinaculum (*white arrowhead*) is intact, because the injury was a pure pronation injury, without a significant rotational component.

lateral collateral ligament injury.[12] A clinical focus on the lateral side of the ankle can lead physicians to overlook associated medial ligamentous injuries, delaying diagnosis of medial injury. Physical examination for the presence of medial injuries is not reliable in the setting of acute lateral ankle injury[11] and so stress radiographs are often used to diagnose deep deltoid injuries. However, one study of stress radiographs and MR imaging in lateral malleolar fractures found that stress radiographs may be falsely positive in patients who have only a partial rupture of the deep deltoid by MR imaging criteria, and who do not need operative treatment.[13]

MR imaging is uncommonly performed for acute ankle sprain, but should be considered in severe cases (**Fig. 5**) because the extent of injuries may not be apparent clinically. In reading MR imaging of cases with multiple injuries, radiologists are in danger of experiencing satisfaction of search. One area where injuries are often overlooked is the proximal origin of the superficial deltoid. This area should be carefully scrutinized on axial images[2] (see **Fig. 5A**).

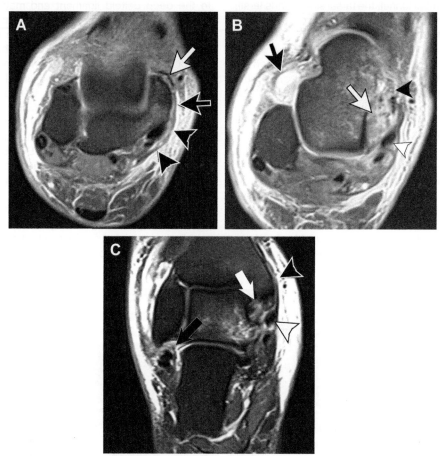

Fig. 5. Traumatic supination–external rotation injury of the deltoid ligament. A 36-year-old woman presented after ankle supination injury complaining of severe medial and lateral ankle pain. Routine ankle series (non–weight bearing because she could not bear weight) showed severe lateral soft tissue swelling, normal alignment, and no fractures. Because of the severity of her pain, MR imaging was performed 1 week after the injury. (*A*) Axial PDFS image at the level of the tibial plafond shows complete avulsion of the medial malleolar fascial sleeve, including the origin of the superficial deltoid ligament (*white arrow*), the medial periosteum (*black arrow*), and the flexor retinaculum (*black arrowheads*). (*B*) Axial PDFS image at the level of the deep deltoid ligament shows amorphous, lax, discontinuous deep deltoid ligament (*white arrow*). The ankle joint effusion (*black arrow*) extends through the completely torn anterior talofibular ligament. The distal bands of the superficial deltoid ligament are torn (*black arrowhead*). The posterior tibial tendon is thinned and irregular in shape, indicating a partial tear (*white arrowhead*). (*C*) Coronal FSE T2FS image at the level of the deep deltoid ligament confirms complete deltoid ligament tear (*white arrow*), medial malleolar fascial sleeve avulsion (*black arrowhead*), and partial tear of the posterior tibial tendon (*white arrowhead*). In addition, a complete tear of the calcaneofibular ligament (*black arrow*) is visible.

Chronic Medial Ankle Instability

There is tremendous variability in reported prevalence of ankle instability after an ankle sprain.[14] So many factors are at play that generalizations concerning prevalence are of doubtful value; it is enough to say that chronic instability is fairly common. A significant number of patients with chronic lateral instability have concomitant medial instability, presenting as medial ankle pain, a feeling of giving way, and a pronation deformity of the hindfoot[15,16] (**Fig. 6**). An MR imaging study found deltoid ligament injuries in 72% of patients with chronic ankle instability.[17] Lateral ankle symptoms and impingement may also develop secondary to chronic medial ligament injuries (**Fig. 7**).

Anteromedial Impingement

The ankle is vulnerable to impingement in multiple locations because of either bony or soft tissue abnormalities.[18] Anteromedial impingement usually occurs because of scar formation in the anteromedial recess, usually caused by chronic injury of the superficial deltoid ligament. MR imaging shows a rounded wad of low to intermediate T2 signal intensity soft tissue anterior to the medial malleolus (**Fig. 8**). Osteophytes in this location may also limit motion.

MR Imaging Criteria

MR imaging has been shown to be reliable in the evaluation of deltoid ligament.[2,19] When the ability of MR imaging to detect injury to any portion of the deltoid complex was studied, reported sensitivity was 84% and specificity was 93%.[19] When the detection of injuries to the superficial and deep deltoid ligament were considered separately, tears of the superficial deltoid were detected with a sensitivity of 83% and specificity of 94%; tears of the deep deltoid were detected with a sensitivity of 96% and specificity of 98%.[2]

The deep deltoid ligament is short, and may show minimal displacement when torn. The ligament inserts on the lower portion of the talar fovea. A torn ligament may displace superiorly (see **Fig. 4**A) and abut the talus above the site of ligament attachment. Knowledge of the normal anatomy enables recognition that this represents a complete ligament tear. Discrete, taut fibers should always be visible in the deep deltoid ligament; a chronic tear may be manifest as an amorphous ligament (see **Fig. 5**B). Frank discontinuity of fibers (see **Fig. 5**C) is the most obvious sign of deltoid tear, but is not always present.

The superficial deltoid may be torn at its origin or more distally. Tears of its origin are best seen on axial images, where the deltoid origin is detached from the medial malleolus (see **Figs. 5**A, **6**A and **7**A). The detachment may be complete, with fluid seen between the deltoid origin and the medial malleolus. Less commonly, the ligament remains attached, but the attachment is posterior to its normal position, along the medial malleolus. Tears more distally can be seen on coronal or axial images, either as discontinuous fibers or absent fibers (see **Figs. 4–6**).

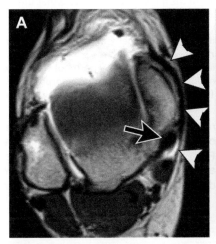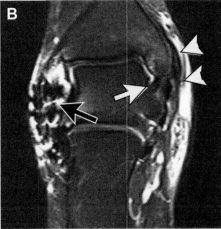

Fig. 6. Chronic lateral and medial ankle instability. Superficial deltoid ligament origin tear in 32-year-old woman with complaints of continued instability and medial pain following lateral ankle ligament reconstruction. (*A*) Axial T1WI postarthrogram at the level of the tibial plafond shows that the entire medial fascial sleeve (*arrowheads*) is avulsed from the medial malleolus. This injury allows arthrographic fluid to extend around the posterior tibial tendon (*arrow*). (*B*) Coronal FSE T2FS image postarthrogram shows that the deep deltoid ligament (*white arrow*) is intact. There is detachment of the origin of the superficial deltoid (*white arrowheads*). Artifact laterally (*black arrow*) is from anchors at ligament reconstruction.

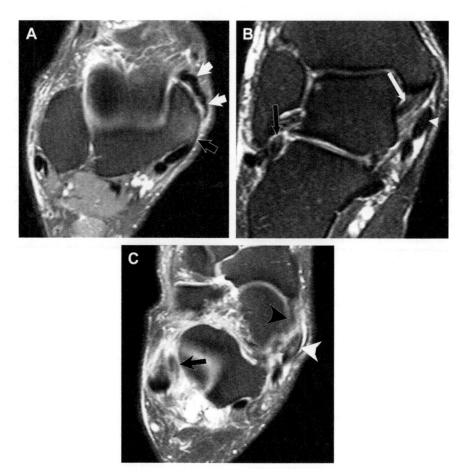

Fig. 7. Chronic medial insufficiency leads to lateral impingement. A 60-year-old man with chronic pes planovalgus complained of increasing deformity and increasing medial and lateral ankle pain. (*A*) Axial PDFS image at the level of the tibial plafond shows complete detachment of the origin of the superficial deltoid ligament (*white arrows*). There is high-signal fluid between the ligament and the cortex of the medial malleolus. Note that the origin of the flexor retinaculum (*black arrow*) is intact. (*B*) Coronal FSE T2FS image shows that the deep deltoid (*white arrow*) is intact. Posterior tibial tendinosis is also evident (*arrowhead*), with mildly increased signal intensity in the posterior tibial tendon. Because of the patient's severe valgus deformity, there is impingement of the peroneal tendons. The calcaneofibular ligament is thick, irregular, and lax (*black arrow*), consistent with chronic tear, perhaps caused by impingement, perhaps because of prior ankle sprain. (*C*) Axial PDFS at level of distal posterior tibial tendon better shows tendinosis (*white arrowhead*). The superomedial spring ligament is thick, lax, and amorphous (*black arrowhead*), and the thickening of the calcaneofibular ligament (*black arrow*) is confirmed.

FLEXOR RETINACULUM INJURIES
Pathophysiology

The flexor retinaculum is often torn in conjunction with a tear of the superficial deltoid ligament (see **Figs. 5** and **6**), or in association with ankle fracture.[20] Tears of the flexor retinaculum are important because they result in posterior tibial tendon subluxation or dislocation.[21–23] An isolated tear of the flexor retinaculum is rare (**Fig. 9**). It may occur because of a twisting injury, often with dorsiflexion.

MR imaging Criteria

MR imaging of isolated flexor retinaculum injury shows focal discontinuity of the retinaculum,

reliably occurring at the insertion of the ligament on the posteromedial corner of the tibia (see **Fig. 9**). The posterior tibial tendon is often but not always subluxated medially. It rarely completely dislocates in the absence of ankle fracture.

SPRING LIGAMENT ABNORMALITIES
Pathophysiology

The spring ligament is often abnormal in patients with flatfoot deformity, whether because of acute injury or chronic deformity. It may be injured in isolation,[24,25] or with talonavicular joint dislocation, but is most commonly seen in concert with abnormalities of the deltoid ligament and posterior

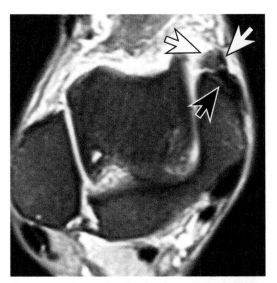

Fig. 8. Anteromedial ankle impingement. A 46-year-old woman with a history of multiple ankle sprains and focal anteromedial pain. Axial PDFS MR imaging at the level of the ankle joint shows focal, rounded scar (*white arrows*) that resulted in pain and limited motion in dorsiflexion and inversion. The origin of the superficial deltoid ligament (*black arrow*) is lax and thick.

tibial tendon.[26] The superomedial band of the spring ligament is the portion of the ligament that is readily surgically accessible and most important for function,[25] and, if a repair is performed, it is of this portion of the ligament. The plantar portion of

the spring ligament is located in the deep plantar compartment of the foot, and is usually not repaired.

MR imaging Criteria

The literature on MR imaging findings of spring ligament abnormalities is sparse. Reported MR imaging signs of spring ligament tear are discontinuity, thickening, abnormal signal intensity, and elongation of 1 or more portions of the ligament.[26,27] Discontinuity of the tibiospring ligament and the superomedial band (**Fig. 10A**) is best seen in the coronal plane, but may be visible on axial images as well (**Fig. 10B**). Thickening of the ligament (**Fig 10C**) is an unreliable sign. It may reflect redundancy adjacent to a tear, but may also occur as a chronic stress response in the presence of an intact ligament. In one MR imaging study,[26] 92% of patients with posterior tibial tendon abnormality also had an abnormal spring ligament, whereas 28% of controls also had an abnormal spring ligament; the high reported prevalence of an abnormal spring ligament in controls raises concern that the MR imaging diagnostic criteria used in the study were overly sensitive and nonspecific. Accuracy of diagnosis is improved if ligament thickening in isolation is not used as a sign of tear, but reported descriptively. Elongation of the spring ligament is a more common finding than focal tear (**Fig. 11**).

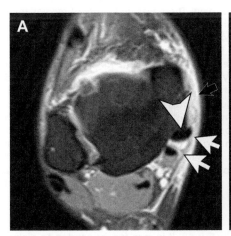
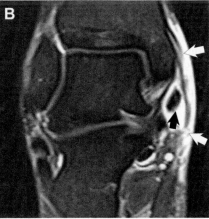

Fig. 9. Traumatic avulsion of the flexor retinaculum. A 30-year-old woman with an acute dorsiflexion injury of the ankle. She complained of posteromedial ankle pain. Based on MR imaging findings, the patient was treated acutely with open repair of the retinaculum. (*A*) Axial PDFS image immediately superior to the ankle joint shows that the flexor retinaculum (*white arrows*) and malleolar periosteum (*black arrow*) are detached from the medial malleolus. The posterior tibial tendon (*white arrowhead*) is subluxated medially; it should never extend medial to the posteromedial corner of the tibia. (*B*) Coronal FSE T2FS image through the midportion of the ankle joint shows injury of the longitudinal fibers of the flexor retinaculum (*white arrows*). The superficial and deep deltoid ligaments are intact. Longitudinal splitting is present in the posterior tibial tendon (*black arrow*) and there is a large amount of fluid in the tendon sheath. The splitting was not repaired at time of surgery, but patient did well after retinacular repair.

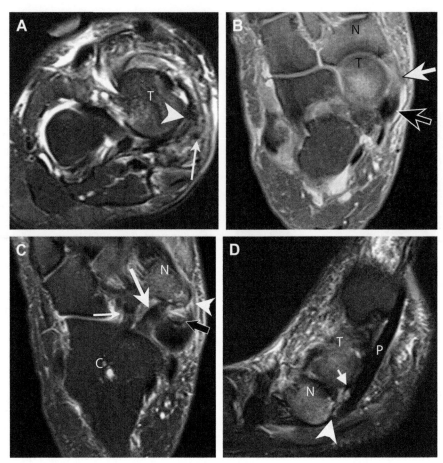

Fig. 10. Traumatic spring ligament tear and posterior tibial tendon tear. A 48-year-old woman fell into a hole, and felt a snap. She complained of severe, acute medial pain. There was no history of medial ankle pain. (*A*) Coronal FSE T2FS image at the level of the talar head shows tears of the superomedial band of the spring ligament (*arrowhead*) and posterior tibial tendon (*arrow*). Spring ligament tear is strongly associated with abnormalities of the posterior tibial tendon. (*B*) Axial PDFS image at the level of the talar head confirms complete disruption of the superomedial spring ligament (*white arrow*). The posterior tibial tendon contains intermediate signal intensity (*black arrow*), which may reflect acute contusion or preexisting tendinosis. (*C*) Axial PDFS image immediately inferior to the sustentaculum tali of the calcaneus shows that the plantar bands of the spring ligament (*large arrow* indicates medioplantar oblique band, *small arrow* indicates inferoplantar band) are thickened but intact. This thickening is consistent with preexisting increased stress before the acute injury. Fluid (*arrowhead*) is seen at the expected insertion of the posterior tibial tendon on the navicular. Careful scrutiny shows the small accessory navicular (*black arrow*), which has been avulsed. Small bone fragments are easily overlooked on MR imaging. (*D*) Sagittal short tau inversion recovery (STIR) image at the medial aspect of the ankle shows the displaced os naviculare (*arrow*) to which an intact posterior tibial tendon (P) is attaching. Arrowhead points to fluid in the disrupted synchondrosis. N, navicular; T, head of talus.

POSTERIOR TIBIAL TENDON TEAR
Pathophysiology of Acute Injury

It is rare for there to be an acute posterior tibial tendon injury, but one may occur because of athletic injury, usually in young patients. Tenosynovitis may develop in running sports.[25] A traumatic avulsion of the flexor retinaculum from the medial malleolus destabilizes the tendon. The destabilized tendon is abraded against the sharp posteromedial corner of the tibia, and develops interstitial

tears, which can progress to complete tear (see **Fig. 8**). It is rare for the tendon to dislocate in the absence of ankle fracture.[28]

Pathophysiology of Chronic Injury

Most posterior tibial tendon abnormalities are a chronic, degenerative phenomenon. Degenerative posterior tibial tendon abnormalities are a common cause of chronic medial ankle pain, almost always associated with abnormalities of the spring

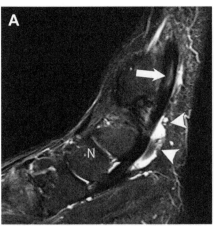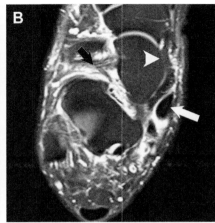

Fig. 11. Chronic thickening and elongation of spring ligament, together with tenosynovitis and longitudinal splitting of the posterior tibial tendon in a 63-year-old woman with increased medial ankle pain and chronic flat-foot deformity. (*A*) Sagittal STIR image through the medial ankle shows the posterior tibial tendon sheath is distended. The sheath has a lobulated contour (*arrowheads*). The fluid in the sheath contains intermediate signal intensity fibrous material consistent with synechiae, indicating chronic tenosynovitis. Longitudinal splitting (*arrow*) of the tendon is evident behind the medial malleolus. (*B*) Axial PDFS image at the level of the talar head shows a thickened posterior tibial tendon (*white arrow*) containing mildly increased signal intensity, and surrounded by fluid. The superomedial spring ligament (*arrowhead*) is thickened and elongated. There is fluid in the tarsal sinus (*black arrow*) reflecting altered stresses in the lateral ankle.

or deltoid ligament or flexor retinaculum.[28] They occur most commonly in middle-aged women who are obese and have preexisting flatfoot deformity, which put chronic stress on the tendon. Rheumatoid arthritis and collagen vascular disease are also associated with posterior tibial tendon tears. Tears follow a predictable progression, starting with tenosynovitis and/or tendinosis, progressing to intrasubstance splitting, partial tear, and complete tear. As the tendon abnormalities progress, the patients also develop elongation and insufficiency of the spring ligament and eventually the deltoid ligament.[26,29] Pes planovalgus develops, and is flexible in the earlier stages, becoming rigid as the deformity decreases. Lateral impingement may occur secondary to the hindfoot valgus (see **Fig. 7**).

Accessory Navicular Injury

A type II accessory navicular, in which the posterior tibial tendon attaches partly to the accessory center of ossification, may be associated with acute or chronic posterior tibial tendon dysfunction. The synchondrosis between an accessory navicular and the parent navicular bone is vulnerable to traction stress by the posterior tibial tendon (**Fig. 10C, D**). The accessory ossicle may displace posteriorly. More often, the synchondrosis is only mildly widened or is normal in width but contains fluid signal intensity.

MR imaging show fluids in the synchondrosis, and bone marrow edema that is centered on the synchondrosis. A small type II ossicle is easily overlooked on fluid-sensitive sequences, especially when bone marrow edema is present (**Fig. 12**).

MR imaging Criteria

MR imaging is reliable in the characterization of posterior tibial tendon abnormalities[30,31] (see **Figs. 4, 7,9–12; Fig. 13**). A small amount of fluid in the tendon sheath is normal, but tenosynovitis is indicated by a large effusion. The sheath often has an irregular, lobulated contour, and there may be synechiae visible within the fluid (see **Fig. 11A**). Tendinosis is characterized on MR imaging by T2 signal intensity that is increased, but less than the signal intensity of fluid (see **Fig. 7B**). Degenerative tears progress from longitudinal splitting to thinning of the tendon to complete tear. As longitudinal splits develop, the tendon becomes thickened, and contains high-signal-intensity streaks between the fibers (see **Fig. 9B**). In more severe partial tears, a decrease in the tendon diameter is seen (see **Fig. 4**A). Complete tears, surprisingly, can be missed at MR imaging (see **Fig. 13**) if the normal flexor digitorum longus tendon is mistaken for the posterior tibial tendon. This error can easily be avoided by always counting the number of tendons posterior to the medial malleolus.

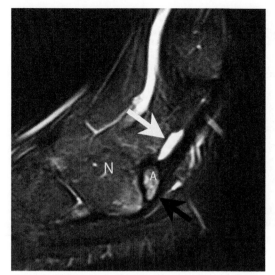

Fig. 12. Acute injury to synchondrosis of accessory navicular. An 18-year-old girl presented with acute onset of medial ankle pain during a basketball game. Sagittal STIR image shows fluid in the posterior tibial tendon sheath (*white arrow*). There is a type II accessory navicular. The posterior tibial tendon inserts on the accessory navicular (*black arrow*). Bone marrow edema in the type II accessory navicular and the parent navicular is consistent with an injury to the synchondrosis of the type II accessory navicular despite the absence of displacement of the ossicle. Abnormalities of the posterior tibial tendon are rare at this age, and usually related either to an accessory ossicle or to an injury of the flexor retinaculum. A, accessory navicular; N, parent navicular.

TARSAL TUNNEL SYNDROME
Pathophysiology

Any space-occupying lesion in the tarsal tunnel may compress the tibial nerve or its branches and result in tarsal tunnel syndrome.[32] A neuropathy may also occur in this location without a space-occupying lesion, probably as the result of chronic traction on the nerve in patients with hindfoot valgus. The clinical symptoms vary depending on which of the branches of the nerve are affected. The treatment is often surgical, but is still debated.[33]

MR imaging Criteria

MR imaging is useful[34,35] to evaluate for a mass lesion and for denervation of affected muscles (**Fig. 14**). Denervation edema is characterized by diffuse high T2 signal within the affected muscle, with preservation of normal muscle architecture. In contrast, muscle contusion or tear has a more heterogeneous appearance, and muscle fibers are disrupted. MR imaging can also be used for evaluation of failed surgical release.[36]

ACCESSORY FLEXOR MUSCLES

Accessory flexor muscles in the tarsal tunnel may compress the tibial nerve and cause tarsal tunnel syndrome. They can also be symptomatic without causing neurologic symptoms. Patients may present with vague, exertional medial ankle

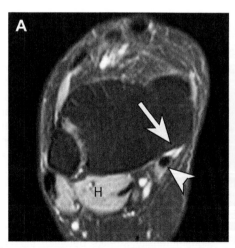
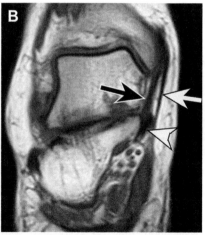

Fig. 13. Chronic, complete posterior tibial tendon tear. A 43-year-old woman had a history of rheumatoid arthritis, and complained of increasing flatfoot deformity. Radiographs showed no evidence of arthritis in the hindfoot, but flatfoot deformity was present. (*A*) Axial PDFS image shows fluid filling expected location of the posterior tibial tendon (*arrow*). The flexor digitorum tendon (*arrowhead*) and flexor hallucis longus (H) are normal. There are no other signs of injury, because the tear is chronic. A chronic, complete tear can easily be overlooked unless the reader has a checklist and systematically evaluates every anatomic structure. (*B*) Coronal PDFS shows the tibiocalcaneal band of the superficial deltoid (*black arrow*) and the flexor retinaculum (*white arrow*). The posterior tibial tendon should lie between these structures but is absent. No tendon was visible on any sequences to the level of the navicular insertion. Scans through distal calf showed the retracted tendon stump. Arrowhead points to flexor digitorum longus tendon.

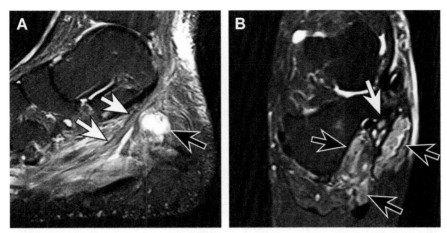

Fig. 14. Tarsal tunnel syndrome caused by malignant peripheral nerve sheath tumor in a 54-year-old woman complaining of burning and tingling pain in the medial foot. (*A*) Sagittal STIR image through the tarsal tunnel shows an irregularly shaped mass (*black arrow*). The irregular borders help distinguish it from a cyst, but there are no specific MR imaging features to identify it as a malignancy. The adjacent medial plantar nerve (*white arrows*) is enlarged. (*B*) Coronal FSE T2FS image through the tarsal tunnel distal to the mass shows denervation edema (*black arrows*) in the quadratus plantae, flexor digitorum brevis, and abductor hallucis muscles, all innervated by the medial plantar nerve. The nerve is mildly enlarged (*white arrow*).

pain. This condition probably reflects increased compartmental pressure caused by the presence of the muscle.[37,38] They are often asymptomatic.

On MR imaging, the accessory muscle has a fusiform shape (**Fig. 15**). A normal pattern of muscle fascicles separated by fat is visible within it. It may appear mildly edematous on fluid-sensitive

sequences, probably reflecting compression within the tarsal tunnel.

TARSAL COALITION

Tarsal coalition is a bony, fibrous, or cartilaginous connection between 2 or more tarsal bones. The coalition restricts motion, and may cause ill-

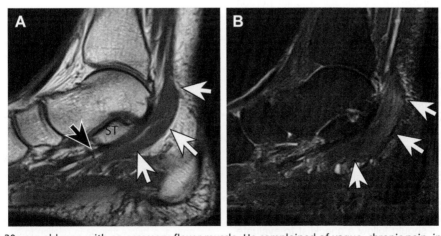

Fig. 15. A 30-year-old man with an accessory flexor muscle. He complained of vague, chronic pain, increased on exertion. (*A*) Sagittal T1WI through the tarsal tunnel shows a fusiform accessory muscle (*white arrows*). It lies adjacent to the flexor hallucis longus tendon (*black arrow*). (*B*) Sagittal STIR image in the same location. The accessory muscle (*white arrows*) is much less conspicuous on fluid-sensitive sequences, and tends to merge visually with the adjacent fat. A small amount of edema in the muscle in this case follows the course of the muscle fibers, and most likely reflects edema caused by muscle compression or overuse. ST, sustentaculum tali.

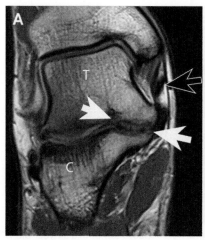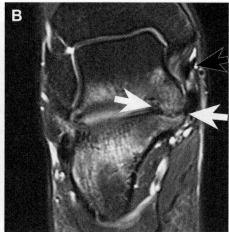

Fig. 16. Talocalcaneal coalition. An 18-year-old man with several-year history of medial and lateral hindfoot pain, and limited motion, but no pes planus. (*A*) Coronal T1WI at the posterior portion of the sustentaculum tali shows a nonbony coalition of the middle subtalar facet. The sustentaculum tali is small and obliquely oriented, there is overgrowth of the adjacent talus, and an irregular junction between the bones, which represents the coalition (*white arrows*). Note that the posterior tibial tendon (*black arrow*) appears thin and irregular.. (*B*) Coronal FSE T2FS at the same location again shows the coalition (*white arrows*). Bone marrow edema caused by altered motion is present around the coalition. The splitting of the posterior tibial tendon (*black arrow*) reflects altered hindfoot biomechanics.

defined pain. Tarsal coalition is generally thought to present in the second decade of life as a rigid flatfoot deformity. However, many patients present later in life, and only about 50% have a flatfoot deformity.[39] The 2 most common types of coalition are subtalar, usually involving the middle subtalar facet, and calcaneonavicular. Subtalar coalitions often present with vague medial pain. They are easily overlooked on radiographs.

MR imaging through the middle subtalar joint shows overgrowth of the medial articular portion of the talus, and a dysmorphic sustentaculum tali (**Fig. 16**). When a nonbony coalition is present, intermediate T2 signal is seen in the obliquely oriented, irregularly marginated cartilaginous or fibrous pseudojoint between the dysmorphic talus and sustentaculum tali. This pseudojoint differs from the normal middle subtalar joint (see **Fig. 1B**) both in its orientation and the irregularity of its margins. The altered biomechanics of the hindfoot often lead to bone marrow edema and to abnormalities of the flexor and peroneal tendons. Posteromedial impingement may also occur.[40]

SUMMARY

Radiologists should follow a checklist to evaluate all the medial structures of the hindfoot. In addition, radiologists need to be aware of the close functional interrelationships of these structures, and their relationships to abnormalities of the lateral ankle.

REFERENCES

1. Mengiardi B, Pfirrmann CW, Vienne P, et al. Medial collateral ligament complex of the ankle: MR appearance in asymptomatic subjects. Radiology 2007;242:817–24.
2. Crim J, Longenecker LG. MRI and surgical findings in deltoid ligament tears. AJR Am J Roentgenol 2015;204:W63–9.
3. Numkarunarunrote N, Malik A, Aguiar RO, et al. Retinacula of the foot and ankle: MRI with anatomic correlation in cadavers. AJR Am J Roentgenol 2007; 188:W348–54.
4. Taniguchi A, Tanaka Y, Takakura Y, et al. Anatomy of the spring ligament. J Bone Joint Surg Am 2003;85-A:2174–8.
5. Desai KR, Beltran LS, Bencardino JT, et al. The spring ligament recess of the talocalcaneonavicular joint: depiction on MR images with cadaveric and histologic correlation. AJR Am J Roentgenol 2011; 196:1145–50.
6. Cromeens BP, Kirchhoff CA, Patterson RM, et al. An attachment-based description of the medial collateral and spring ligament complexes. Foot Ankle Int 2015;36:710–21.
7. Kaye RA, Jahss MH. Tibialis posterior: a review of anatomy and biomechanics in relation to support of the medial longitudinal arch. Foot Ankle 1991;11:244–7.
8. Kelikian AS, Sarrafian SK, Sarrafian SK. Sarrafian's anatomy of the foot and ankle: descriptive, topographical, functional. 3rd edition. Philadelphia: Wolters Kluwer Health; Lippincott Williams & Wilkins; 2011.

9. Hintermann B, Knupp M, Pagenstert GI. Deltoid ligament injuries: diagnosis and management. Foot Ankle Clin 2006;11:625–37.

10. Lotscher P, Lang TH, Zwicky L, et al. Osteoligamentous injuries of the medial ankle joint. Eur J Trauma Emerg Surg 2015;41:615–21.

11. van den Bekerom MP, Mutsaerts EL, van Dijk CN. Evaluation of the integrity of the deltoid ligament in supination external rotation ankle fractures: a systematic review of the literature. Arch Orthop Trauma Surg 2009;129:227–35.

12. Roemer FW, Jomaah N, Niu J, et al. Ligamentous injuries and the risk of associated tissue damage in acute ankle sprains in athletes: a cross-sectional MRI study. Am J Sports Med 2014;42:1549–57.

13. Koval KJ, Egol KA, Cheung Y, et al. Does a positive ankle stress test indicate the need for operative treatment after lateral malleolus fracture? A preliminary report. J Orthop Trauma 2007;21:449–55.

14. van Rijn RM, van Os AG, Bernsen RM, et al. What is the clinical course of acute ankle sprains? A systematic literature review. Am J Med 2008;121:324–31.e6.

15. Hintermann B, Valderrabano V, Boss A, et al. Medial ankle instability: an exploratory, prospective study of fifty-two cases. Am J Sports Med 2004;32:183–90.

16. Knupp M, Lang TH, Zwicky L, et al. Chronic ankle instability (medial and lateral). Clin Sports Med 2015;34:679–88.

17. Crim JR, Beals TC, Nickisch F, et al. Deltoid ligament abnormalities in chronic lateral ankle instability. Foot Ankle Int 2011;32:873–8.

18. Donovan A, Rosenberg ZS. MRI of ankle and lateral hindfoot impingement syndromes. AJR Am J Roentgenol 2010;195:595–604.

19. Chun KY, Choi YS, Lee SH, et al. Deltoid ligament and tibiofibular syndesmosis injury in chronic lateral ankle instability: magnetic resonance imaging evaluation at 3T and comparison with arthroscopy. Korean J Radiol 2015;16:1096–103.

20. Crim J, Enslow M, Smith J. CT assessment of the prevalence of retinacular injuries associated with hindfoot fractures. Skeletal Radiol 2013;42:487–92.

21. Godino M, Vides M, Guerado E. Traumatic dislocation of posterior tibial tendon by avulsion of flexor retinacular release. Reconstruction with suture anchors. Rev Esp Cir Ortop Traumatol 2015;59:211–4.

22. Mitchell K, Mencia MM, Hoford R. Tibialis posterior tendon dislocation: a case report. Foot (Edinb) 2011;21:154–6.

23. Rolf C, Guntner P, Ekenman I, et al. Dislocation of the tibialis posterior tendon: diagnosis and treatment. J Foot Ankle Surg 1997;36:63–5.

24. Orr JD, Nunley JA 2nd. Isolated spring ligament failure as a cause of adult-acquired flatfoot deformity. Foot Ankle Int 2013;34:818–23.

25. Ribbans WJ, Garde A. Tibialis posterior tendon and deltoid and spring ligament injuries in the elite athlete. Foot Ankle Clin 2013;18:255–91.

26. Balen PF, Helms CA. Association of posterior tibial tendon injury with spring ligament injury, sinus tarsi abnormality, and plantar fasciitis on MR imaging. AJR Am J Roentgenol 2001;176:1137–43.

27. Williams G, Widnall J, Evans P, et al. MRI features most often associated with surgically proven tears of the spring ligament complex. Skeletal Radiol 2013;42:969–73.

28. Gluck GS, Heckman DS, Parekh SG. Tendon disorders of the foot and ankle, part 3: the posterior tibial tendon. Am J Sports Med 2010;38:2133–44.

29. Deland JT, de Asla RJ, Sung IH, et al. Posterior tibial tendon insufficiency: which ligaments are involved? Foot Ankle Int 2005;26:427–35.

30. Khoury NJ, el-Khoury GY, Saltzman CL, et al. MR imaging of posterior tibial tendon dysfunction. AJR Am J Roentgenol 1996;167:675–82.

31. Chhabra A, Soldatos T, Chalian M, et al. 3-Tesla magnetic resonance imaging evaluation of posterior tibial tendon dysfunction with relevance to clinical staging. J Foot Ankle Surg 2011;50:320–8.

32. Pomeroy G, Wilton J, Anthony S. Entrapment neuropathy about the foot and ankle: an update. J Am Acad Orthop Surg 2015;23:58–66.

33. McSweeney SC, Cichero M. Tarsal tunnel syndrome–A narrative literature review. Foot (Edinb) 2015;25:244–50.

34. Kerr R, Frey C. MR imaging in tarsal tunnel syndrome. J Comput Assist Tomogr 1991;15:280–6.

35. Donovan A, Rosenberg ZS, Cavalcanti CF. MR imaging of entrapment neuropathies of the lower extremity. Part 2. The knee, leg, ankle, and foot. Radiographics 2010;30:1001–19.

36. Zeiss J, Fenton P, Ebraheim N, et al. Magnetic resonance imaging for ineffectual tarsal tunnel surgical treatment. Clin Orthop Relat Res 1991;264:264–6.

37. Al-Himdani S, Talbot C, Kurdy N, et al. Accessory muscles around the foot and ankle presenting as chronic undiagnosed pain. An illustrative case report and review of the literature. Foot (Edinb) 2013;23:154–61.

38. Sookur PA, Naraghi AM, Bleakney RR, et al. Accessory muscles: anatomy, symptoms, and radiologic evaluation. Radiographics 2008;28:481–99.

39. Crim J. Imaging of tarsal coalition. Radiol Clin North Am 2008;46:1017–26, vi.

40. Song W, Liu W, Chen B, et al. Posteromedial ankle impingement caused by hypertrophy of talocalcaneal coalition: a report of five cases and introduction of a novel index system. J Foot Ankle Surg 2016. [Epub ahead of print].

MR Imaging Findings in Heel Pain

Ching-Di Chang, MD[a], Jim S. Wu, MD[b],*

KEYWORDS

- Heel pain • MR imaging • Achilles tendon • Plantar fasciitis • Tarsal tunnel
- Calcaneal stress fracture • Retrocalcaneal bursitis

KEY POINTS

- Knowledge of the anatomic structures that form the heel is important in understanding the various osseous and soft tissue causes of heel pain.
- Common causes of heel pain include disorders of the Achilles tendon, plantar fascia, calcaneus, bursae, nerves in the tarsal tunnel, and heel pad.
- MR imaging is the best imaging modality to assess heel pain due to its superior soft tissue contrast and ability to localize the site end extent of disease.

INTRODUCTION

Heel pain is common and accounts for more than 1 million doctor visits annually in the United States.[1] Several osseous and soft tissue disorders can lead to heel pain and it is important for both radiologists and clinicians to be familiar with the relevant hindfoot anatomy to arrive at a correct diagnosis. Moreover, it is important to understand the relationship of the various structures with one another because this can have implications for treatment. For instance, abnormalities of the Achilles tendon can lead to a higher incidence of plantar fasciitis.[2] Causes of heel pain can be classified based on the structure in which it arises and can be divided into 6 major anatomic categories[3]: (1) Achilles tendon (tendinopathy, tear, and paratenonitis), (2) plantar fascia (fasciitis, fascial tear, and fibromatosis), (3) calcaneus (stress fracture, osteomyelitis, tumors, and Sever disease), (4) bursae (retrocalcaneal and retro-Achilles bursitis, and Haglund syndrome), (5) nerves (tarsal tunnel syndrome and Baxter neuropathy) (6) and heel pad (fat pad syndrome) (Table 1). Other less common causes of heel pain include avascular necrosis, tarsal coalition, arthritic disorders (osteoarthritis, gout, rheumatoid arthritis, and reactive arthritis), and posterior impingement.[3–5]

Diagnosis of heel pain can be challenging based only on clinical history and physical examination. Imaging can be useful, with MR imaging the most useful imaging modality.[3,6] MR imaging has great soft tissue contrast and excellent anatomic detail, which allow for assessment of the location and extent of the hindfoot disorder, which can also assist with preoperative planning.[6] This article discusses the most common conditions that cause heel pain based on their anatomic location and emphasizes their MR imaging appearances.

HEEL ANATOMY

The heel refers to the posterior aspect of the foot, which includes the posterior calcaneus and adjacent soft tissue structures (Fig. 1). It functions to dissipate the compressive forces that occur during gait especially during the stance phase.[7] Together with the metatarsal heads, the heel supports the

Disclosure Statement: The authors have nothing to disclose.
[a] Department of Radiology, Kaohsiung Chang Gung Memorial Hospital, Chang Gung University College of Medicine, 123 Ta-Pei Road, Niao-Sung District, Kaohsiung City 833, Taiwan; [b] Department of Radiology, Beth Israel Deaconess Medical Center, Harvard Medical School, 330 Brookline Avenue, Boston, MA 02215, USA
* Corresponding author.
E-mail address: jswu@bidmc.harvard.edu

Table 1 Causes of heel pain	
Anatomic Structure	**Disorder**
Achilles tendon	Achilles tendinopathy (midportion or insertional) Achilles partial tear Achilles complete tear Paratendinopathy or paratenonitis of Achilles tendon
Plantar fascia	Plantar fasciitis Plantar fascia tear Plantar fibromatosis
Calcaneus	Stress fracture Osteomyelitis Sever disease Tumor (intraosseous lipoma, simple bone cyst, aneurysmal bone cyst, etc.)
Bursae	Retrocalcaneal bursitis Retro-Achilles bursitis Haglund syndrome
Nerve	Tarsal tunnel syndrome Baxter neuropathy
Heel pad	Heel pad syndrome

full weight of the body; thus, it can be subjected to high repetitive forces leading to certain injuries.[4,8] The heel is comprised of the Achilles tendon, plantar fascia, calcaneus, bursa, nerves in the tarsal tunnel, and inferior heel pad. The Achilles tendon attaches to the calcaneal tuberosity and is the longest and strongest tendon in the body, formed by the gastrocnemius and soleus muscles.[9] The plantar aponeurosis, or plantar fascia, is a thick band of connective tissue that supports the arch of foot.[2] It consists of 3 bands (medial, lateral, and central) and originates from the medial tuberosity of calcaneus and extends anteriorly to insert on the base of the proximal phalanges. A fascial connection exists between the distal

Achilles tendon and the posterior aspect of the plantar fascia; thus, forces exerted on the Achilles can affect the plantar fascia.[2] This fascial connection diminishes with age.[10] The calcaneus is the bony foundation of the heel and serves as the attachment site for several structures. The retrocalcaneal and retro-Achilles bursa are located anterior and posterior to the Achilles tendon, respectively, and can become inflamed by various disorders, leading to bursitis.[11] The tarsal tunnel is a fibro-osseous tunnel located at the medial ankle, which is bounded by the flexor retinaculum (roof) and medial surface of talus and calcaneus (floor). It contains the flexor tendons and a neurovascular bundle (posterior tibial artery, vein and tibial

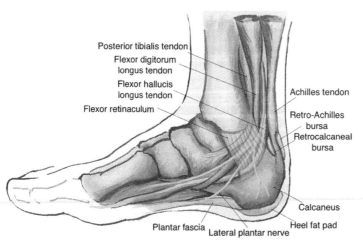

Fig. 1. Illustration showing the normal anatomy of the heel.

Posterior tibialis tendon
Flexor digitorum longus tendon
Flexor hallucis longus tendon
Flexor retinaculum
Achilles tendon
Retro-Achilles bursa
Retrocalcaneal bursa
Calcaneus
Heel fat pad
Plantar fascia
Lateral plantar nerve

nerve). Compression of the regional neural structures may cause numbness, paresthesia, and heel pain.[12,13] Lastly, a fat pad is present along the inferior aspect of the posterior calcaneus that helps to cushion the weight of the body. Injury or inflammation to this fat pad can lead to heel pain.[14]

ACHILLES TENDON

Disorders of the Achilles tendon are often due to repetitive microtrauma from overuse in athletes or in patients with abnormal alignment, such as flatfeet.[4,15,16] The Achilles tendon represents the union of the gastrocnemius and soleus muscles and attaches onto the posterior calcaneus. It lacks a true tendon sheath but is surrounded by thin connective tissue, paratenon.[17] Moreover, there is a critical zone within the tendon representing a segment of the tendon with decreased vascularity, located 2 cm to 7 cm proximal to the calcaneal insertion. Injuries at this location heal poorly due to poor blood flow and tendon ruptures commonly occur in this location.[18]

Terminology used to describe overuse injuries of the Achilles tendon can be confusing and inconsistent.[16] Because there is often no chronic inflammation, the term, *tendinosis*, should be used instead of *tendinitis*; however, both terms refer to the histopathologic appearance of the tendon. *Tendinopathy*, on the other hand, includes the clinical syndrome of tendon pain, swelling, and impaired performance; thus, it has been suggested as the ideal term to use when describing Achilles tendon injuries.[16,19] These injuries can be classified into 4 types: midportion tendinopathy, insertional tendinopathy, paratendinopathy, and tendon tear/rupture.[16]

Midportion tendinopathy is the clinical syndrome of pain, swelling, and impaired performance located 2 cm to 7 cm above the calcaneal insertion and manifests as tendon thickening with loss of the normal anterior concave margin on axial images (**Fig. 2**) and increased intrasubstance signal on edema-sensitive (T2 and short tau inversion recovery [STIR]) sequences.[9,16] The normal Achilles tendon should be dark on T1 and T2 MR imaging pulse sequences and should measure 5 mm to 8 mm in thickness, depending on the size of the patient.[6,17] With tendinopathy, tendon contrast enhancement can be present and is consistent with intratendinous neovascularization from the body's attempt and failure at tendon repair.[9,16] Occasionally, normal intratendinous high signal intensity can be seen in the Achilles tendon, which can be attributed to magic angle effect related to rotation of the tendon fibers.[17] This artifact can be avoided by using long echo time sequences, such as T2-weighted sequences.[17,20]

Insertional tendinopathy presents with enthesophyte formation and tendon thickening at the distal calcaneal insertion.[16] Calcifications and ossifications in the distal tendon occur with this condition and can be associated with retrocalcaneal and/or retro-Achilles bursitis.[16] Bone spur and tendon calcifications can be seen on radiographs; and on MR imaging; there is often marrow edema in the calcaneus and distal Achilles tendon substance (**Fig. 3**).[3,16] CT aids in surgical planning by detailing the bony anatomy for removal of the posterior spur.[16,21] Peritendinopathy or peritenonitis of the Achilles tendon refers to acute or chronic inflammation of the thin membrane, peritenon, surrounding the Achilles tendon.[6] It can result from seronegative arthropathy, infection, or overuse injury.[6,9,16] On MR imaging, the Achilles tendon can have normal low signal and size; however, there is partially circumferential edema or fluid around the Achilles tendon on fluid-sensitive sequences and enhancement after contrast administration (**Fig. 4**).[6,9,16] Isolated fluid and/or edema in Kager fat pad should be termed, *paratendonitis*, because the abnormality is adjacent to the tendon

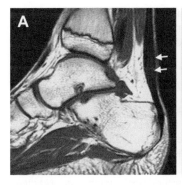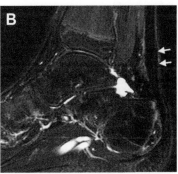

Fig. 2. Midportion Achilles tendinopathy in a 27-year-old man. Sagittal (*A*) T1-weighted and (*B*) STIR MR images show intrasubstance isointense signal intensity and fusiform enlargement (*arrows*) of the midportion of the Achilles tendon.

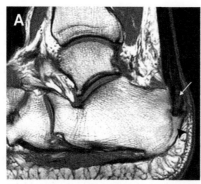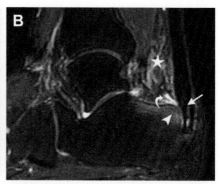

Fig. 3. Insertional Achilles tendinopathy in a 32-year-old man. (*A*) Sagittal T1-weighted MR image shows thickening and increased signal intensity in the distal Achilles tendon (*arrow*) and a large calcaneal enthesophyte (*black arrowhead*). (*B*) Sagittal T2 fat-saturated MR image shows marrow edema in the posterior superior calcaneus (*arrowhead*) and Kager fat pad (*star*). The high signal intensity in distal Achilles tendon (*arrow*) representing an interstitial tear. Also noted fluid in retrocalcaneal bursa (*curved arrow*).

and not surrounding it.[6] The potential space between the peritenon and tendon can fill with fluid and exudate, leading to thickening of the peritenon and the patient can present with palpable crepitus.[16]

The Achilles tendon is the most common tendon in the body to rupture and is often seen in middle-aged men engaged in sports activities, such as basketball or tennis.[6,16,22] Most tears occur in the avascular zone or midportion of the tendon during an acute traumatic event.[9] Tears can also occur, however, from progression of chronic Achilles tendinopathy, steroid injection, and fluoroquinolone antibiotics.[9,15,16] On MR imaging, the presence of fluid within the tendon on fluid-sensitive sequences indicates a tear.[6,17] There can also be tendon thickening, heterogeneous signal intensity, and disruption of tendon fibers (**Fig. 5**).[3,6,17,23] When no intact tendon fibers are seen, then a complete tear has occurred. In cases of partial or complete tear, it is crucial to describe the exact location and size of the tendon tear, because treatment options vary depending on the location of the tear.[24,25] Achilles tendon rupture can occur at the midsubstance (75%), distal insertion (10%–20%), and myotendinous junction (5%–15%).[24,25] Tears in the tendon midsubstance are typically easier to fix surgically than tears at the myotendinous junction or distal insertion.[22] Moreover, it is important to describe size of the tendon gap and character of the tendon free edge, such as fraying or tapering (**Fig. 6**). In addition, tears at the myotendinous junction may not been included on the field of view in standard protocols for imaging the ankle; thus, larger sagittal field of view images could be considered in these cases.

PLANTAR FASCIA
Plantar Fasciitis

Plantar fasciitis is the most common cause of heel pain and can be due to variety of conditions, including long-distance running, obesity, pes cavus (high arch), pes planus (flat feet), prolonged standing, and arthritidies, such as reactive

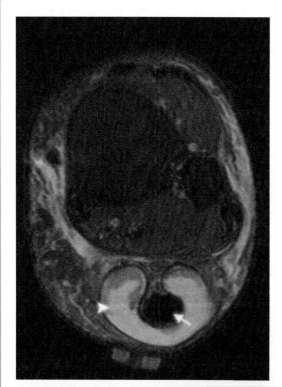

Fig. 4. Achilles paratenonitis in a 52-year-old woman. Axial T2-weighted fat-saturated MR image shows partial circumferential fluid signal (*arrowhead*) surrounding the Achilles tendon (*arrow*).

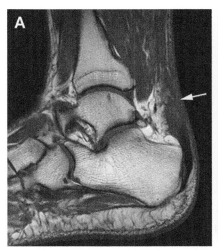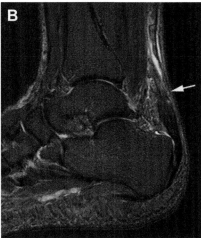

Fig. 5. Complete Achilles tendon tear in a 37-year-old man from playing soccer. (*A*) Sagittal T1-weighted and (*B*) T2-weighted fat-saturated MR images show a complete tear of the Achilles tendon (*arrow*) at the critical zone 6 cm above the calcaneal insertion.

arthritis (formerly termed Reiter disease) or psoriatic arthritis.[26–28] Similar to the development of Achilles tendon injury, repetitive trauma can induce microtears in the plantar fascia leading to degeneration and/or inflammatory changes, often in the central cord and at the calcaneal insertion.[27,28] Patients typically experience pain

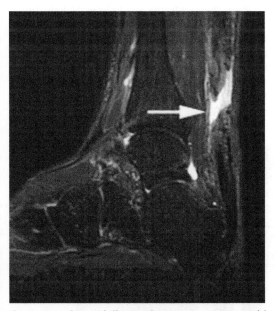

Fig. 6. Complete Achilles tendon tear in a 24-year-old man with 2-cm tendon gap. Sagittal T2-weighted fat-saturated MR image shows a complete tear of the midportion of the Achilles tendon with a 2-cm tendon gap filled with fluid (*arrow*). Commenting on the location and dimensions of the tendon gap is important for surgical planning.

at the inferior heel that is worse with their initial steps in the morning or after a period of inactivity.[29] The plantar fascia is best seen on coronal and sagittal images MR images and appears as a uniform low signal intensity structure extending from the inferior calcaneal tuberosity to the base of the proximal phalanges measuring 2 mm to 3 mm in thickness.[27,30] MR imaging findings of plantar fasciitis include thickening of plantar fascia (>4 mm in the craniocaudal dimension), increased intrasubstance signal intensity on T1-weighted and T2-weighted images, and perifascial and bone marrow edema at the calcaneal insertional area (**Fig. 7**).[5,27,29,31,32] Occasionally, an inferior calcaneal spur is seen. The association of an inferior calcaneal spur with plantar fasciitis is controversial, however, with some studies indicating no association[28,30] and other studies indicating a higher association of planter fasciitis with calcaneal spurs.[5,33,34] A recent study by Zhou and colleagues[34] finds that there are 2 types of calcaneal spurs. The type A spur extends superior to the plantar fascia insertion whereas a type B spur is enclosed by the plantar fascia and correlates with more severe symptoms.[34] MR imaging can be helpful in these cases by delineating the anatomy of the plantar fascia relative to the spur.

Plantar Fascia Tear

Tear of the plantar fascia can occur from progression of chronic plantar fasciitis or acute sports-related injury in athletes or be related to local corticosteroid injections.[4,35,36] Patients are often unable to perform a single-stance heel raise and have plantar ecchymosis.[37] Most plantar

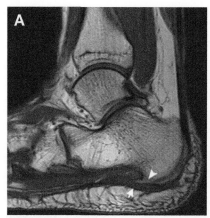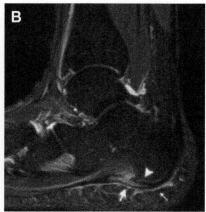

Fig. 7. Plantar fasciitis in a 32-year-old man. (*A*) Sagittal T1 and (*B*) sagittal T2 fat-saturated MR images demonstrate heterogeneous thickening (7 mm, normal is ≤4 mm) of the posterior plantar fascia (*arrow*) and perifascial edema (*small arrow*) at the medial calcaneal tuberosity. There is a calcaneal spur (*arrowhead*). (*Courtesy of Dr Jennifer Ni Mhuircheartaigh, Boston, MA.*)

fascia tears are located at proximal part of the plantar fascia, near calcaneal insertion, and in the central cord.[38] Similar to tendon rupture, MR imaging can reveal a fluid-filled gap within the disrupted plantar fascia, best seen on fluid-sensitive sequences (**Fig. 8**).[6] Additional findings include adjacent soft tissue edema, hemorrhage, and injury of the flexor digitorum brevis muscle in acute cases.[6,38] Fusiform or nodular thickening with low signal intensity on T1-weighted and T2-weighted images can be seen in chronic cases with hypertrophic scar.[38] Delineating the location of the tear and fascial gap on MR imaging is important in surgical planning.

Plantar Fibromatosis

Plantar fibromatosis is a benign but locally aggressive superficial fibroblastic proliferation in the plantar fascia, similar to Dupuytren disease in the hand and desmoid tumors, which involve deeper soft tissue structures.[39,40] Physical examination often reveals 1 or several palpable nodules along the plantar aspect of foot and can be bilateral in 25% of cases.[41] The nodules can lead to pain, contracture, and even walking disability.[3,42,43] Plantar fibromatosis usually involves the central or medial cords of plantar fascia.[39] On MR imaging, plantar fibromatosis typically demonstrates low to intermediate signal intensity on both T1-weighted and T2-weighted images due the dense fibrous content of the nodules (**Fig. 9**).[39,42] Occasionally fibromatosis can have high signal intensity on T2-weighted images, if there is a paucity of collagen or fibrous tissue content.[39] Postcontrast MR imaging shows internal, but variable, enhancement in

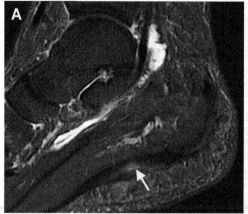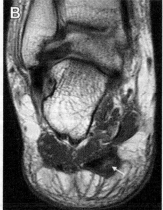

Fig. 8. Plantar fascia tear in a 25-year-old man, sustained while playing basketball. (*A*) Sagittal T2 fat-saturated and (*B*) coronal proton density MR images demonstrate heterogeneous thickening (7 mm) and high signal (*arrow*) in the central cord of the plantar fascia consistent with a partial tear.

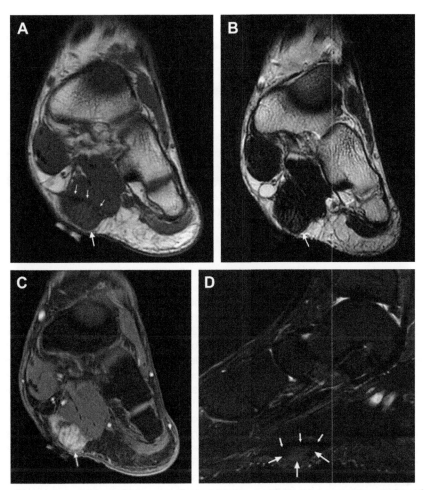

Fig. 9. Plantar fibroma in a 43-year-old woman. Coronal (*A*) T1 and (*B*) T2, (*C*) coronal T1-weighted fat-saturated postcontrast, and (*D*) sagittal T2-weighted fat-saturated MR images show a 2.2 cm lesion (*arrows*) arising from the plantar aponeurosis (*small arrows*). The lesion is isointense to the adjacent muscle on both the T1-weighted and T2-weighted images due to its fibrous content and demonstrates solid internal enhancement on the postcontrast image.

the lesion.[39,42] Linear regions of enhancement extending from the lesion and along the plantar aponeurosis, called a fascial tail, can be seen and is best seen on postcontrast images.[43] Due to the characteristic appearance of plantar fibromas, MR imaging is helpful in the diagnosis and assessing the anatomic location of the lesions, especially those with deep extension, for surgical removal.[39,40,43]

CALCANEUS
Stress Fracture

Stress fractures in the calcaneus are most often fatigue fractures (abnormal stress to normal bone) and oppose to insufficiency fracture (normal stress to weakened bone).[6,8] This injury is often seen in sedentary patients who initiate a new bout of physical activity or in runners who rapidly increase their level of training.[6,8] In both cases, the bone does not have sufficient time to adjust to the rapid increase in stress.[8,44,45] Radiographs can show subtle sclerosis often with a vertical orientation; however, they can be negative in 24% of calcaneal stress fractures.[44] MR imaging has better sensitivity in detecting calcaneal stress fracture and can identify the injury earlier than radiographs or CT.[46,47] On MR imaging, a low signal fracture line on T1-weighted and T2-weighted images usually extends to the cortex and is surrounded by bone marrow edema, which appears as low signal on T1-weighted images and high signal on T2-weighted images (**Fig. 10**).[47,48] A recent study by Cronlein and colleagues[49] suggests that PET–MR imaging can be useful in the diagnosis of calcaneal stress fractures and stress

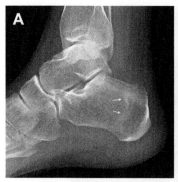
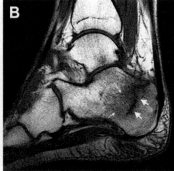
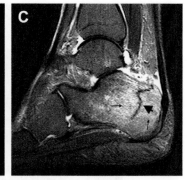

Fig. 10. Stress fracture in a 34-year-old female runner. (*A*) Lateral radiograph of the ankle shows a vertical linear region of sclerosis in the posterior calcaneus (*arrows*). (*B*) Sagittal T1-weighted MR image shows a hypointense fracture line (*short arrows*) with adjacent hypointense marrow edema (*thin arrows*). (*C*) On the STIR MR image, the fracture line is low signal (*short arrow*) and there is surrounding high signal marrow edema (*thin arrows*).

reaction, especially when conventional plain radiographs are normal.

Osteomyelitis

Osteomyelitis of the calcaneus can be a cause of heel pain in both children and adults. In children, calcaneal osteomyelitis is most often the result of hematogenous spread and typically begins at the calcaneal metaphysis, in the posterior calcaneus, adjacent and anterior to the growth plate (**Fig. 11**).[50] In adults, calcaneal osteomyelitis is invariably the result of adjacent soft tissue infection from skin ulcers, especially in a patient with diabetes.[51] Infection by *Staphylococcus aureus* is the most common organism in both children and adults.[50,52] MR imaging provides superior soft tissue contrast, which allows for the detection of early osteomyelitis and depicts the extent of the disease, crucial in preoperative planning.[50,51,53]

Similar to other disorders, such as trauma and avascular necrosis, osteomyelitis results in marrow edema, which appears as hypointensity on T1-weighted images and hyperintensity on T2-weighted images. A useful reference is to compare the marrow intensity to the normal muscle. If the marrow signal is isointense or hypointense to muscle, then osteomyelitis is more likely especially if the clinical picture is suspicious for infection.[50,51,53] It can be helpful to give intravenous gadolinium contrast to identify soft tissue and intraosseous abscesses as well as subperiosteal fluid collections for surgical planning (**Fig. 12**).[50,53,54] An intraosseous abscess appears as focal intramedullary hypointensity on the T1-weighted images and hyperintensity on T2-weighted images and demonstrates peripheral rim enhancement.[50,51,53] In the setting of chronic osteomyelitis, MR imaging can be useful in detecting a sequestrum or sinus tract. A sequestrum is a

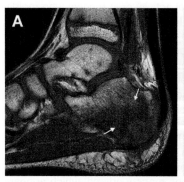
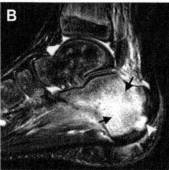
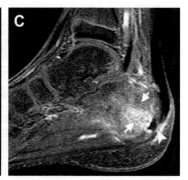

Fig. 11. Calcaneal osteomyelitis with Brodie abscess presenting with heel pain and fever in a 11-year-old boy. (*A*) Sagittal T1-weighted MR image reveals diffuse decrease signal intensity in the posterior calcaneus (*arrows*). (*B*) Sagittal T2 fat-saturated MR image shows extensive marrow edema (*arrows*) in the calcaneus and a focal area of fluid signal in the posterior apophysis (*arrowhead*). (*C*) Sagittal T1 fat-saturated postcontrast MR image shows enhancement of the bone marrow (*arrows*) and a small nonenhancing Brodie abscess in the calcaneal apophysis (*arrowhead*).

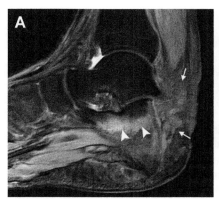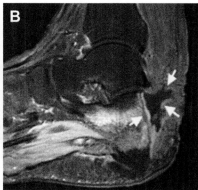

Fig. 12. Recurrent calcaneal osteomyelitis and soft tissue abscess in a 47-year-old woman with diabetes and prior resection of the posterior calcaneus. (*A*) Sagittal T2-weighted fat-saturated MR image shows abnormal marrow edema (*arrowheads*) in the calcaneal remnant and edema in the adjacent soft tissues (*arrows*). (*B*) On the sagittal T1-weighted fat-saturated postcontrast MR image, there is a region of nonenhancement (*arrows*) consistent with a soft tissue abscess.

fragment of necrotic bone usually exhibiting hypo-intensity on both T1-weighted and T2-weighted images without enhancement.[50,51,53]

Sever Disease

Sever disease, also known as calcaneal apophysitis, is one of the most common causes of heel pain in the pediatric population.[55] The average age at presentation is 11 years and the entity is more common in boys.[56] It is commonly seen in an active child engaged in sports activity and is bilateral in 61% of cases.[56] Calcaneal apophysitis is a repetitive overuse injury with abnormal stress applied to the growing apophysis (secondary ossification center) and is not a true inflammatory process.[57] Sever disease is often diagnosed clinically without imaging study. Imaging, however, can exclude other causes of heel pain. Radiographs classically demonstrate osseous irregularity, sclerosis and fragmentation of the calcaneal apophysis but can be difficult to distinguish from normal osseous changes in this age group.[58,59] On MR imaging, Sever disease appears hyopintense on T1-weighted and hyperintense on T2-weighted images at the calcaneal apophysis.[6,57]

Tumors

A full discussion of tumors that can occur in the calcaneus is beyond the scope of the article; however, lesions in the calcaneus can be an unusual cause of heel pain and mimic more common non-neoplastic disorders. In these cases, imaging is of high importance. Approximately 3% of osseous tumors are found in the foot and ankle, with the calcaneus the second most common site after the metatarsals.[60,61] Most tumors are benign and found

incidentally; however, many lesions can cause pain, swelling, or pathologic fracture.[60] The key to the correct diagnosis depends on the patient's clinical history and imaging studies. A list of the most common tumors in the calcaneus is provided in **Table 2**.[60,62] Simple bone cysts, intraosseous lipoma, and aneurysmal bone cyst are the most common benign tumors, and osteosarcoma and chondrosarcoma are the most common malignant tumors seen in calcaneus.[60,62] Moreover, because the calcaneus is an epiphyseal equivalent bone, lesions that occur in the epiphysis, such as chondroblastoma and giant cell tumor, can also occur.[60,61] Radiographs should be in the initial imaging study. An indeterminate lesion may need to undergo biopsy or additional imaging with CT or MR imaging. MR imaging can be particularly helpful in certain cases, such as distinguishing an intraosseous lipoma from a simple bone cyst. Intraosseous lipomas have fatty hyperintensity on T1-weighted images and often contain a central low T1 dystrophic calcification (**Fig. 13**), whereas simple bone

Table 2	
Common bone tumors of the calcaneus	
Type	**Common Tumors**
Benign	Simple bony cyst
	Intraosseous lipoma
	Aneurysmal bone cyst
	Chondroblastoma
	Giant cell tumor of bone
	Osteoid osteoma
Malignant	Osteosarcoma
	Chondrosarcoma
	Metastasis

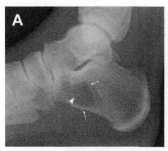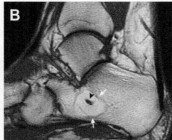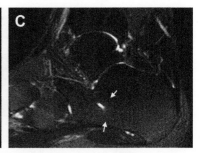

Fig. 13. Calcaneal intraosseous lipoma in a 29-year-old woman. (*A*) Lateral radiograph of the ankle shows a geographic lucent lesion (*arrows*) with central calcification (*arrowhead*) in the anterior calcaneus. On the (*B*) T1-weighted MR image the lesion (*arrows*) has high signal intensity with central low signal calcification (*arrowhead*). On the (*C*) T2-weighted fat-saturated MR image the lesion (*arrows*) has low signal intensity, indicating fat content.

cysts have hypointense T1 and hyperintense T2 fluid signal intensity.[60,61] Aneurysmal bone cysts can have characteristic fluid-fluid level and honeycomb-like cystic changes on T1-weighted and T2-weighted sequences representing the different stages of blood products in the lesion.[60,61]

BURSA
Retrocalcaneal and Retro-Achilles Bursitis

Two different bursae are located in the heel — the retrocalcaneal bursa and the retro-Achilles bursa. The retrocalcaneal bursa lies anterior to the distal insertion of the Achilles tendon onto the calcaneus and the retro-Achilles bursa lies posterior to the distal Achilles tendon, just anterior to the skin.[3,6,11] Both bursae can become irritated, leading to bursitis, and this can occur in conjunction with insertional Achilles tendinopathy.[6,16] Retrocalcaneal bursitis may also occur with inflammatory arthropathies, such as rheumatoid arthritis.[3] Normally, the dimensions of the retrocalcaneal bursa are transverse (0–11 mm), craniocaudal (0–7 mm), and anteroposterior (1–2 mm) and the bursa is easily seen on MR imaging.[11] If the bursa is enlarged, a bursitis should be considered. A weight-bearing lateral radiograph can help in the diagnosis of retrocalcaneal bursitis, with obliteration of the posteroinferior corner of Kager triangle.[63] On MR imaging, retrocalcaneal bursitis is seen as an enlarged fluid-filled structure that has low signal intensity on T1-weighted imaging and high signal intensity on fluid-sensitive sequences.[9,64] There can be associated marrow edema in the adjacent calcaneus or distal Achilles tendon indicating chronic mechanical irritation.[6] Retro-Achilles bursitis is typically seen in women wearing ill-fitting shoes that cause mechanical irritation of the posterior heel soft tissue sand can have associated redness and hyperkeratosis of the skin.[3,64] On MR imaging, there is fluid signal posterior (superficial) to the Achilles tendon at its calcaneal insertion.[3,6] After contrast administration, varying combinations of fluid and thicknened synovium can be seen in the bursae. When the retrocalcaneal bursa is associated with bone erosions, a diagnosis of inflammatory arthropathy should be considered.

Haglund Syndrome

Haglund syndrome (or Haglund disease) is the triad of retrocalcaneal bursitis, insertional Achilles tendinosis, and posterior soft tissue prominence from retro-Achilles bursitis.[6,16,65] It results in posterior ankle pain often the result of mechanical irritation from wearing low-back rigid shoes.[6,65] On physical examination, a pump-bump can be seen, which refers to soft tissue swelling of the posterior heel at the Achilles tendon insertion.[65] This syndrome can be associated with a Haglund deformity, which refers to an osseous prominence at the posterior superior aspect of calcaneus, which develops from irritation of the distal Achilles tendon and adjacent soft tissues.[65,66] The enlarged osseous bump is diagnosed by drawing 2 parallel pitch lines along superior and inferior aspect of calcaneus on a lateral radiograph.[6,65] The lower pitch line is tangent to the anterior calcaneal tubercle and the upper pitch line is parallel to the lower pitch line at the level of subarticular facet. A Haglund deformity is present if a bony spur extends above the superior pitch line (**Fig. 14**).[6,65] Lateral radiographs can show the typical osseous bump and obliteration of retrocalcaneal recess, which is situated between calcaneus and Achilles tendon.[63] On MR imaging, there can be edema in the osseous bump and MR imaging signs of bursitis in the retrocalcaneal and retro-Achilles soft tissues (see **Fig. 14**).[3,6,7]

NERVES OF THE HINDFOOT
Tarsal Tunnel Syndrome

Tarsal tunnel syndrome refers to a compression or entrapment neuropathy of the tibial nerve and its

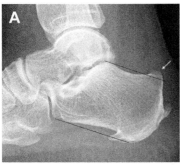
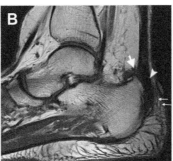
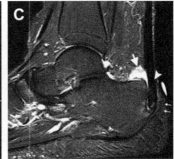

Fig. 14. Haglund syndrome with a Haglund deformity in a 47-year-old woman. (*A*) Lateral ankle radiograph show an osseous bump, or Haglund deformity (*arrow*), at the posterior superior aspect of the calcaneus. The presence of a Haglund deformity can be assessed by drawing 2 parallel pitch lines (*black lines*) along the superior and inferior aspect of calcaneus. The lower pitch line is tangent to the anterior calcaneal tubercle and the upper pitch line is parallel to the lower pitch line at the level of subarticular facet. A Haglund deformity is present if a bony spur extends above the superior pitch line. (*B*) Sagittal T1 and (*C*) T2 fat-saturated MR images show fluid in the retocalcaneal bursa (*arrow*), insertional Achilles tendon edema (*arrowhead*), and edema in the retro-Achilles soft tissues (*thin arrows*), consistent with the triad of Haglund syndrome.

branches within the tarsal tunnel.[67] The tibial nerve generally divides into the medial calcaneal nerve, medial plantar nerve, and lateral plantar nerve (LPN) at the level of tarsal tunnel.[13,68] Common causes of tarsal tunnel syndrome include fracture deformity, anomalous muscles, tenosynovitis of the flexor tendons, and ganglia or large vessels that compress the nerves in the tunnel.[3,67,69] Less common causes include solid masses, such as lipomas, giant cell tumors of the tendon sheath, and synovial sarcomas. Patients can experience numbness, dyskinesia, parethesia, and heel pain.[70] The Tinel sign is a frequently used physical examination test in which lightly tapping of the affected nerve elicits neurologic sensory deficits.[70] On MR imaging, the nerves can be enlarged and have high T2 or STIR hyperintensity, contour deformity, a deviated course, loss of normal fascicular pattern, and/or enlarged fascicles; however, the nerves are often not directly visualized.[71,72] Thus, a space-occupying lesion in the tarsal tunnel causing nerve compression should be carefully looked for, such as a ganglion or nerve sheath tumor (**Fig. 15**).[3,69] In addition, strandlike T1 and T2 hypointense scar tissue can be seen surrounding and deforming the nerves.[72] MR imaging can also show signs of denervation, such as muscle edema or fatty muscle atrophy in the

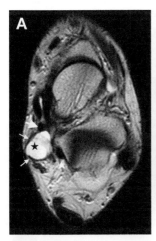
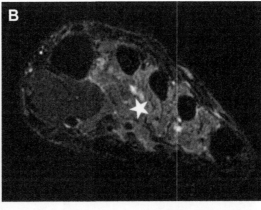

Fig. 15. Tarsal tunnel syndrome caused by a ganglion in a 35-year-old man with pain and tingling sensation in the foot. (*A*) Axial T2-weighted MR image shows a lobulated hyperintense ganglion (*star*) in the tarsal tunnel located posterior to the flexor digitorum longus tendon (*arrow*) and deep to the flexor retinaculum (*thin arrows*). (*B*) Coronal T2 fat-saturated MR image shows edema (*star*) in the intrinsic muscles of the forefoot likely due to compression of the LPN by the ganglion in the tarsal tunnel.

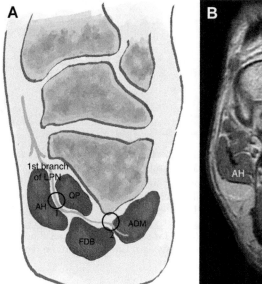
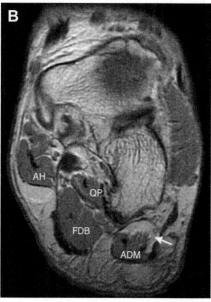

Fig. 16. (A) Illustration indicates the normal course of Baxter nerve, the first branch of the LPN. Circles indicate common sites of nerve entrapment: (1) between the abductor hallucis (AH) and medial aspect of quadratus plantae (QP) muscles and (2) between the medial calcaneal tuberosity and ADM and flexor digitorum brevis (FDB) muscles. (B) Coronal T1-weighted MR image in a 43-year-old man with heel pain show atrophy and fatty infiltration of ADM muscle (arrow).

distribution of the nerves, in chronic cases.[3,71,72] High-resolution magnetic resonance neurography has been shown to improve detection of nerve abnormalities in the tarsal tunnel in a small group of patients.[72]

Baxter Neuropathy

Entrapment of the first branch of the LPN (Baxter nerve) is known as Baxter neuropathy and is believed to account for 20% of cases of heel pain but is often not considered.[12,73] The LPN is a mixed sensory and motor nerve, which innervates the abductor digiti minimi (ADM) muscle (also known as the abductor digiti quinti muscle). The nerve exits the tarsal tunnel and travels along the plantar aspect of the foot.[74] There are 2 common sites of entrapment of the LPN: (1) between the abductor hallucis muscle and medial aspect of quadratus plantae muscles and (2) adjacent to the medial calcaneal tuberosity.[12,73,74]

There is an association of Baxter neuropathy with plantar spurs and plantar fasciitis.[73] Chronic heel pain is the most common complaint, because weakness of the ADM muscle is hard to detect clinically; however, MR imaging is helpful in

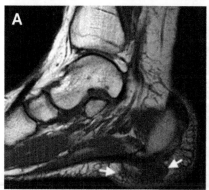
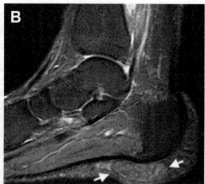

Fig. 17. Heel fat pad syndrome in a 45-year-old female long-distance runner. (A) Sagittal T1-weighted MR image shows low signal intensity in the inferior heel fat pad (arrows) and (B) slight increase signal intensity in the fat pad (arrows) on the sagittal T2 fat-saturated MR image.

providing evidence for the diagnosis. In the subacute setting, the affected ADM muscle is edematous, slightly enlarged, and may have high signal on T2-weighted or STIR MR images.[75] In the chronic setting, the ADM muscle is replaced by fatty tissue, reflecting fatty atrophy, which is best seen as interdigitation of high fatty T1-weighted signal throughout the muscle **(Fig. 16)**.[12,75,76]

HEEL PAD FAT

The heel fat pad is a subcalcaneal fibroadipose structure with shock-absorbing properties.[77] This fat pad can become injured or inflamed leading to atrophy and has been associated with running, obesity, rheumatoid arthritis, and steroid injections.[78–80] Pain is located at the central portion of the heel fat pad and is usually aggravated by hard-sole shoes and walking on hard surfaces.[70] Although the diagnosis can often be made clinically, the clinical symptoms and location of pain are often confused with plantar fasciitis; thus, imaging can be helpful. On MR imaging, the heel fat pad can appear as low signal intensity on T1-weighted images and heterogeneous high signal in T2-weighted images **(Fig. 17)**.[3] There can be also be low-signal-intensity bands representing fibrosis and decreased height of the fat pad, although this height can be variable depending on the size of the patient.[3,78]

SUMMARY

Heel pain is common and is due to a wide variety of osseous and soft tissues disorders. This article reviews the most common disorders that caused heel pain. These include disorders of the Achilles tendon, plantar fascia, calcaneus, bursae, nerves in the tarsal tunnel, and the heel pad. Although careful history taking and physical examination are often useful, MR imaging can be important in equivocal cases where the differential diagnosis is broad. MR imaging is the most helpful imaging modality in evaluating heel pain because it can highlight the relevant anatomy and reveal the extent of the disease.

ACKNOWLEDGMENTS

We thank Hsiang-Ling Hsu for assistance in creating the diagrams.

REFERENCES

1. Riddle DL, Schappert SM. Volume of ambulatory care visits and patterns of care for patients diagnosed with plantar fasciitis: a national study of medical doctors. Foot Ankle Int 2004;25(5):303–10.

2. Stecco C, Corradin M, Macchi V, et al. Plantar fascia anatomy and its relationship with Achilles tendon and paratenon. J Anat 2013;223(6):665–76.

3. Narvaez JA, Narvaez J, Ortega R, et al. Painful heel: MR imaging findings. Radiographics 2000;20(2):333–52.

4. Hunt KJ, Anderson RB. Heel pain in the athlete. Sports Health 2009;1(5):427–34.

5. McMillan AM, Landorf KB, Barrett JT, et al. Diagnostic imaging for chronic plantar heel pain: a systematic review and meta-analysis. J Foot Ankle Res 2009;2:32.

6. Lawrence DA, Rolen MF, Morshed KA, et al. MRI of heel pain. AJR Am J Roentgenol 2013;200(4):845–55.

7. Chimutengwende-Gordon M, O'Donnell P, Singh D. Magnetic resonance imaging in plantar heel pain. Foot Ankle Int 2010;31(10):865–70.

8. Mayer SW, Joyner PW, Almekinders LC, et al. Stress fractures of the foot and ankle in athletes. Sports Health 2014;6(6):481–91.

9. Pierre-Jerome C, Moncayo V, Terk MR. MRI of the Achilles tendon: a comprehensive review of the anatomy, biomechanics, and imaging of overuse tendinopathies. Acta Radiol 2010;51(4):438–54.

10. Snow SW, Bohne WH, DiCarlo E, et al. Anatomy of the Achilles tendon and plantar fascia in relation to the calcaneus in various age groups. Foot Ankle Int 1995;16(7):418–21.

11. Bottger BA, Schweitzer ME, El-Noueam KI, et al. MR imaging of the normal and abnormal retrocalcaneal bursae. AJR Am J Roentgenol 1998;170(5):1239–41.

12. Rodrigues RN, Lopes AA, Torres JM, et al. Compressive neuropathy of the first branch of the lateral plantar nerve: a study by magnetic resonance imaging. Radiol Bras 2015;48(6):368–72.

13. Kim BS, Choung PW, Kwon SW, et al. Branching patterns of medial and inferior calcaneal nerves around the tarsal tunnel. Ann Rehabil Med 2015;39(1):52–5.

14. Cheung YY, Doyley M, Miller TB, et al. Magnetic resonance elastography of the plantar fat pads: Preliminary study in diabetic patients and asymptomatic volunteers. J Comput Assist Tomogr 2006;30(2):321–6.

15. Johansson K, Lempainen L, Sarimo J, et al. Macroscopic anomalies and pathological findings in and around the achilles tendon: observations from 1661 operations during a 40-year period. Orthop J Sports Med 2014;2(12):2325967114562371.

16. van Dijk CN, van Sterkenburg MN, Wiegerinck JI, et al. Terminology for Achilles tendon related disorders. Knee Surg Sports Traumatol Arthrosc 2011;19(5):835–41.

17. Schweitzer ME, Karasick D. MR imaging of disorders of the Achilles tendon. AJR Am J Roentgenol 2000;175(3):613–25.

18. Chen TM, Rozen WM, Pan WR, et al. The arterial anatomy of the Achilles tendon: anatomical study

and clinical implications. Clin Anat 2009;22(3): 377–85.

19. Maffulli N, Khan KM, Puddu G. Overuse tendon conditions: time to change a confusing terminology. Arthroscopy 1998;14(8):840–3.

20. Erickson SJ, Prost RW, Timins ME. The "magic angle" effect: background physics and clinical relevance. Radiology 1993;188(1):23–5.

21. Sundararajan PP, Wilde TS. Radiographic, clinical, and magnetic resonance imaging analysis of insertional Achilles tendinopathy. J Foot Ankle Surg 2014;53(2):147–51.

22. Rosenzweig S, Azar FM. Open repair of acute Achilles tendon ruptures. Foot Ankle Clin 2009;14(4):699–709.

23. Agyekum EK, Ma K. Heel pain: a systematic review. Chin J Traumatol 2015;18(3):164–9.

24. Gwynne-Jones DP, Sims M, Handcock D. Epidemiology and outcomes of acute Achilles tendon rupture with operative or nonoperative treatment using an identical functional bracing protocol. Foot Ankle Int 2011;32(4):337–43.

25. Ahmad J, Repka M, Raikin SM. Treatment of myotendinous Achilles ruptures. Foot Ankle Int 2013;34(8): 1074–8.

26. Cutts S, Obi N, Pasapula C, et al. Plantar fasciitis. Ann R Coll Surg Engl 2012;94(8):539–42.

27. Berkowitz JF, Kier R, Rudicel S. Plantar fasciitis: MR imaging. Radiology 1991;179(3):665–7.

28. Ehrmann C, Maier M, Mengiardi B, et al. Calcaneal attachment of the plantar fascia: MR findings in asymptomatic volunteers. Radiology 2014;272(3): 807–14.

29. Buchbinder R. Clinical practice. plantar fasciitis. N Engl J Med 2004;350(21):2159–66.

30. Osborne HR, Breidahl WH, Allison GT. Critical differences in lateral X-rays with and without a diagnosis of plantar fasciitis. J Sci Med Sport 2006;9(3):231–7.

31. Jeswani T, Morlese J, McNally EG. Getting to the heel of the problem: plantar fascia lesions. Clin Radiol 2009;64(9):931–9.

32. Theodorou DJ, Theodorou SJ, Kakitsubata Y, et al. Plantar fasciitis and fascial rupture: MR imaging findings in 26 patients supplemented with anatomic data in cadavers. Radiographics 2000;20 Spec No: S181–97.

33. Moroney PJ, O'Neill BJ, Khan-Bhambro K, et al. The conundrum of calcaneal spurs: do they matter? Foot Ankle Spec 2014;7(2):95–101.

34. Zhou B, Zhou Y, Tao X, et al. Classification of calcaneal spurs and their relationship with plantar fasciitis. J Foot Ankle Surg 2015;54(4):594–600.

35. Leach R, Jones R, Silva T. Rupture of the plantar fascia in athletes. J Bone Joint Surg Am 1978;60(4): 537–9.

36. Sellman JR. Plantar fascia rupture associated with corticosteroid injection. Foot Ankle Int 1994;15(7): 376–81.

37. Saxena A, Fullem B. Plantar fascia ruptures in athletes. Am J Sports Med 2004;32(3):662–5.

38. Roger B, Grenier P. MRI of plantar fasciitis. Eur Radiol 1997;7(9):1430–5.

39. Morrison WB, Schweitzer ME, Wapner KL, et al. Plantar fibromatosis: a benign aggressive neoplasm with a characteristic appearance on MR images. Radiology 1994;193(3):841–5.

40. English C, Coughlan R, Carey J, et al. Plantar and palmar fibromatosis: characteristic imaging features and role of MRI in clinical management. Rheumatology (Oxford) 2012;51(6):1134–6.

41. Haedicke GJ, Sturim HS. Plantar fibromatosis: an isolated disease. Plast Reconstr Surg 1989;83(2): 296–300.

42. Veith NT, Tschernig T, Histing T, et al. Plantar fibromatosis–topical review. Foot Ankle Int 2013;34(12):1742–6.

43. Murphey MD, Ruble CM, Tyszko SM, et al. From the archives of the AFIP: musculoskeletal fibromatoses: radiologic-pathologic correlation. Radiographics 2009;29(7):2143–73.

44. Wilson ES Jr, Katz FN. Stress fractures. An analysis of 250 consecutive cases. Radiology 1969;92(3): 481–6. passim.

45. Greaney RB, Gerber FH, Laughlin RL, et al. Distribution and natural history of stress fractures in U.S. Marine recruits. Radiology 1983;146(2):339–46.

46. Anderson MW, Greenspan A. Stress fractures. Radiology 1996;199(1):1–12.

47. Lee JK, Yao L. Stress fractures: MR imaging. Radiology 1988;169(1):217–20.

48. Tins BJ, Garton M, Cassar-Pullicino VN, et al. Stress fracture of the pelvis and lower limbs including atypical femoral fractures-a review. Insights Imaging 2015;6(1):97–110.

49. Cronlein M, Rauscher I, Beer AJ, et al. Visualization of stress fractures of the foot using PET-MRI: a feasibility study. Eur J Med Res 2015;20(1):99.

50. Pugmire BS, Shailam R, Gee MS. Role of MRI in the diagnosis and treatment of osteomyelitis in pediatric patients. World J Radiol 2014;6(8):530–7.

51. Malhotra R, Chan CS, Nather A. Osteomyelitis in the diabetic foot. Diabet Foot Ankle 2014;5.

52. Tiemann AH, Hofmann GO, Steen M, et al. Adult calcaneal osteitis: incidence, etiology, diagnostics and therapy. GMS Interdiscip Plast Reconstr Surg DGPW 2012;1:Doc11.

53. Marcus CD, Ladam-Marcus VJ, Leone J, et al. MR imaging of osteomyelitis and neuropathic osteoarthropathy in the feet of diabetics. Radiographics 1996; 16(6):1337–48.

54. Craig JG, Amin MB, Wu K, et al. Osteomyelitis of the diabetic foot: MR imaging-pathologic correlation. Radiology 1997;203(3):849–55.

55. Kim CW, Shea K, Chambers HG. Heel pain in children. Diagnosis and treatment. J Am Podiatr Med Assoc 1999;89(2):67–74.

56. Micheli LJ, Ireland ML. Prevention and management of calcaneal apophysitis in children: an overuse syndrome. J Pediatr Orthop 1987;7(1):34–8.

57. Ogden JA, Ganey TM, Hill JD, et al. Sever's injury: a stress fracture of the immature calcaneal metaphysis. J Pediatr Orthop 2004;24(5):488–92.

58. Sitati FC, Kingori J. Chronic bilateral heel pain in a child with Sever disease: case report and review of literature. Cases J 2009;2:9365.

59. Ishikawa SN. Conditions of the calcaneus in skeletally immature patients. Foot Ankle Clin 2005;10(3): 503–13, vi.

60. Young PS, Bell SW, MacDuff EM, et al. Primary osseous tumors of the hindfoot: why the delay in diagnosis and should we be concerned? Clin Orthop Relat Res 2013;471(3):871–7.

61. Kilgore WB, Parrish WM. Calcaneal tumors and tumor-like conditions. Foot Ankle Clin 2005;10(3): 541–65, vii.

62. Weger C, Frings A, Friesenbichler J, et al. Osteolytic lesions of the calcaneus: results from a multicentre study. Int Orthop 2013;37(9):1851–6.

63. van Sterkenburg MN, Muller B, Maas M, et al. Appearance of the weight-bearing lateral radiograph in retrocalcaneal bursitis. Acta Orthop 2010; 81(3):387–90.

64. Canoso JJ, Liu N, Traill MR, et al. Physiology of the retrocalcaneal bursa. Ann Rheum Dis 1988;47(11): 910–2.

65. Pavlov H, Heneghan MA, Hersh A, et al. The Haglund syndrome: initial and differential diagnosis. Radiology 1982;144(1):83–8.

66. Bulstra GH, van Rheenen TA, Scholtes VA. Can we measure the heel bump? radiographic evaluation of haglund's deformity. J Foot Ankle Surg 2015; 54(3):338–40.

67. Bailie DS, Kelikian AS. Tarsal tunnel syndrome: diagnosis, surgical technique, and functional outcome. Foot Ankle Int 1998;19(2):65–72.

68. Torres AL, Ferreira MC. Study of the anatomy of the tibial nerve and its branches in the distal medial leg. Acta Ortop Bras 2012;20(3):157–64.

69. Antoniadis G, Scheglmann K. Posterior tarsal tunnel syndrome: diagnosis and treatment. Dtsch Arztebl Int 2008;105(45):776–81.

70. Alshami AM, Souvlis T, Coppieters MW. A review of plantar heel pain of neural origin: differential diagnosis and management. Man Ther 2008;13(2): 103–11.

71. Lopez-Ben R. Imaging of nerve entrapment in the foot and ankle. Foot Ankle Clin 2011;16(2):213–24.

72. Chhabra A, Subhawong TK, Williams EH, et al. High-resolution MR neurography: evaluation before repeat tarsal tunnel surgery. AJR Am J Roentgenol 2011;197(1):175–83.

73. Chundru U, Liebeskind A, Seidelmann F, et al. Plantar fasciitis and calcaneal spur formation are associated with abductor digiti minimi atrophy on MRI of the foot. Skeletal Radiol 2008;37(6):505–10.

74. Recht MP, Grooff P, Ilaslan H, et al. Selective atrophy of the abductor digiti quinti: an MRI study. AJR Am J Roentgenol 2007;189(3):W123–7.

75. Fleckenstein JL, Watumull D, Conner KE, et al. Denervated human skeletal muscle: MR imaging evaluation. Radiology 1993;187(1):213–8.

76. May DA, Disler DG, Jones EA, et al. Abnormal signal intensity in skeletal muscle at MR imaging: patterns, pearls, and pitfalls. Radiographics 2000;20 Spec No:S295–315.

77. Falsetti P, Frediani B, Acciai C, et al. Ultrasonography and magnetic resonance imaging of heel fat pad inflammatory-oedematous lesions in rheumatoid arthritis. Scand J Rheumatol 2006;35(6): 454–8.

78. Rome K, Campbell R, Flint A, et al. Heel pad thickness–a contributing factor associated with plantar heel pain in young adults. Foot Ankle Int 2002; 23(2):142–7.

79. Falsetti P, Frediani B, Acciai C, et al. Heel fat pad involvement in rheumatoid arthritis and in spondyloarthropathies: an ultrasonographic study. Scand J Rheumatol 2004;33(5):327–31.

80. Tu P, Bytomski JR. Diagnosis of heel pain. Am Fam Physician 2011;84(8):909–16.

MR Imaging of the Midfoot Including Chopart and Lisfranc Joint Complexes

Monica Tafur, MD[a], Zehava Sadka Rosenberg, MD[b],*,
Jenny T. Bencardino, MD[b]

KEYWORDS

- MR imaging • Midfoot • Chopart joint complex • Lisfranc joint complex

KEY POINTS

- The navicular, cuboid, and 3 cuneiform bones form the midfoot, the anatomic region located between the Chopart and Lisfranc joints.
- Midfoot pathology, involving the osseous and soft tissue structures at the midfoot and at the junction of the midfoot with the hindfoot (Chopart joint complex) and forefoot (Lisfranc joint complex), is a common, albeit elusive cause for pain.
- Navicular, cuboid and cuneiform fractures represent radiographically occult causes of foot pain that often require evaluation with MR imaging.
- MR imaging is the modality of choice for detection of several tendon and ligamentous pathology about the midfoot.

INTRODUCTION

The midfoot, composed of the navicular, cuboid, the 3 cuneiform bones and their interconnecting articulations and ligaments, is located between the Chopart (talonavicular and calcaneocuboid articulations) and the Lisfranc (tarsometatarsal) joints.[1] Forces generated during normal gait are transmitted from the hindfoot to the forefoot through the midfoot.[2] The midfoot remains mobile during the first phase of heel strike and first 15% of the gait cycle and converts to a rigid lever during the toe-rise or push-off phase. Injuries to the midfoot are less common than those of the hindfoot and forefoot and can be easily missed because of lack of obvious radiographic findings in up to 33% of such injuries.[3,4]

Following a brief description of the normal anatomy and biomechanics of the midfoot, this article focuses on imaging features, with emphasis on MR imaging of common osseous, tendon, and ligament abnormalities that affect the midfoot. Discussion of Chopart joint complex and Lisfranc joint complex, both of which play important roles in linking the midfoot to the hindfoot and the forefoot respectively, also is included. Charcot arthropathy, even though it commonly occurs in the midfoot, is beyond the scope of this article, and will not be discussed.

NORMAL ANATOMY OF THE MIDFOOT

The midfoot is located between the Chopart and Lisfranc joints and includes the navicular, cuboid,

The authors have nothing to disclose.
[a] Joint Department of Medical Imaging, University of Toronto, 399 Bathurst Street, 3rd Fl Room 3MC-410, Toronto, Ontario M5T 2S8, Canada; [b] Department of Radiology, NYU School of Medicine, NYU Hospital for Joint Diseases, 301 East 17th Street, New York, NY 10003, USA
* Corresponding author.
E-mail address: zehava.rosenberg@nyumc.org

Magn Reson Imaging Clin N Am 25 (2017) 95–125
http://dx.doi.org/10.1016/j.mric.2016.08.006
1064-9689/17/© 2016 Elsevier Inc. All rights reserved.

mri.theclinics.com

and the 3 cuneiform bones (**Fig. 1**). The Chopart joint, also known as the Chopart joint complex, or midtarsal or transverse tarsal joint, consists of the calcaneocuboid and talocalcaneonavicular joints (**Fig. 2**). These 2 joints lie in a plane perpendicular to the longitudinal arch of the foot, and act as a single unit with respect to the hindfoot.[3] The Lisfranc joint complex, also called the tarsometatarsal joint, represents the junction of the midfoot and the forefoot. It consists of several articulations between the 3 cuneiforms, the metatarsals, and the cuboid bone (**Fig. 3**).[1]

Many tendons traverse or insert at the midfoot, and, thus, are susceptible to injury in this region. The most important tendons include the posterior tibial, the anterior tibial, the peroneus longus, and the flexor hallucis longus tendons. The dorsalis pedis artery traverses the midfoot, on its way distally, between the first and second metatarsal bases, to the plantar surface of the foot to form the plantar arch. The artery may be injured or thrombosed in a midfoot/forefoot fracture-dislocation, resulting in hematoma or compartment syndrome. The deep peroneal nerve follows the dorsalis pedis artery, providing innervation to the extensor digitorum brevis muscle and to the first dorsal web space. Thus, the nerve is also susceptible to entrapment at the dorsal aspect of the midfoot. The medial and plantar nerves contribute to innervation of the plantar region and forefoot.[1]

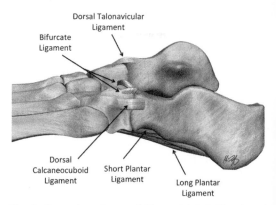

Fig. 2. Normal anatomy of Chopart joint. The dorsal talonavicular, bifurcate, and dorsal calcaneocuboid ligaments are important passive stabilizers of Chopart joint. The short and long plantar ligament help to stabilize the midfoot to the hindfoot.

Biomechanical Properties

Normal biomechanics of the foot are best understood with the use of the column theories. The Chopart joint consists of flexible medial (talus and navicular bones) and lateral (calcaneus and cuboid bones) columns. The more distal medial column, including the cuneiforms and the first, second, and third metatarsals, is limited in motion, providing stability to the transverse and longitudinal arches. The more distal lateral column, consisting of the cuboid fourth and fifth metatarsal joints, is highly mobile accommodating walking on varied surfaces.[3]

The midfoot locks the hindfoot to the forefoot, during the normal gait cycle. Talonavicular motion

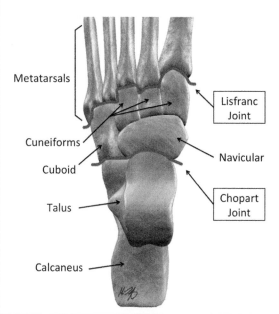

Fig. 1. Normal anatomy of the midfoot. The midfoot contains osseous, ligamentous, and tendinous structures located between the Chopart and the Lisfranc joints.

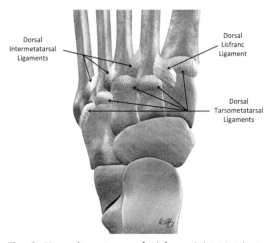

Fig. 3. Normal anatomy of Lisfranc joint. Intricate ligamentous insertions help to stabilize the Lisfranc joint, including the Lisfranc ligament complex, and intermetatarsal and tarsometatarsal ligaments. Only the dorsal ligaments are noted in this drawing.

is related to subtalar and calcaneocuboid motion, allowing the foot to invert and evert during gait. The head of the talus rotates in its articulation with the navicular surface during motion, thus, the talonavicular joint is essential for normal foot biomechanics.[2] The naviculocuneiform joints have limited motion and provide stability for the transverse tarsal arch and the longitudinal medial column. Articulations between the cuboid and the fourth and fifth metatarsal bases are mobile and help the foot to accommodate to different surfaces.[2]

MR IMAGING OF THE MIDFOOT
MR Imaging Protocol

An MR imaging protocol, dedicated to the midfoot, is essential for high-quality, diagnostic images, although portions of the midfoot may be glanced at during ankle and forefoot MR imaging.[5] Midfoot imaging in the prone position has been advocated but is uncomfortable and is usually unnecessary for adequate midfoot imaging.[6] Supine imaging, in 3 planes, and a field of view of 12 cm or smaller are routinely used. Placement of localizing markers at the symptomatic site should be encouraged.[7] To avoid confusion of terms, short-axis and long-axis planes are often used, instead of oblique coronal and axial planes, when imaging the midfoot and forefoot. Sagittal MR images are obtained from a short-axis (oblique coronal)

localizer at the level of mid-metatarsals, with images acquired perpendicular to a best-fit transmetatarsal line (**Fig. 4A**). Long-axis (oblique axial) MR images are obtained from a short-axis (oblique coronal) localizer at the level of mid-metatarsals with images acquired parallel to a best-fit transmetatarsal line (**Fig. 4B**). Short-axis (oblique coronal) MR images are obtained from a sagittal localizer, at the level of the second or third metatarsal, with images acquired perpendicular to a line parallel to the second or third metatarsal (**Fig. 4C**).[5,6]

Typically performed sequences include T1-weighted non–fat-suppressed (NFS), fat-suppressed (FS) T2 or proton density (PD) and short tau inversion recovery (STIR). T1-weighted NFS sequences are useful to assess radiographically occult fractures or bone marrow abnormalities. Fat-suppressed (FS) T2-weighted and STIR sequences facilitate visualization of pathologic processes such as joint effusion and bone marrow and soft tissue edema. STIR sequences are of particular importance in the midfoot and forefoot because they provide more uniform fat suppression and are less susceptible to metallic-related artifacts, as compared with PD or FS T2-weighted sequences.

Magic angle effect typically occurs when highly organized structures (ie, tendons and ligaments) are oriented at an angle of 55° with respect to the main magnetic vector (B_0) in MR sequences with short echo times (TEs) of 10 to 20 ms. This

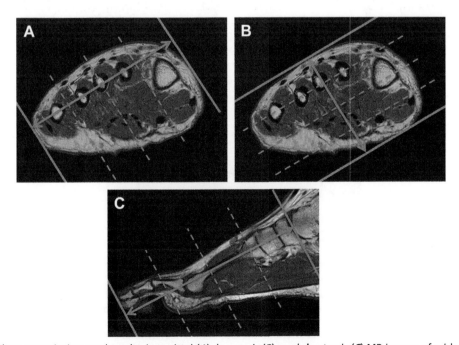

Fig. 4. Plane prescription used to obtain sagittal (A), long-axis (B), and short-axis (C) MR images of mid and forefoot. Plane prescription should be modified if the clinical indication involves the first ray.

results in increased T2 signal mimicking pathology. In the midfoot, magic angle affects the extensor tendons, in particular the extensor hallucis longus tendon, as they curve along the dorsum of the foot, as well as the posterior tibial tendon (PTT) at its navicular insertion. The peroneus longus tendon may also be susceptible to magic angle effect, as it curves around the cuboid toward its distal plantar insertion. Sequences with TEs greater than 35 ms, such as STIR or T2-weighted sequences, eliminate the effect and should be evaluated along with shorter TE sequences to avoid misinterpretation.[7,8]

Chopart Joint and Its Supporting Ligamentous Structures

Osseous structures
The Chopart joint, also called the Chopart joint complex, is formed by the calcaneocuboid and talocalcaneonavicular joints. It is a flexible joint, which, with the aid of the subtalar joints, functions to evert and invert the foot. It also provides pivoting motion of the hindfoot, while the forefoot remains stationary. When the Chopart joint is locked (the calcaneocuboid joint and talonavicular joints are not parallel to each other), it stabilizes the midfoot during push-off phase of the gait cycle.

The calcaneocuboid joint is formed by the quadrilateral facets of the calcaneus and cuboid bones. It is a saddle-shaped joint that allows both incongruous and congruous fit between the 2 bones during eversion and inversion of the foot. There are 4 ligaments connecting the calcaneus and cuboid: the medial calcaneocuboid ligament, which is a component of the bifurcate ligament; the dorsal calcaneocuboid ligament; the plantar calcaneocuboid ligament, or short plantar ligament; and the long plantar ligament (see **Fig. 2**; **Fig. 5**).[9]

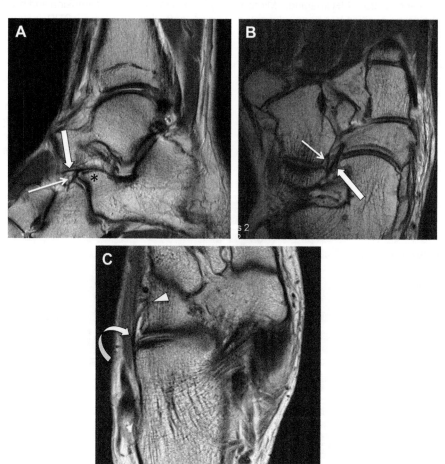

Fig. 5. Normal anatomy of the Chopart joint. (*A, B*) Sagittal T1-weighted (*A*) and long-axis PD (*B*) MR images show the lateral calcaneonavicular component of the bifurcate ligament (*thick arrow*) extending from the anterior process of the calcaneus (*asterisk*) toward the navicular bone. The medial calcaneocuboid component of the bifurcate ligament (*thin arrow*) originates lateral to the lateral calcaneonavicular component and inserts onto the cuboid. (*C*) Long-axis PD MR image demonstrates the dorsal calcaneocuboid ligament (*curved arrow*). Note that the ligament inserts onto the cuboid at least 5 mm distal to the articulation (*arrowhead*).

The talocalcaneonavicular joint comprises the rounded head of the talus, the concave posterior surface of the navicular bone, and the anterior articular surface of the calcaneus. It is a condyloid joint stabilized in part by the acetabulum pedis, the deep socket of the navicular bone that contains the head of the talus.[2,3] The dorsal talonavicular ligament and the lateral calcaneonavicular ligament (portion of the bifurcate ligament) reinforce the articular capsule superolaterally (see **Fig. 2**). The plantar calcaneonavicular ligament, also called the spring ligament complex, reinforces the capsule inferomedially.[10]

Ligamentous structures
The Chopart joint complex is stabilized by multiple ligaments, the strongest of which includes the spring ligament, the Y-shaped bifurcate ligament, and the short and long plantar ligaments. Smaller ligaments include the previously mentioned dorsal calcaneocuboid and dorsal talonavicular ligaments.

The Bifurcate Ligament

The bifurcate ligament, or Chopart ligament, is a major stabilizer of the Chopart joint and is formed by 2 ligaments: the medial calcaneonavicular ligament and lateral calcaneocuboid ligament. These ligaments extend from the anterior calcaneal process to the lateral side of the navicular and the dorsal surface of the cuboid, respectively (see **Fig. 2**).[10,11] The 2 components of the bifurcate ligament can typically be visualized on sagittal MR images of the ankle or midfoot as thin low to intermediate signal structures, highlighted by fat, but can be more difficult to discern on short-axis and long-axis images of the midfoot (see **Fig. 5**).

Spring Ligament Complex

The spring ligament, also called the plantar calcaneonavicular ligament, has 2 important functions: to support the head of the talus within the acetabulum pedis, providing stability to the talocalcaneonavicular joint and midfoot, and to act as a static agonist of the PTT and static stabilizer of the medial longitudinal arch.[10,12,13]

The spring ligament complex has 3 distinct components: the superomedial (SM), the medioplantar oblique (MPO), and the inferoplantar longitudinal (IPL) (**Fig. 6**).

The SM component represents the medial part of the spring ligament complex, is triangular and hammock-shaped, with its deep surface covered with fibrocartilage to form an articular surface for the head of the talus. The ligament extends from the sustentaculum tali of the calcaneus to the

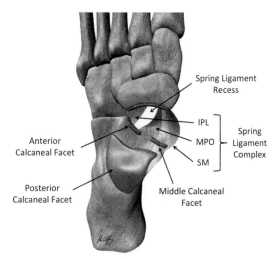

Fig. 6. Illustration of the normal anatomy of the spring ligament complex. From medial to lateral, the 3 components of the spring ligament complex are: the SM, the MPO, and the IPL. The spring ligament recess and the anterior, middle, and posterior calcaneal facets are also depicted.

superomedial aspect of the navicular tuberosity and to the tibiospring component of the deltoid ligament complex. The SM component is the widest and strongest of the 3 ligaments and contains both collagen and fibrocartilage.[13–15]

The SM component of the spring ligament complex is consistently seen on ankle and midfoot MR imaging images. In an MR imaging study of cadaveric feet by Mengiardi and colleagues[15] the SM component of the spring ligament complex was visible in all of the subjects, whereas the MPO and IPL components were visible in 77% and 91% of the cases, respectively. The SM component of the spring ligament complex is best seen on coronal or axial ankle MR images and on short-axis and long-axis midfoot MR images and appears as an intermediate signal intensity structure on T1-weighted sequences in 99% of cases, and as a low signal intensity structure on T2-weighted MR images in 96% of cases (**Fig. 7**A). The mean thickness of the SM component is 3.2 mm (mean range of 2.5–4.7 mm). Studies have found a moderate interobserver agreement for mean thickness measurements of the SM component due to difficulty in differentiating the PTT, the gliding layer, and the SM component on MR images.[15,16]

The most variable MPO component of the spring ligament complex originates from the coronoid fossa, a notch between the anterior and middle facets of the calcaneus, and terminates at the tuberosity of the navicular.[13,14] On MR imaging, the MPO component of the spring ligament complex

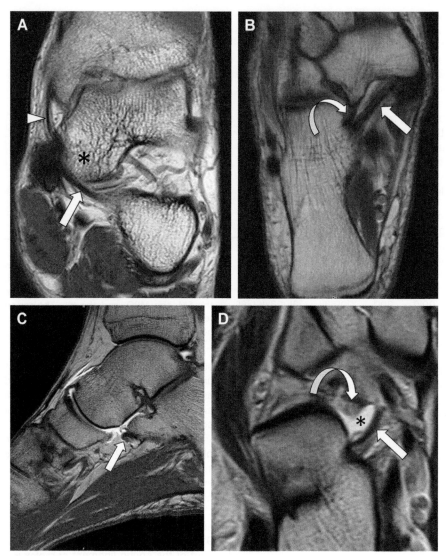

Fig. 7. Normal MR appearance of the spring ligament complex. Coronal PD (*A*), axial PD (*B*), and sagittal (*C*) T2-weighted ankle MR images. (*A*) The superomedial (SM) component is seen as an oblique band (*arrow*) medial to the talar head (*asterisk*). The attachment of the SM component to the tibiospring component (*arrowhead*) of the deltoid ligament complex is appreciated. (*B*) The MPO component (*arrow*) has a striated pattern and extends between the coronoid fossa of the calcaneus and the navicular. The IPL component (*curved arrow*) also is seen, inserting into the beak of the navicular. (*C*) The MPO component (*arrow*) is partially shown on the sagittal image. (*D*) The spring ligament recess is seen as a teardrop-shaped, fluid-filled structure (*asterisk*) interposed between the partially visualized IPL (*curved arrow*) and MPO (*arrow*) components of the spring ligament complex on the long-axis T2-weighted MR image.

is best seen on axial ankle or long-axis midfoot planes and has a striated appearance on both T1-weighted and T2-weighted MR images (**Fig.** 7B, C). The mean thickness of the MPO component is 2.8 mm (mean range of 1–5 mm). It also can be identified on coronal ankle and short-axis midfoot MR images. Due to its oblique course, the MPO is typically not seen on a single sagittal image.[15]

The IPL component of the spring ligament complex is a short, cordlike bundle and constitutes the lateral plantar part of the spring ligament. The IPL ligament originates anterior to the middle calcaneal facet and attaches at the inferior beak of the navicular bone.[13,14] The IPL component is best seen on axial and coronal ankle MR images and on long-axis or short-axis midfoot images, and has intermediate signal intensity on T1-weighted and variable signal intensity on T2-weighted MR images (**Fig. 7**B, D). The mean thickness of the IPL component is 4 mm (mean range of 2–6 mm).[15]

The spring ligament recess of the talonavicular joint is a synovium-lined, teardrop-shaped recess that communicates with the talocalcaneonavicular joint and is located between the plantar MPO and IPL components of the spring ligament complex (see **Fig. 7**D). A fluid distended spring ligament recess does not equate to spring ligament injury and should not be confused with a tear of the plantar components of the spring ligament complex. A fluid distended spring ligament recess is commonly associated with talar head impaction injuries, ankle sprains, and talonavicular osteoarthrosis (**Fig. 8**).[13]

Long and Short Plantar Ligaments

The plantar calcaneocuboid ligament is subdivided into the short and long plantar ligaments. The short plantar ligament, also called the short plantar calcaneocuboid ligament, is more medial than the long plantar ligament. It originates from the anterior tubercle of the calcaneus and inserts on the entire posterior plantar surface and beak of the cuboid. The long plantar ligament originates from the more proximal aspect of the anterior

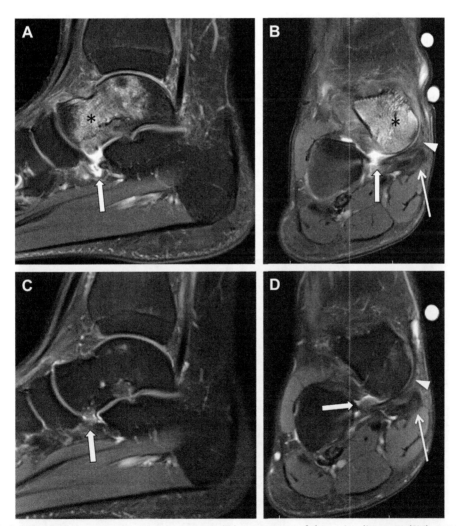

Fig. 8. Spring ligament recess and sprained superomedial component of the spring ligament (SM) post inversion injury, with follow-up. Baseline sagittal (*A*) and coronal (*B*) FS T2-weighted ankle MR images show distention of the spring ligament recess (*thick arrow*) and talar head contusion (*asterisks*). The SM is thickened and ill defined, compatible with a sprain (*arrowhead*). On follow-up sagittal (*C*) and coronal (*D*) FS T2-weighted ankle MR images, fluid in the spring ligament recess (*thick arrows*), signal alterations of the SM, and talar bone contusions have resolved. Increased PTT signal is consistent with a type I partial tear (*thin arrows*).

calcaneal tubercle and from the intertubercular segment of the posterior calcaneal tuberosity. The deeper fibers of the long plantar ligament represent the bulk of the ligament and insert on the cuboid crest. Its superficial fibers form a thinner layer, which form the roof of the cuboid tunnel of the peroneus longus tendon, and insert on the second to fifth metatarsal bases.[10,17]

The plantar calcaneocuboid ligaments are easily seen on sagittal and long-axis MR images of the midfoot as highly striated, thick bands of intermediate to low signal along the plantar aspect of the foot (**Fig. 9**).

Chopart Joint Injuries

Injuries involving the Chopart joint, also called midtarsal injuries, range from pure ligamentous injuries to small avulsion fractures, to the rare fracture: dislocation. They can be missed in up to 41% of cases. Chopart fracture-dislocations are frequently caused by high-energy trauma, such as motor vehicle accidents or fall from height (11%) and may require surgical intervention. Conversely, midfoot avulsion fractures are most often due to low-energy trauma, such as inversion injury or sports injury (89%) and usually improve with conservative measures. They may be isolated, or may be associated with lateral collateral ligament sprains, in up to 24% and 33% of ankle inversion injuries, respectively. The clinical manifestations of these injuries, particularly the low-energy ones, may mimic and thus be mistaken for the more common lateral ankle ligament injury. A proper diagnosis of the more advanced injuries involving the Chopart joint is crucial to avoid permanent disability and functional limitations of weight-bearing.[18]

Based on location, osseous traumatic lesions of the Chopart joint can be divided into those affecting the medial column, including talar head and navicular injuries, and those involving the lateral column, including cuboid and anterior calcaneal process fractures. Disruption of the Cyma line, a congruent lazy S-shaped line, along Chopart joint, as seen on anteroposterior (AP) and lateral radiographs of the foot, should alert the radiologist to the presence of this injury. Tiny avulsion fragments lateral to the anterior process of the calcaneus or proximal cuboid, on AP radiograph of the foot, indicate a tear of the dorsal calcaneocuboid ligament; this may occur in isolation but may reflect a clue to a more extensive Chopart joint injury. Similarly, navicular fractures or avulsions of the dorsal talar head or navicular, at the dorsal talonavicular ligament, often related to a plantarflexion injury, and of the bifurcate ligament, at the anterior process of the calcaneus, may reflect isolated injuries, but should alert the radiologist to the possibility of a more serious disruption of Chopart joint. Computed tomography (CT) may further demonstrate occult fractures, not clearly

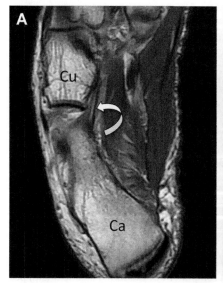 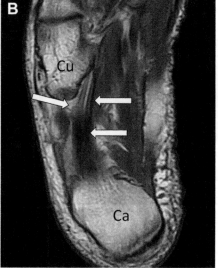

Fig. 9. Normal anatomy of the long and short plantar ligaments. (A, B) Axial PD MR images demonstrate the short plantar ligament (*curved arrow*), which originates from the anterior tubercle of the calcaneus and inserts onto the posterior plantar surface and beak of the cuboid. The long plantar ligament (*straight arrows*) is lateral and plantar to the short plantar ligament. The long plantar ligament originates from the anterior tubercle and from the posterior calcaneal tuberosity and inserts onto the cuboid crest. Ca, calcaneus; Cu, cuboid.

visualized on the radiographs. Marrow contusions and ligamentous disruptions at Chopart joint can be optimally visualized on MR imaging (**Figs. 10 and 11**). Talar head fractures, causing significant shortening of the medial column, or talar head contusion may also be associated with talonavicular dislocations.

Isolated disruption of the plantar calcaneocuboid ligaments is uncommon and may be present in isolated stress fractures of the cuboid bone. Edema within these ligaments on MR imaging should raise a red flag, however, to the possibility of a Chopart joint injury.[19] Increased signal within the plantar calcaneocuboid ligaments may also reflect enthesopathy, particularly in the setting of seronegative disorders.

Spring Ligament Complex Injuries

Pathology of the spring ligament may be degenerative, in the setting of PTT dysfunction, or may be traumatic, secondary to either eversion injury or to the less common fracture-dislocation injury of the Chopart joint.

Both the PTT and spring ligament complex act to support the medial longitudinal arch of the foot. Furthermore, the functional role of the spring ligament complex becomes more crucial when the PTT, the primary dynamic stabilizer of the longitudinal arch, fails, adding stress on the ligament. Thus, spring ligament abnormality is a very frequent finding, in association with advanced primary PTT injury, typically causing tearing of the SM component and thickening of the plantar components of the spring ligament complex. Disruption of the spring ligament results in similar pathology to that of PTT dysfunction, with loss of the medial longitudinal arch, talar vertical tilt, hindfoot valgus, and acquired flatfoot deformity.[16,20]

PTT insufficiency has long been implicated as the initial cause of adult acquired flat foot. Recently, however, there has been a debate in the literature as to whether PTT insufficiency primarily develops and then leads to increased strain on the spring ligament complex, or whether an attenuated spring ligament complex contributes to increased strain on the PTT and eventually to its insufficiency.[21,22] Sectioning of the spring ligament complex in cadaveric models creates instability in the foot, with malalignment among the talus, navicular, and calcaneus, for which the PTT is unable to compensate.[21]

In recent years, surgical repair of the spring ligament complex has become an important adjunct to treating PTT abnormalities, allowing for more anatomic repair of the stabilizing medial structures and obviating postsurgical stiffness.[23] The treatment of acquired flat foot associated with PTT dysfunction will vary depending on the flexibility and severity of flat foot deformity. In early stages before any rigid deformity or tendon rupture has occurred, the treatment consists of debridement

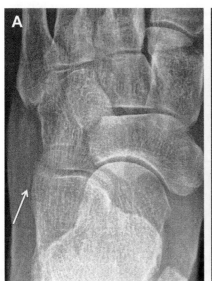
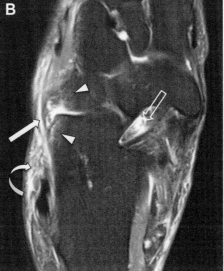

Fig. 10. Partial Chopart injury with lateral column disruption in a 62-year-old woman post inversion injury. (*A*) AP radiograph shows a small avulsion fragment (*arrow*) adjacent to the calcaneus. (*B*) Long-axis FS T2-weighted MR image demonstrates a torn dorsal calcaneocuboid ligament (*arrow*) with fraying and signal heterogeneity of its fibers and opposing bone marrow edema (*arrowheads*). Note the periligamentous soft tissue edema (*curved arrow*), fluid in the spring ligament recess (*open arrow*), and small calcaneocuboid joint effusion.

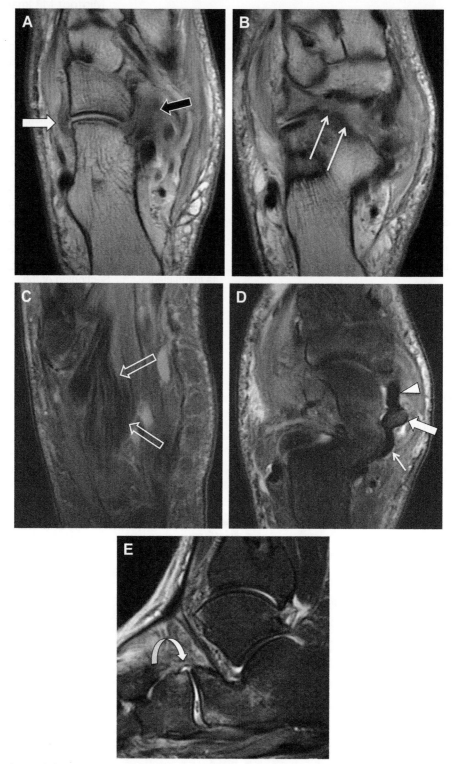

Fig. 11. Advanced Chopart injury in a diabetic patient with tearing/sprains of the dorsal calcaneocuboid, bifurcate ligament, spring ligament, and short and long plantar ligaments. (*A*) Axial PD image demonstrates sprained dorsal calcaneocuboid (*white arrow*) and short plantar ligaments (*black arrow*). (*B*) Axial PD image demonstrates absence of the MPO and IPL components of the spring ligament (*thin arrows*) consistent with complete tears. (*C*) Axial FS PD image demonstrates a thickened, heterogeneous, sprained long plantar ligament (*open arrows*). (*D*) Axial FS PD image demonstrates a torn and retracted SM component of the spring ligament (*thick arrow*), located between the posterior tibial (*arrowhead*) and flexor digitorum longus (*short thin arrow*) tendons. (*E*) Sagittal FS T2-weighted image shows widened calcaneocuboid joint, contusions and heterogeneous, sprained calcaneocuboid component of the bifurcate ligament (*curved arrow*). (*Courtesy of* A. Ross Sussmann, MD, East Brunswick, New Jersey.)

and synovectomy of the PTT. In 74% of patients complete pain relief is achieved and PTT function will return in 84% of cases after the procedure.[24] Ruptured tendons can be repaired but there are no good results to prove that tendon repair improves either the pain or the flat foot deformity.[25] Most surgical cases of chronic PTT rupture, with flatfoot deformity, are treated with a calcaneal osteotomy (lengthening of the lateral column) and reconstruction of the medial soft tissue, including tendon transfer and spring ligament repair. The results of the procedure are good to excellent in 79% of patients (walking on uneven surfaces).[18]

Acquired flat foot due to isolated, traumatic spring ligament complex insufficiency, with a normal PTT, also can occur, typically in young adults, as a result of ankle eversion trauma or Chopart joint injury. In this condition, there is forefoot abduction and hind foot valgus, with spared ability to single-leg tiptoe (heel rise).[26,27] Subsequent development of flat foot deformity can be quick, therefore early diagnosis is crucial to avoid irreversible complications of the injury. On MR imaging, this condition presents with tearing of the plantar components (MPO and IPL) of the spring ligament complex, with an intact PTT.[26]

Toye and colleagues[28] found a full-thickness gap in the spring ligament complex on MR imaging in 79% of 14 cases with surgically proven spring ligament complex tears (see **Fig. 11**). Other MR findings that can be found in spring ligament complex tears include disruption, increased caliber (>4 or 5 mm), attenuation, abnormal signal intensity, and waviness of the ligament as well as PTT dysfunction (**Fig. 12**).

The Lisfranc Joint Complex

The Lisfranc joint complex has 3 separate synovial compartments. The first tarsometatarsal joint forms the medial compartment. The central and largest compartment includes the second and third tarsometatarsal joints, and the intercuneiform and naviculocuneiform joints. The lateral compartment is formed by the articulations of the cuboid with the fourth and fifth metatarsals. The 3 compartments correlate with the columnar description of the foot: the medial column is formed by the first ray and medial cuneiform, the middle column includes the second and third metatarsals and cuneiforms, and the lateral column includes the fourth and fifth rays and the cuboid.[17,29]

The stability of the Lisfranc joint complex is derived from osseous relationships and ligamentous support. The position of the second metatarsal base is an essential component of osseous stability. In the short axis, the osseous components form an arch with the second metatarsal at the dorsal-most position. In the long axis, the second metatarsal base is recessed between the medial and lateral cuneiforms, forming a mortise. The Lisfranc joint complex is further supported by the morphology of the cuneiforms and bases of the metatarsals (wide dorsal bases and tapered plantar apices), forming a roman-arch–like configuration, and by the protruding third

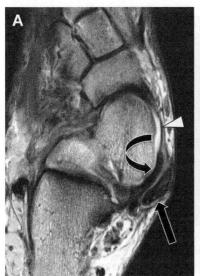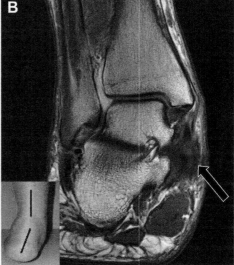

Fig. 12. Degenerative tearing of the spring ligament in a middle-aged woman with PTT dysfunction. Axial (A) and coronal (B) PD ankle MR images show a type I tear of the PTT (*black arrows*). The SM component of the spring ligament is proximally retracted (*curved arrow*), with minimal residual fibers versus capsule (*arrowhead*) extending to the navicular. Flat foot deformity and hindfoot valgus (B) are present.

cuneiform, wedged between the second and third metatarsal bases.[30]

The osseous structures and capsules are reinforced by highly variable ligamentous structures, which can be subdivided into 3 groups, the dorsal, interosseous, and plantar (see **Fig. 3**). Each division contains longitudinally oriented oblique and transverse ligaments and can be further subdivided into tarsometatarsal, intertarsal, and intermetatarsal ligaments. In general, the dorsal ligaments tend to be thin and weaker than their interosseous and plantar counterparts. Similarly, the medial ligaments tend to be stronger than the lateral ones. Thus, the interosseous Lisfranc ligament is the largest and strongest of the tarsometatarsal ligaments and the plantar Lisfranc is the strongest of the plantar ligaments.[17,31,32]

The importance of the Lisfranc ligament in supporting the arch of the foot is increased due to the lack of intermetatarsal ligaments between the first and second metatarsals. The Lisfranc ligament has been divided into 3 parts: the interosseous ligament, which is often referred to as the Lisfranc ligament, and the relatively weak dorsal component, both of which extend from the first cuneiform to the base of the second metatarsal, and the strong plantar component, which extends from the first cuneiform to the bases of the second and third metatarsals (**Fig. 13**).[33,34]

Lisfranc Joint Complex Injury

Pathology involving the Lisfranc joint can be degenerative or traumatic. Congenital and acquired deformities can contribute to midfoot or Lisfranc degenerative disease. Hallux valgus, with a short first ray, may result in transfer of peak pressures to the lesser metatarsals, which can cause joint instability, plantar plate tears,

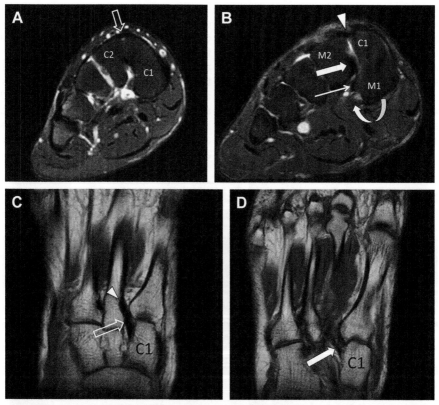

Fig. 13. Normal anatomy of Lisfranc ligament complex. (*A, B*) Short-axis FS T2-weighted MR image at the level of the first cuneiform (C1) shows the dorsal intercuneiform ligament (*open arrow*). (*B*) Short-axis FS T2-weighted MR image at the level of the second metatarsal (M2) demonstrates the 3 components of Lisfranc ligament: interosseous or Lisfranc ligament proper (*thick arrow*), dorsal component (*arrowhead*), and plantar component (*thin arrow*). Note striated insertion of the peroneus longus tendon (*curved arrow*) at the first metatarsal base (M1). (*C, D*) Long-axis PD MR images show the interosseous (*open arrow*) and plantar (*white arrow*) components of Lisfranc ligament complex extending between the first cuneiform (C1) and second metatarsal base (*arrowhead*) and between the first cuneiform and third metatarsal base.

stress fractures, and degenerative joint disease of the tarsometatarsal articulations. Flat foot deformity and pes equinus are other conditions that may contribute to the development of midfoot osteoarthrosis (OA).[31]

Traumatic injuries at the tarsometatarsal joints, or Lisfranc joint complex, may occur in the setting of high-energy and low-energy trauma. High-energy trauma injuries are usually secondary to direct forces and are associated with motor vehicle collisions or falls from a height. These lesions are often associated with crush injuries and multiple fractures within the foot and at distant sites. Extensive soft tissue edema may delay the diagnosis in these patients.[29,30,35] Low-energy trauma injuries, also called midfoot sprains, are most frequently sports-related and can be due to indirect forces.[30,36]

In 1909, Quenu and Kuss classified Lisfranc injuries into 3 categories: homolateral, isolated, and divergent. In homolateral injuries, all 5 metatarsals are displaced in 1 direction. In divergent-type injuries, metatarsals are displaced in different directions in the sagittal and coronal planes. In isolated injuries, 1 or more metatarsals may be intact.[29] This classification was later modified by Hardcastle and colleagues[37] in 1982 and 3 types of injuries were defined: type A, indicating total incongruity; type B, partial incongruity; and type C, divergent. In 1986 Myerson and colleagues[38] further divided types B and C. Type B1 indicating partial incongruity with medial displacement; type B2, partial incongruity with lateral displacement; type C1, divergent pattern with partial displacement; and type C2, total displacement. Most of these classifications apply to the more severe Lisfranc injuries and were found to provide little guidance in treatment and in predicting outcome and prognosis.[39]

Nunley and Vertullo[40] developed a 3-stage classification system for low-energy midfoot sprains. Stage I injuries represent a low-grade sprain of the Lisfranc ligament complex and a dorsal capsular tear with intact joint stability. Stage II injuries demonstrate elongation or disruption of the Lisfranc ligament complex with maintenance of the plantar capsular structures. In stage III injuries, there is loss of arch height and the interosseous and plantar Lisfranc ligaments are disrupted. Stages II and III present with different grades of instability and abnormal findings on radiographs.[41]

Initial radiographic evaluation in Lisfranc injuries usually includes an AP, lateral, and 30° internally rotated oblique images. Weight-bearing films are crucial because subtle malalignment may be missed on non–weight-bearing views. Findings in conventional radiography include small avulsion fractures (the fleck-sign) at the base of the second metatarsal or the first cuneiform, and cuboid fractures and signs of subtle malalignment at the second tarsometatarsal joint (a distance of >2 mm between the first and second tarsometatarsal articulations) (**Figs. 14** and **15**).[41]

MR imaging allows direct evaluation of the Lisfranc ligament complex and associated osseous and soft tissue injury. Primary signs of ligamentous injury include fluid surrounding the Lisfranc ligament, ligament irregularity or frank disruption, and abnormal signal intensity within the ligament (see **Fig. 15**). Disruption of the intertarsal and intermetatarsal ligaments can also be diagnosed on

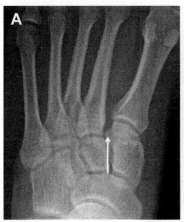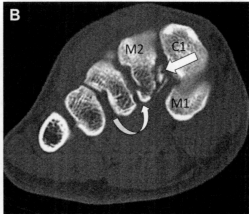

Fig. 14. Lisfranc joint injury in a 21-year-old man following a fall off a bike. (*A*) AP radiograph shows widening of the C1–M2 interval and proximally displaced small avulsion fracture (*thin arrow*) (the fleck-sign). (*B*) The fleck-sign is better appreciated on the short-axis CT scan (*thick arrow*). Note also a fracture at the base of M2 (*curved arrow*). C1, first cuneiform; M1, first metatarsal; M2, second metatarsal.

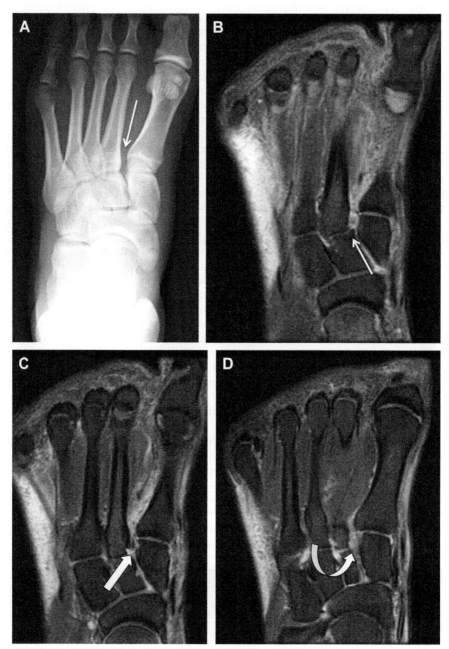

Fig. 15. (*A–D*) Lisfranc joint injury in a 33-year-old man with history of twisting injury. (*A*) AP radiograph shows diastasis of the first cuneiform–second metatarsal interval (*thin arrow*). (*B–D*) Long-axis FS T2-weighted MR images demonstrate malalignment at the second cuneiform–second metatarsal and tearing of the interosseous Lisfranc ligament (*thick arrow*). The plantar component is not seen due to complete tear (*curved arrow*).

MR images. Small avulsion fractures at the insertion sites are difficult to detect on radiographs and MR imaging and are more advantageously noted on CT (see **Fig. 14**B). Secondary signs that aid in predicting ligamentous injury include fractures along the second cuneometatarsal joint, or soft tissue edema surrounding the second metatarsal and strain of the first dorsal interosseous muscle between the first and second metatarsals.[29,31,42,43] Contusions at the tarsometatarsal joints should always raise the possibility of an occult Lisfranc joint injury. Isolated or multiple metatarsal fractures are common findings in injuries of the Lisfranc joint and occur most frequently at the second metatarsal base (see **Fig. 14**; **Fig. 16**).[44] Thickening of the interosseous

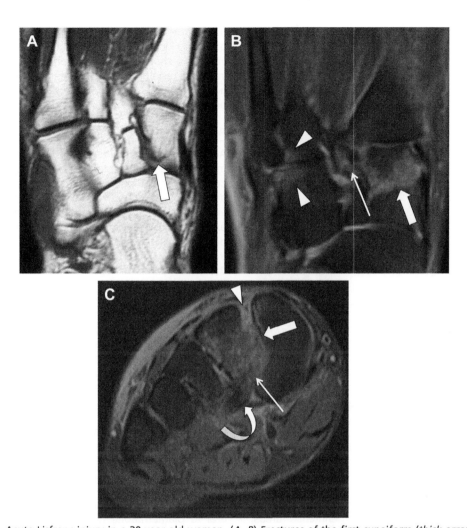

Fig. 16. Acute Lisfranc injury in a 30-year-old woman. (*A, B*) Fractures of the first cuneiform (*thick arrows*) and base of the second metatarsal (*thin arrow*) and bone contusions in the third cuneiform and base of the third metatarsal (*arrowheads*) are seen on long-axis PD (*A*) and FS T2-weighted (*B*) images. (*C*) Short-axis FS T2-weighted MR image shows a complete tear of the Lisfranc ligament complex (dorsal = *arrowhead*; interosseous = *thick arrow*; plantar = *thin arrow*). Intact distal fibers of the peroneus longus tendon are observed (*curved arrow*).

Lisfranc ligament, particularly in the setting of osteoarthrosis at the tarsometatarsal joint, typically indicate old midfoot sprain (**Fig. 17**).

OSSEOUS INJURIES AT THE MIDFOOT
Navicular Stress Fractures

Stress fractures occur when normal bone is subjected to abnormal stress (fatigue fracture) or when abnormal bone undergoes stress associated with activities of daily living (insufficiency fracture). Stress fractures result from repetitive stress load (less than that required to cause a fracture in a single event), which, over time, leads to fatigue and fracture.[12] Although stress fractures have been described in all midfoot bones, the most commonly involved is the navicular bone. Navicular fractures represent up to 35% of all stress fractures in the body. Delayed union, nonunion, avascular necrosis, osteoarthrosis, and chronic pain are all potential consequences of navicular stress fractures. Because of its sparse blood supply, the middle third of the navicular bone is most frequently affected.

Radiographs have a low sensitivity for detecting stress fractures of the navicular (33%) and CT or MR imaging have shown improved sensitivity (**Fig. 18**).[45–47] MR imaging is sensitive and specific in the evaluation of bone marrow edema, periosteal reaction, and detection of subtle

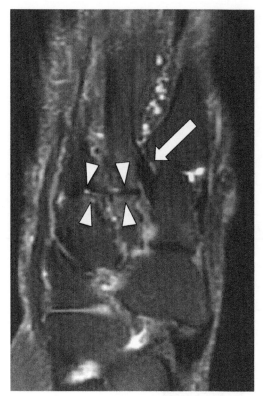

Fig. 17. Old Lisfranc joint injury with secondary osteoarthrosis. A thickened interosseous Lisfranc ligament (*arrow*) and narrowing and edema at the second and third tarsometatarsal joints (*arrowheads*) are observed on the long-axis FS T2-weighted MR image.

fracture lines. As with other stress fractures, early osseous edema, seen as hyperintense areas, without a definite fracture line, may be detected on fluid-sensitive MR sequences (**Fig. 19**). A discrete, hypointense, fracture line may be observed on T1-weighted and T2-weighted MR images. Periosteal reaction, frequently observed in stress fractures of the metatarsal bones, is not seen in tarsal bones due to lack of periosteum.[12,42]

Acute Navicular Fractures

Acute fractures of the navicular bone are rare but more frequent than fractures of the cuboid and cuneiforms. Radiographic images miss or typically underestimate the magnitude of injury, and CT or MR imaging are useful to assess the extent of injury. Navicular acute fractures include dorsal avulsion, tuberosity avulsion, and body fractures (**Fig. 20**). Dorsal avulsion fractures are the most common fractures of the navicular bone (47%) and result from tension forces, typically related to plantarflexion injury, at the talonavicular ligaments, capsule, or tibionavicular band of the deltoid ligament attachment sites (see **Fig. 20A**). They may be associated with a more severe injury to the Chopart joint complex. Fractures at the tuberosity are usually related to PTT avulsion pull, often associated with eversion injury (see **Fig. 20B**). Navicular body fractures are uncommon and are usually associated with high-energy crushing and axial-load mechanisms (see **Fig. 20C, D**). Sangeorzan and colleagues[48] classified navicular body fractures into 3 types: type 1, transverse fracture with a dorsal fragment that is less than 50% of the body; type 2, oblique fracture line from dorsolateral to plantarmedial with a main dorsomedial bone fragment; and type 3, central or lateral comminution.

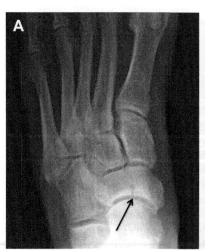

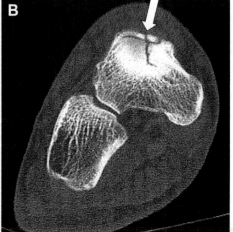

Fig. 18. Navicular stress fracture in a 66-year-old man. (*A*) AP radiograph demonstrates an irregular fracture line in the navicular body with intra-articular extension (*thin arrow*). (*B*) The short-axis CT scan performed a few months later allows further characterization of the comminuted stress fracture (*thick arrow*).

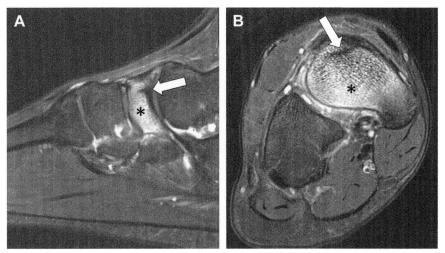

Fig. 19. Navicular stress fracture in an 18-year-old woman. (*A*, *B*) Sagittal (*A*) and short-axis (*B*) FS T2-weighted MR images demonstrate a thin hypointense line in the navicular bone with intra-articular extension (*arrows*) and extensive bone marrow edema (*asterisks*).

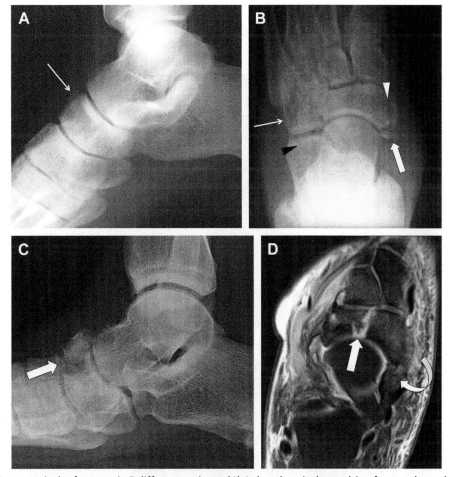

Fig. 20. Acute navicular fractures in 3 different patients. (*A*) A dorsal navicular avulsion fracture (*arrow*) on lateral radiograph. (*B*) A navicular tuberosity avulsion fracture (*thick arrow*), related to a pull by the posterior tibial tendon. Faint fracture lines in the navicular body (*white arrowhead*), calcaneus (*black arrowhead*), and cuboid (*thin arrow*) are also demonstrated. Comminuted navicular body fracture with fragment distraction (*straight arrows*) on lateral radiograph (*C*) and on long-axis FS T2-weighted MR image (*D*). Note the edematous SM component of the spring ligament complex (*curved arrow* in *D*), suggesting a more significant Chopart injury.

Mueller-Weiss Syndrome

Mueller-Weiss syndrome was touted to be spontaneous osteonecrosis of the tarsal navicular bone in the adult, but this theory is less favored in recent literature. The precise mechanism remains unclear, and different theories have been described, such as congenital malformation, osteochondritis, chronic stress fracture, and necrosis secondary to traumatic or biomechanical etiologies.[49] A repetitive traumatic injury, with or without secondary necrosis, is the most likely etiology. Radiographic findings include comma-shaped navicular, manifested as tapering of the lateral AP diameter of the bone, and dorsal subluxation (**Fig. 21A, B**). Advanced disease may depict navicular fragmentation and osteoarthrosis at the articulation with the talar head and/or cuneiforms. MR imaging parallels the radiographic findings with the additional marrow signal abnormalities as well as occasional T1-weighted subchondral sclerosis suggestive of superimposed necrosis (**Fig. 21C**). Treatment usually consists of non–weight-bearing cast immobilization and anti-inflammatory and analgesic medications.[45,49]

Osteonecrosis of the Navicular Bone

Osteonecrosis may develop as a consequence of injury to the adult tarsal navicular and traumatic disruption of its vascular supply. The limited arterial and venous vascularity of the navicular bone is related to its extensive articular cartilage coverage.[45] Lateral navicular collapse following osteonecrosis allows a hindfoot varus to develop, which is similar to that seen in Mueller-Weiss syndrome. Arthrodesis may ultimately be necessary to alleviate symptoms from this posttraumatic complication.[50]

Atraumatic osteonecrosis is an unusual pathology of the foot. A number of associated risk factors have been identified, including corticosteroids, smoking, alcohol, and rheumatologic, hematologic and metabolic disorders. The most common systemic disease that causes infarcts in the ankle and foot is systemic lupus erythematosus.[51,52]

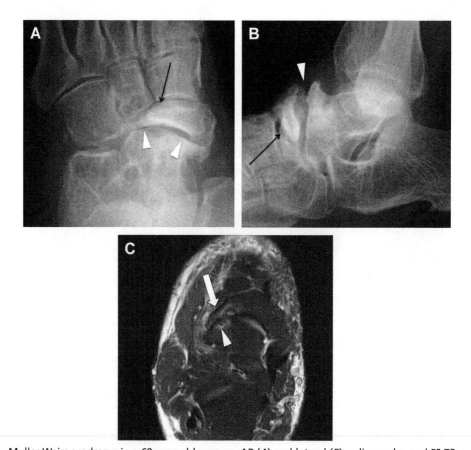

Fig. 21. Muller-Weiss syndrome in a 68-year-old woman. AP (*A*) and lateral (*B*) radiographs, and FS T2-weighted MR image (*C*) demonstrate lateral tapering and sclerosis of the navicular (*arrows*) with secondary osteoarthrosis and remodeling at the talonavicular joint (*white arrowheads*).

The bone marrow signal is characteristically of low signal intensity on T1-weighted images with or without increased signal intensity on T2-weighted images. The characteristic "double-line sign" of osteonecrosis can be seen and, when present, suggests systemic disorders, as most post-traumatic osteonecroses lack this sign.[52]

Accessory Navicular (Os Naviculare)

Accessory navicular ossicles are the most common accessory bones of the foot, occurring in 4% to 21% of the population (**Fig. 22**). They are more common in women and are bilateral in 50% to 90% of cases.[50] Dorsal navicular accessory ossifications are not infrequently seen on lateral radiographs and are known to predispose to navicular fractures (see **Fig. 22**B). Grogan and colleagues[53] described 3 types of navicular accessory bones. Type I is a small and rounded ossicle, usually 2 to 6 mm in diameter, located proximal to the navicular tuberosity. The ossicle, a sesamoid bone, embedded within the PTT distal fibers and completely separate from the navicular bone, is rarely symptomatic. Type II ossicles represent the most common (70%) type, are triangular or heart-shaped, range from 8 to 12 mm in diameter, and are attached to the navicular tuberosity by a cartilaginous synchondrosis. Type II ossicles are the most likely to become symptomatic due to post-traumatic synchondrosis degeneration, related to a pull of the PTT (see **Fig. 22**A). Type III accessory navicular, or cornuate navicular, is a proximal, hooklike, prominence of the navicular tuberosity, possibly reflecting a fused type II os naviculare.

Type III bones may cause midfoot pain due to pressure and bunion formation in the adjacent soft tissues.[45,53] Accessory navicular bones can also have a multiossicle appearance in 14% of cases.[54]

Type II and, at times, type III accessory navicular may be associated with PTT dysfunction, typically in middle-aged or older patients who present with insidious medial foot pain, following a minor trauma, and progressive flat foot deformity (see later in this article for discussion of anomalous PTT distal insertions). Younger patients with type II accessory navicular, and without PTT dysfunction, typically present with complaints of foot pain that is exacerbated during physical activity. MR imaging has replaced nuclear bone scans and has the highest sensitivity and specificity for diagnosing symptomatic accessory navicular syndrome. MR imaging findings include marrow edema at the opposing surfaces of the os and navicular bone as well as irregularity, widening, and fluid within the synchondrosis, suggestive of disruption or micromotion (see **Fig. 22**A). MR features of distal PTT dysfunction may also be encountered.[45,50,55]

Cuboid Fractures

Isolated acute cuboid fractures are rare, generally caused by low-energy mechanism of injury. In the setting of high-energy trauma, cuboid fractures have complex patterns and may result in shortening of both medial and lateral columns of the midfoot. Cuboid fractures may occur with eversion or inversion injuries. A nutcracker mechanism has been described in the setting of an eversion injury

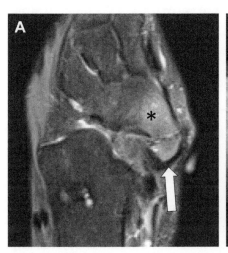
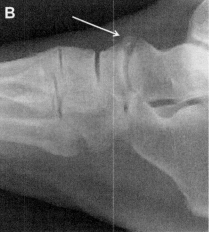

Fig. 22. Accessory navicular ossicles in 2 different patients. (*A*) Type II accessory navicular (*arrow*) in a 31-year-old woman with painful prominence along the medial side of the midfoot seen on long-axis FS T2-weighted image. There is marrow edema (*asterisk*) at the navicular proper and at the os. (*B*) A dorsal os naviculare (*arrow*) is shown on the lateral radiograph.

in which the cuboid is crushed between the fourth and fifth metatarsal bases and the anterior process of the calcaneus. These fractures are usually diagnosed on plain films and CT or MR imaging can be performed to further evaluate fracture extension and displacement (**Fig. 23A**).[2] Cuboid avulsion fracture at the dorsal calcaneocuboid ligament may be an isolated injury, typically related to an inversion injury, or may less commonly occur in the setting of advanced midtarsal (Chopart) joint fracture-dislocation.

Isolated stress fractures of the cuboid are rare and are usually radiographically occult causes of foot pain, requiring further evaluation with MR imaging. As with other stress fractures, marrow edema is observed and may be the initial sign of subtle stress fractures (**Fig. 23B**). The fractures are usually associated with abnormal findings in adjacent structures, such as the plantar fascia, the peroneal tendons, and the PTT. The plantar calcaneocuboid ligament may be disrupted, resulting in widening on the inferior aspect of the calcaneocuboid joint.[19]

Careful examination of the cuboid is necessary when marrow edema is encountered on MR imaging examination, particularly when no fracture line is appreciated. Attention should be given to the surrounding ligaments, particularly the dorsal calcaneocuboid and bifurcate, so as not to miss a partial or complete Chopart joint injury. Conversely, edema along the plantar aspect of the cuboid, at the cuboid tunnel or groove, is typically reactive, secondary to increased friction by the peroneus longus tendon, rather than indicating a fracture or contusion. Adjacent peroneus longus tenosynovitis

and tendinosis will typically clue in the diagnosis. Concomitantly, an enlarged peroneal tubercle and, thus, lateral displacement and inevitable change in the course of the tendon, is often a predisposing factor for increased friction of the tendon against the plantar cuboid. The peroneus longus tendon glides along the proximal wall of the cuboid tunnel.[56] Pathology of the undersurface of the cuboid tunnel and cuboid tubercle may also predispose to increased peroneal tendon friction and plantar cuboid marrow edema (**Fig. 24**).

Cuneiform Fractures

Acute fractures of the cuneiforms rarely occur in isolation but rather as part of a more complex injury with other associated fractures and/or dislocations (see **Fig. 16**).[2] Of all tarsal stress fractures, fractures affecting the cuneiforms are the rarest. Fractures of the cuneiforms, particularly stress fractures, are often occult on plain films and are more easily diagnosed on MR imaging. MR imaging features of cuneiform stress fractures are similar to those of stress fractures elsewhere in the body, and include abnormal marrow signal, with or without a fracture line. Periosteal reaction is not present. It has been reported that cuneiform, metatarsal, and cuboid stress fractures may be present more frequently in patients with plantar fasciitis due to the altered biomechanics.[57]

TENDON ABNORMALITIES
Posterior Tibial Tendon

The PTT divides into anterior, middle, and posterior components, approximately 1.5 to 2.0 cm

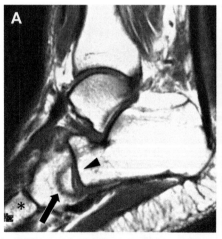
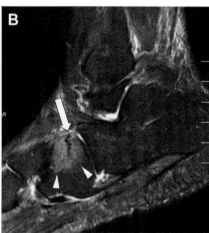

Fig. 23. Cuboid fractures in 2 different patients. (*A*) Osteochondral cuboid fracture (*arrow*) secondary to eversion injury and the nutcracker effect, seen on sagittal T1-weighted MR image. In this type of fracture, the cuboid is crushed between the fourth and fifth metatarsal bases (*asterisk*) and the anterior process of the calcaneus (*arrowhead*). (*B*) Stress fracture of the cuboid (*arrow*) is demonstrated on the sagittal FS T2-weighted MR image. Bone marrow edema (*arrowheads*) on fluid-sensitive MR images helps to outline subtle stress fractures.

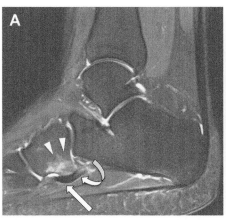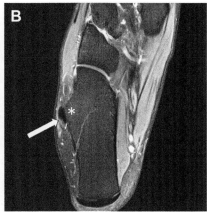

Fig. 24. Cuboid plantar marrow edema in a 32-year-old woman with enlarged peroneal tubercle. Sagittal (*A*) and long-axis (*B*) FS T2-weighted MR images show the peroneus longus tendon (*straight arrow*) riding an edematous cuboid tubercle (*arrowheads*). Lateral displacement of the tendon by a prominent peroneal tubercle (*asterisk*) likely predisposes to increased friction of the tendon against the cuboid. Note small os peroneum (*curved arrow*).

proximal to its navicular insertion (**Fig. 25**). The anterior, largest component, which is a direct extension of the more proximal PTT, attaches to the navicular tuberosity, the inferior capsule of the medial navicular-cuneiform joint, and the inferior surface of the medial cuneiform. The middle component, or plantar cuneometatarsal extension of the PTT, extends to the second and third cuneiforms, the cuboid bone, and bases of the second, third, and fourth metatarsals. This component

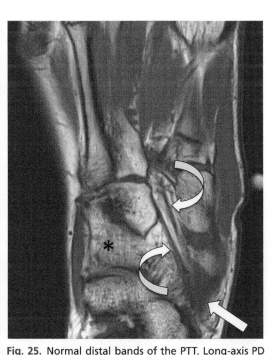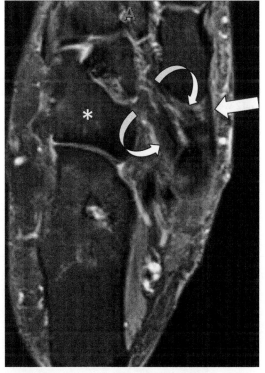

Fig. 25. Normal distal bands of the PTT. Long-axis PD MR image shows the normal terminal divisions of the distal posterior tibial tendon. Anterior division inserts on the navicular tuberosity (*straight arrow*) and 2 visualized slips of the middle, tarsometatarsal division (*curved arrows*) insert on the cuneiforms and metatarsal bases. Asterisk = cuboid.

Fig. 26. Thickened distal bands of the PTT in a 34-year-old woman with PTT tearing more proximally (not shown). Long-axis FS T2-weighted MR image shows marked increased size of the anterior division (*straight arrow*) and 2 slips of the middle, tarsometatarsal division of the PTT (*curved arrows*). Asterisk = cuboid.

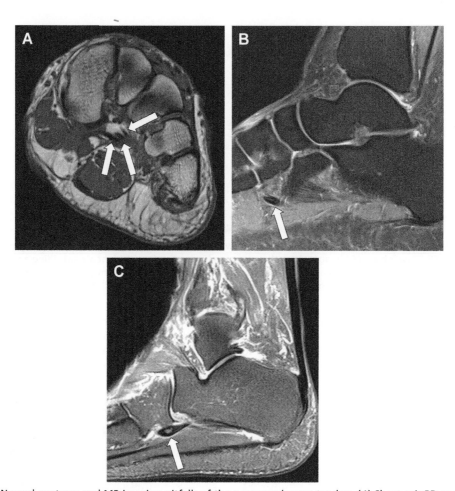

Fig. 27. Normal anatomy and MR imaging pitfalls of the peroneus longus tendon. (*A*) Short-axis PD and sagittal FS T2-weighted (*B*) MR images demonstrate the normal fan-shaped distal divisions of the peroneus longus tendon (*arrows*), simulating a split tear. (*C*) Sagittal FS T2-weighted MR image shows an os peroneum embedded on the tendon fibers (*arrow*), not to be confused with a focal tear.

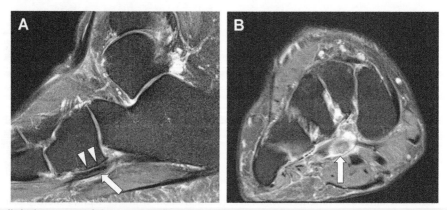

Fig. 28. Full-thickness tear of the peroneus longus tendon associated with abnormal cuboid tunnel in a 51-year-old woman. Sagittal (*A*) FS T2-weighted MR image shows a torn, retracted peroneus longus tendon (*arrow*), abutting against a shallow, irregular cuboid tubercle (*arrowheads*), a predisposing factor to tendon injury. Short-axis MR image (*B*) shows near complete absence of the tendon (*arrow*) in the midfoot.

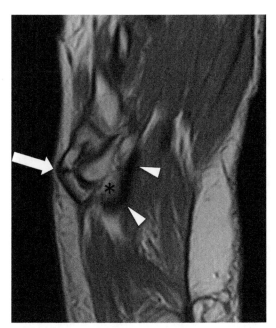

Fig. 29. Proximal subluxation of the peroneus longus tendon in a 41-year-old woman. The tendon (*arrowheads*) is proximal to the cuboid tuberosity (*asterisk*), as seen on a long-axis PD MR image. Comminuted fifth metatarsal fracture (*arrow*) may have predisposed to the subluxation.

provides an attachment also to the Y-shaped origin of the flexor hallucis brevis muscle. The posterior component of the PTT inserts as a band into the anterior aspect of the sustentaculum tali. Other insertion sites to the fifth metatarsal and cuboid bone also have been described.

The distal tendon slips of the PTT, highlighted by fat, are optimally seen as thin, linear, tendon slips, along the plantar aspect of the foot, on axial ankle and long-axis midfoot MR images. Knowledge of the complex anatomy of the PTT distal insertions will also preclude misinterpreting these anatomic variants as distal tendon tears on MR imaging (**Fig. 26**).

When a type I accessory navicular is present, the tendon may directly insert into the ossicle and only a thin slip attaches to the medial aspect of the navicular bone.[58] Furthermore, in the cases of type II and type III accessory navicular bones, the PTT may function as 2 separate tendons, with the proximal portion inserting fully into the accessory bone, while a separate tendon, originating from the os, continues to its distal cuneiform and metatarsal insertion sites. These anomalous insertions of the PTT can result in further stress on the synchondrosis (type II os) and can predispose to flat foot deformity, as they weaken the powerful inversion and plantarflexion roles of the PTT.[59]

In the athletic population, PTT dysfunction typically presents as symptomatic tenosynovitis and tendinosis, typically involving the inframalleolar, distal, and insertional PTT fibers. Rare, acute ruptures, when they occur in the younger population, are also usually located near the navicular insertion. MR imaging is particularly well suited to help localize tears of the distal PTT and distal insertional slips at the level of the cuneiforms and metatarsal bases.[60,61]

The distal PTT is best assessed on axial ankle and long-axis midfoot MR images. The sagittal MR images are also useful. Normal increased T2 signal at the insertion of the PTT to the navicular bone, however, is commonly seen, not to be mistaken for disease. This is in part related to magic angle effect, as the tendon changes direction, and to fibrocartilaginous area at the

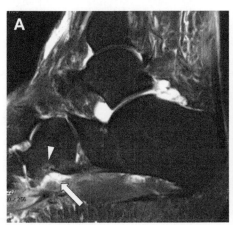
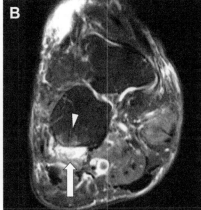

Fig. 30. Torn distal peroneus longus tendon. Sagittal (*A*) and short-axis (*B*) FS T2-weighted MR images in a 59-year-old man with history of twisting injury demonstrate absence of peroneus longus tendon (*arrow*) at the cuboid tunnel. Note the mild plantar cuboid marrow edema (*arrowheads*).

navicular's tendon insertion.[59] The tendon sheath of the PTT ends just proximal to the distal insertion site. Therefore, fluid at the tendon insertion is usually pathologic; care should be taken, however, not to confuse partial volume averaging from adjacent vessels for distal PTT disease on the sagittal images. Thickening of the middle tendon slips has been noted in the setting of PTT dysfunction.[61,62]

Peroneus Longus Tendon, Os Peroneum, and Painful Os Peroneum Syndrome

The peroneus longus tendon traverses the midfoot within the cuboid tunnel or groove, along the plantar surface of the cuboid, to insert onto the first metatarsal base and the plantar aspect of the first cuneiform. As the tendon crosses from its lateral position in the ankle to its medial, plantar insertion on the midfoot, it dynamically supports the transverse and longitudinal arches of the foot.[3]

The peroneus longus tendon glides within the cuboid tunnel during plantar and dorsiflexion of the foot: the tendon can perch on the plantar aspect of the cuboid tubercle, with an apparent pseudosubluxation on MR imaging or ultrasound, during dorsiflexion, best seen on sagittal MR images (see **Fig. 24**).[56]

The distal plantar insertion of the peroneus longus tendon is typically fan-shaped and striated on short-axis and long-axis midfoot MR images, not to be mistaken for a tear. The distal divisions of the insertional fibers may be visualized proximally, up to the level of the calcaneocuboid joint. This proximal division can sometimes mimic a proximal split of the peroneus longus tendon (**Fig. 27**A, B).[61] Furthermore, vessels along the plantar path of the tendon should not be confused with pathology. A small ganglion in close proximity to the insertion of the tendon is not uncommonly seen.

The peroneus longus tendon contains a sesamoid, the os peroneum, at the level of the cuboid bone, radiographically visible in up to 25% of cases.[63] On MR imaging, an os peroneum is depicted as a focal increased signal within the peroneus longus tendon, in the region of the calcaneocuboid joint. This should not be mistaken for a focal tear of the tendon (see **Fig. 24**A; **Fig. 27**C).[61–63]

Peroneus longus tendon disease at the midfoot is not common but should be perused for when patients present with plantar midfoot pain (**Figs. 28–32**). Tearing of the tendon may be attritional or may be associated with an acute trauma, such as strong peroneal muscle contraction, associated with dorsiflexion of the foot. Anatomic predisposing factors include changes in direction of the tendon and increased friction against a

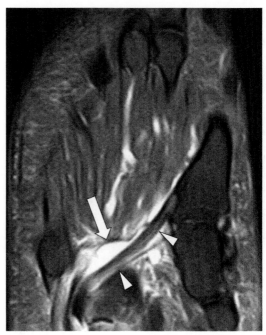

Fig. 31. Tenosynovitis and partial tearing of the plantar peroneus longus tendon. Long-axis FS T2-weighted MR image of a 53-year-old woman with midfoot pain shows plantar tenosynovitis (*arrow*), delamination, and intrasubstance signal heterogeneity of the peroneus longus tendon (*arrowheads*).

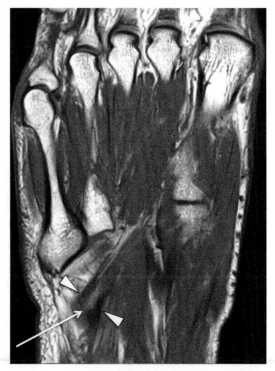

Fig. 32. A split tear of the peroneus longus tendon. There are tendon fibers (*arrowheads*) distal and proximal to the cuboid tubercle (*arrow*).

hypertrophied peroneal tubercle, irregularly shaped cuboid tunnel, and, possibly, an os peroneum (see **Figs. 24, 28,** and **29**). As stated previously, peroneus longus tendon disease in the midfoot may be associated with plantar cuboid marrow edema on MR imaging.

Painful os peroneum syndrome (POPS) is a clinical syndrome of lateral foot pain and tenderness over the cuboid, in the setting of an os peroneum. POPS reflects a spectrum of conditions, including os peroneum fracture or diastasis of multipartite os peroneum. Either of the aforementioned causes may predispose to partial or complete tears of the peroneus longus tendon, tenosynovitis, and tendinosis.[64] Proximal migration of the os peroneum, indicative of a peroneus longus full-thickness tear, can be noted, oftentimes in retrospect, on routine radiographs of either the foot or the ankle. More than 1 cm proximal migration of the os relative to the calcaneocuboid joint and greater than 6-mm diastasis between os peroneum fragments are typically diagnostic of POPS and peroneus longus tendon disease. On MR imaging, abnormal findings include a fragmented or edematous os peroneum, proximal migration of the ossicle or one of its fragments, and peroneus longus tearing (**Fig. 33**).[12,64]

Anterior Tibial Tendon

In the ankle, the anterior tibial muscle (ATT) passes beneath the superomedial and inferomedial bands

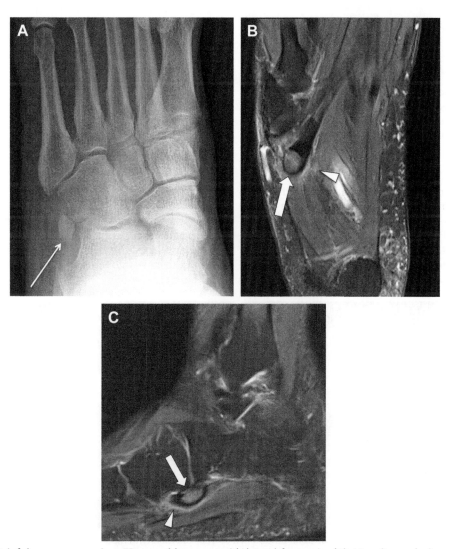

Fig. 33. Painful os peroneum in a 73-year-old woman with lateral foot pain. (*A*) AP radiograph shows a large, multipartite os peroneum (*arrow*). (*B, C*) Long-axis (*B*) and sagittal (*C*) FS T2-weighted MR images show marrow edema in the os (*arrows*) and adjacent soft tissue edema (*arrowheads*).

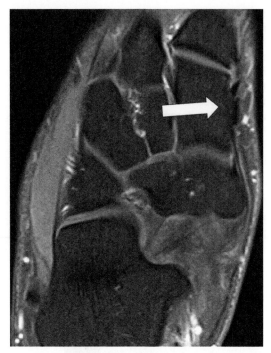

Fig. 34. Normal anterior tibial tendon. Long-axis FS T2-weighted MR image demonstrates the normal striated appearance of the anterior tibial tendon (*arrow*), close to its distal insertion, not to be confused with a split tear.

of the inferior extensor retinaculum and the transverse retinacular band and inserts into the dorsum of the first metatarsal base and medial cuneiform.

The ATT provides stability to the first tarsometatarsal joint. It receives its blood supply exclusively from the anterior tibial artery and therefore is susceptible to ischemia. Most injuries are related to hypoxic degenerative tendinosis or mucoid degeneration. Tears can be complete or partial and can be classified as acute or chronic in nature. Many of the tears occur as an acute event superimposed on a long-standing process and might be designated as acute-on-chronic in nature. In the midfoot, rupture of the ATT usually occurs between the extensor retinaculum and the distal insertion, typically within 3 cm of the distal insertion.

Assuming there is no full-thickness tear, with proximal migration of the tendon stump to the dorsal ankle level, abnormalities of the anterior tibial tendon in the midfoot often can be missed on ankle MR imaging, because they may be detected only on a single, far medial sagittal, or far distal axial image. Thus, midfoot imaging is quite useful for detecting tendinosis and tenosynovitis of the tendon. The 2 major distal divisions of the anterior tibial tendon, as it inserts into the first cuneiform and base of first metatarsal, can be best seen on short-axis and long-axis images and should not be misinterpreted as tears (**Fig. 34**). MR imaging findings in ATT injuries include heterogeneity and thickening of the tendon, fluid-filled gaps in cases of full-thickness rupture, fluid in the tendon sheath, and bone marrow edema and enthesopathy at the distal insertions of the tendon (**Figs. 35 and 36**).[12,65]

Flexor Hallucis Longus Tendon

The flexor hallucis longus (FHL) tendon crosses the plantar aspect of the foot, deep to the flexor digitorum longus tendon (at the master knot of Henry), to insert into the base of the distal phalanx of the great toe (**Fig. 37A**).[62] In the midfoot, the

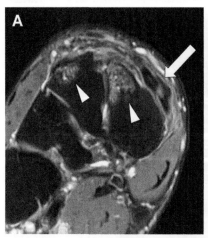

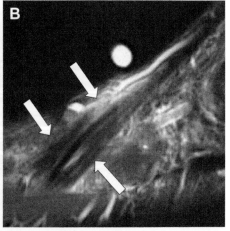

Fig. 35. Partial tearing of the anterior tibial tendon in a 68-year-old man with medial midfoot pain. There is thickening and heterogeneity of the anterior tibial tendon (*arrow*) observed on short-axis (*A*) and sagittal (*B*) T2-weighted FS MR images. Note dorsal osteophytosis of the medial and middle cuneiforms (*arrowheads*), which may have predisposed to the tear. Marker is in close proximity to the diseased tendon.

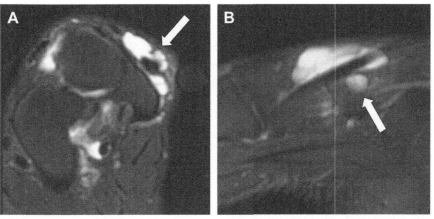

Fig. 36. Ganglion cyst originating from the distal anterior tibial tendon sheath (*arrows*) is demonstrated on the short-axis (*A*) and sagittal (*B*) FS T2-weighted MR images of a 42-year-old woman with a palpable mass at medial foot.

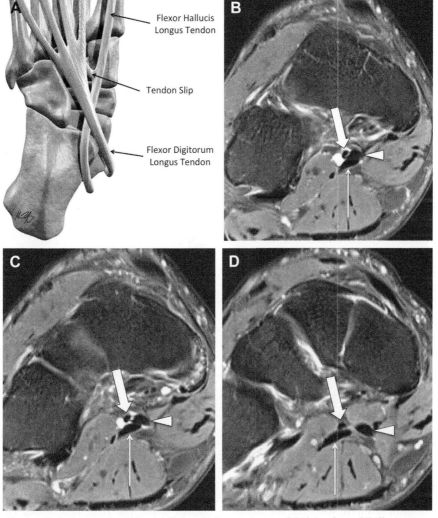

Fig. 37. Tendinous slip between the FHL and flexor digitorum longus (FDL) tendons. (*A*) Illustration of the most common variation of the slip. (*B–D*) Proximal to distal sequential short-axis FS T2-weighted MR images show a hypointense, thin tendinous slip (*thick arrow*) that originates from the FHL tendon (*arrowheads*) and approximating the FDL tendon (*thin arrows*). The tendon sheath is distended with fluid, allowing a better visualization of the tendon slip.

FHL tendon sends a tendon slip to the flexor digitorum longus tendon. The slip plays an important role in anchoring the 2 tendons together, so as to prevent proximal migration of the FHL, when it is torn distal to the knot of Henry. The slip, which varies in size, proximal origin, and distal insertion, is optimally seen on short-axis images of the midfoot, particularly when fluid distends the FHL tendon sheath. Occasionally, the origin of the slip is noted as proximal as the level of the sustentaculum tali. Perusal of sequential images will avoid misinterpreting the slip as a longitudinal split tear of the FHL (**Fig. 37**B–D).

Tenosynovitis remains the most frequent pathology of the FHL tendon (**Fig. 38**). Ruptures of the FHL tendon can occur in the midfoot, although are reported more commonly at the distal insertion of the tendon (**Fig. 39**).[66] In the midfoot, tenosynovitis usually occurs at the master knot of Henry. Because of normal communication between the tendon sheath of the FHL and the ankle joint, it may be difficult to determine whether fluid within the tendon sheath is indeed pathologic. Fluid loculation, synovitis, and debris may aid in distinguishing a normal decompression of fluid from the ankle joint from a true pathology.

Nerves

The medial plantar nerve is located posteromedial to the FHL and courses between the quadratus plantae and abductor hallucis muscles (**Fig. 40**). Due to its close proximity to the tendon, tenosynovitis of the FHL tendon at the master knot of

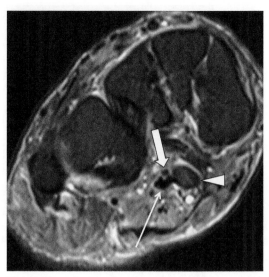

Fig. 39. Torn FHL tendon in a 42-year-old man with sudden onset of plantar foot pain. A partial tear of the FHL tendon with thickening and signal hyperintensity (*arrowhead*) is seen on the short-axis FS T2-weighted MR image. The tendon slip (*thick arrow*) and FDL tendon (*thin arrow*) have a normal appearance.

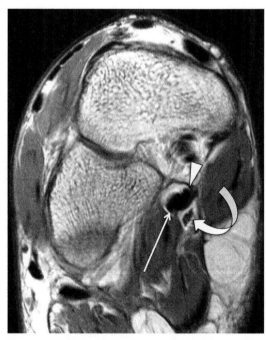

Fig. 40. Normal FHL tendon at the master knot of Henry. Short-axis PD MR image of an asymptomatic patient shows the close relationship between the medial plantar neurovascular bundle (*curved arrow*), the FDL (*arrowhead*), and FHL (*thin arrow*) tendons. The FHL has not yet crossed over to the medial side of the foot.

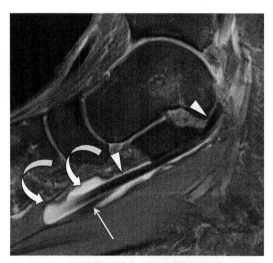

Fig. 38. Tenosynovitis of the FHL tendon at the master knot of Henry. Sagittal FS T2-weighted MR image shows loculated fluid (*curved arrows*) distending the sheath of the FHL tendon (*arrowheads*). Note the more plantar FDL (*thin arrow*).

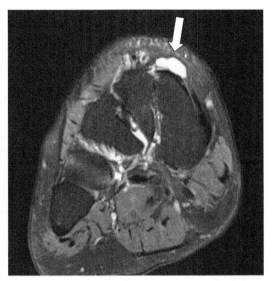

Fig. 41. Impingement on the medial branch of the deep peroneal nerve in a 42-year-old woman with tingling in the first web space. A small ganglion (*arrow*) is noted along the dorsal medial aspect of the foot on short-axis T2 FS image.

Henry can cause medial plantar nerve entrapment. Jogger's foot, a recognized condition in runners, is caused by repetitive eversion of the foot. In jogger's foot, the medial plantar nerve may become compressed as it passes adjacent to the master knot of Henry. Symptoms include burning, shooting, sharp pain, or numbness radiating from the arch toward the plantar aspect of the second and great toe.[67,68]

The deep peroneal nerve divides into 2 branches at the dorsal ankle, with a motor, lateral branch innervating the extensor digitorum brevis and a medial branch, coursing along the medial axis of the midfoot, providing motor and sensory innervation to the first web space structures. Entrapment of the medial branch of the deep peroneal nerve should be entertained when a dorsal mass, such as a ganglion, is encountered in the medial aspect of the midfoot (**Fig. 41**) or in the setting of degenerative dorsal navicular-cuneiform or medial Lisfranc joint osteophytosis.

SUMMARY

Midfoot injuries represent increasingly recognized causes of foot pain, leading to permanent disability if not promptly diagnosed and treated. Many of these injuries can be easily missed on conventional radiographs and may require advanced imaging. MR imaging represents the modality of choice for the detection of radiographically occult fractures of the navicular, cuboid, and cuneiform bones and of tendon and ligamentous injuries affecting the midfoot.

This article focused on the MR imaging features of various osseous, tendon, and ligament abnormalities affecting the midfoot, as well as on Chopart and Lisfranc joints. The complex anatomy and MR imaging pitfalls that may mimic pathology in the midfoot was also emphasized so as to avoid misdiagnosis.

REFERENCES

1. Williams PL, Warwick R. Gray's anatomy, vol. I. Madrid: Churchill Livingstone; 1992.
2. Swords MP, Schramski M, Switzer K, et al. Chopart fractures and dislocations. Foot Ankle Clin 2008; 13(4):679–93, viii.
3. Benirschke SK, Meinberg E, Anderson SA, et al. Fractures and dislocations of the midfoot: Lisfranc and Chopart injuries. J Bone Joint Surg Am 2012; 94(14):1325–37.
4. Baker JC, Hoover EG, Hillen TJ, et al. Subradiographic foot and ankle fractures and bone contusions detected by MRI in elite ice hockey players. Am J Sports Med 2016;44(5):1317–23.
5. Arnold G, Vohra S, Marcantonio D, et al. Normal magnetic resonance imaging anatomy of the ankle & foot. Magn Reson Imaging Clin N Am 2011; 19(3):655–79.
6. Moeller TB, Reif E. MRI parameters and positioning. Stuttgart (Germany): Thieme; 2003.
7. Shortt CP. Magnetic resonance imaging of the midfoot and forefoot: normal variants and pitfalls. Magn Reson Imaging Clin N Am 2010;18(4):707–15.
8. Gyftopoulos S, Bencardino JT. Normal variants and pitfalls in MR imaging of the ankle and foot. Magn Reson Imaging Clin N Am 2010;18(4):691–705.
9. Kelikian A, Sarrafian SK. Sarrafian's anatomy of the foot and ankle. 3rd edition. Philadelphia: Lippincott Williams & Wilkins - Wolters Kluwer; 2011.
10. Melao L, Canella C, Weber M, et al. Ligaments of the transverse tarsal joint complex: MRI-anatomic correlation in cadavers. AJR Am J Roentgenol 2009; 193(3):662–71.
11. Sconfienza LM, Orlandi D, Lacelli F, et al. Dynamic high-resolution US of ankle and midfoot ligaments: normal anatomic structure and imaging technique. Radiographics 2015;35(1):164–78.
12. Ting AY, Morrison WB, Kavanagh EC. MR imaging of midfoot injury. Magn Reson Imaging Clin N Am 2008;16(1):105–15.
13. Desai KR, Beltran LS, Bencardino JT, et al. The spring ligament recess of the talocalcaneonavicular joint: depiction on MR images with cadaveric and histologic correlation. AJR Am J Roentgenol 2011; 196(5):1145–50.

14. Taniguchi A, Tanaka Y, Takakura Y, et al. Anatomy of the spring ligament. J Bone Joint Surg Am 2003;85-A(11):2174–8.

15. Mengiardi B, Zanetti M, Schöttle PB, et al. Spring ligament complex: MR imaging–anatomic correlation and findings in asymptomatic subjects. Radiology 2005;237(1):242–9.

16. Yao L, Gentili A, Cracchiolo A. MR imaging findings in spring ligament insufficiency. Skeletal Radiol 1999;28(5):245–50.

17. Manaster BJ, Roberts CC, Andrews CL, et al. Musculoskeletal imaging anatomy. In: SRK, editor. Diagnostic and Surgical Imaging Anatomy: Musculoskeletal. Hagerstown (MD): Lippincott Williams & Wilkins; 2006. p. 1034–128.

18. van Dorp KB, de Vries MR, van der Elst M, et al. Chopart joint injury: a study of outcome and morbidity. J Foot Ankle Surg 2010;49(6):541–5.

19. Yu SM, Dardani M, Yu JS. MRI of isolated cuboid stress fractures in adults. AJR Am J Roentgenol 2013;201(6):1325–30.

20. Nazarenko A, Beltran LS, Bencardino JT. Imaging evaluation of traumatic ligamentous injuries of the ankle and foot. Radiol Clin North Am 2013;51(3):455–78.

21. Jennings MM, Christensen JC. The effects of sectioning the spring ligament on rearfoot stability and posterior tibial tendon efficiency. J Foot Ankle Surg 2008;47(3):219–24.

22. Arnoldner MA, Gruber M, Syré S, et al. Imaging of posterior tibial tendon dysfunction–comparison of high-resolution ultrasound and 3T MRI. Eur J Radiol 2015;84(9):1777–81.

23. Gazdag AR, Cracchiolo A 3rd. Rupture of the posterior tibial tendon. Evaluation of injury of the spring ligament and clinical assessment of tendon transfer and ligament repair. J Bone Joint Surg Am 1997;79(5):675–81.

24. Teasdall RD, Johnson KA. Surgical treatment of stage I posterior tibial tendon dysfunction. Foot Ankle Int 1994;15(12):646–8.

25. Deland JT. The adult acquired flatfoot and spring ligament complex. Patholology and implications for treatment. Foot Ankle Clin 2001;6(1):129–35.

26. Tryfonidis M, Jackson W, Mansour R, et al. Acquired adult flat foot due to isolated plantar calcaneonavicular (spring) ligament insufficiency with a normal tibialis posterior tendon. Foot Ankle Surg 2008;14(2):89–95.

27. Shuen V, Prem H. Acquired unilateral pes planus in a child caused by a ruptured plantar calcaneonavicular (spring) ligament. J Pediatr Orthop B 2009;18(3):129–30.

28. Toye LR, Helms CA, Hoffman BD, et al. MRI of spring ligament tears. AJR Am J Roentgenol 2005;184(5):1475–80.

29. Hatem SF. Imaging of Lisfranc injury and midfoot sprain. Radiol Clin North Am 2008;46(6):1045–60.

30. Burge AJ, Gold SL, Potter HG. Imaging of sports-related midfoot and forefoot injuries. Sports Health 2012;4(6):518–34.

31. Chaney DM. The Lisfranc joint. Clin Podiatr Med Surg 2010;27(4):547–60.

32. Castro M, Melão L, Canella C, et al. Lisfranc joint ligamentous complex: MRI with anatomic correlation in cadavers. AJR Am J Roentgenol 2010;195(6):W447–55.

33. de Palma L, Santucci A, Sabetta SP, et al. Anatomy of the Lisfranc joint complex. Foot Ankle Int 1997;18(6):356–64.

34. Hirano T, Niki H, Beppu M. Anatomical considerations for reconstruction of the Lisfranc ligament. J Orthop Sci 2013;18(5):720–6.

35. Kalia V, Fishman EK, Carrino JA, et al. Epidemiology, imaging, and treatment of Lisfranc fracture-dislocations revisited. Skeletal Radiol 2012;41(2):129–36.

36. Haverstock BD. Foot and ankle imaging in the athlete. Clin Podiatr Med Surg 2008;25(2):249–62, vi–vii.

37. Hardcastle PH, Reschauer R, Kutscha-Lissberg E, et al. Injuries to the tarsometatarsal joint. Incidence, classification and treatment. J Bone Joint Surg Br 1982;64(3):349–56.

38. Myerson MS, Fisher RT, Burgess AR, et al. Fracture dislocations of the tarsometatarsal joints: end results correlated with pathology and treatment. Foot Ankle 1986;6(5):225–42.

39. Mahmoud S, Hamad F, Riaz M, et al. Reliability of the Lisfranc injury radiological classification (Myerson-modified Hardcastle classification system). Int Orthop 2015;39(11):2215–8.

40. Nunley JA, Vertullo CJ. Classification, investigation, and management of midfoot sprains: Lisfranc injuries in the athlete. Am J Sports Med 2002;30(6):871–8.

41. Siddiqui NA, Galizia MS, Almusa E, et al. Evaluation of the tarsometatarsal joint using conventional radiography, CT, and MR imaging. Radiographics 2014;34(2):514–31.

42. Gorbachova T. Midfoot and forefoot injuries. Top Magn Reson Imaging 2015;24(4):215–21.

43. Raikin SM, Elias I, Dheer S, et al. Prediction of midfoot instability in the subtle Lisfranc injury. J Bone Joint Surg Am 2009;91(4):892–9.

44. Preidler KW, Brossmann J, Daenen B, et al. MR imaging of the tarsometatarsal joint: analysis of injuries in 11 patients. AJR Am J Roentgenol 1996;167(5):1217–22.

45. Scott-Moncrieff A, Forster BB, Andrews G, et al. The adult tarsal navicular: why it matters. Can Assoc Radiol J 2007;58(5):279–85.

46. Fowler JR, Gaughan JP, Boden BP, et al. The non-surgical and surgical treatment of tarsal navicular stress fractures. Sports Med 2011;41(8):613–9.

47. Burne SG, Mahoney CM, Forster BB, et al. Tarsal navicular stress injury: long-term outcome and clinicoradiological correlation using both computed tomography and magnetic resonance imaging. Am J Sports Med 2005;33(12):1875–81.

48. Sangeorzan BJ, Benirschke SK, Mosca V, et al. Displaced intra-articular fractures of the tarsal navicular. J Bone Joint Surg Am 1989;71(10):1504–10.

49. Tosun B, Al F, Tosun A. Spontaneous osteonecrosis of the tarsal navicular in an adult: Mueller-Weiss syndrome. J Foot Ankle Surg 2011;50(2):221–4.

50. Tuthill HL, Finkelstein ER, Sanchez AM, et al. Imaging of tarsal navicular disorders: a pictorial review. Foot Ankle Spec 2014;7(3):211–25.

51. Greenhagen RM, Crim BE, Shinabarger AB, et al. Bilateral osteonecrosis of the navicular and medial cuneiform in a patient with systemic lupus erythematosus: a case report. Foot Ankle Spec 2012;5(3):180–4.

52. Weishaupt D, Schweitzer ME. MR imaging of the foot and ankle: patterns of bone marrow signal abnormalities. Eur Radiol 2002;12(2):416–26.

53. Grogan DP, Gasser SI, Ogden JA. The painful accessory navicular: a clinical and histopathological study. Foot Ankle 1989;10(3):164–9.

54. Perdikakis E, Grigoraki E, Karantanas A. Os naviculare: the multi-ossicle configuration of a normal variant. Skeletal Radiol 2011;40(1):85–8.

55. Choi YS, Lee KT, Kang HS, et al. MR imaging findings of painful type II accessory navicular bone: correlation with surgical and pathologic studies. Korean J Radiol 2004;5(4):274–9.

56. Stone TJ, Rosenberg ZS, Velez ZR, et al. Subluxation of the peroneus long tendon in the cuboid tunnel: is it normal or pathologic? An ultrasound and magnetic resonance imaging study. Skeletal Radiol 2016;45(3):357–65.

57. Bui-Mansfield LT, Thomas WR. Magnetic resonance imaging of stress injury of the cuneiform bones in patients with plantar fasciitis. J Comput Assist Tomogr 2009;33(4):593–6.

58. Pastore D, Dirim B, Wangwinyuvirat M, et al. Complex distal insertions of the tibialis posterior tendon: detailed anatomic and MR imaging investigation in cadavers. Skeletal Radiol 2008;37(9):849–55.

59. Kiter E, Günal I, Karatosun V, et al. The relationship between the tibialis posterior tendon and the accessory navicular. Ann Anat 2000;182(1):65–8.

60. Teitz CC, Garrett WE Jr, Miniaci A, et al. Tendon problems in athletic individuals. Instr Course Lect 1997;46:569–82.

61. Donovan A, Rosenberg ZS, Bencardino JT, et al. Plantar tendons of the foot: MR imaging and US. Radiographics 2013;33(7):2065–85.

62. Fernandes R, Aguiar R, Trudell D, et al. Tendons in the plantar aspect of the foot: MR imaging and anatomic correlation in cadavers. Skeletal Radiol 2007;36(2):115–22.

63. Rademaker J, Rosenberg ZS, Delfaut EM, et al. Tear of the peroneus longus tendon: MR imaging features in nine patients. Radiology 2000;214(3):700–4.

64. Oh SJ, Kim YH, Kim SK, et al. Painful os peroneum syndrome presenting as lateral plantar foot pain. Ann Rehabil Med 2012;36(1):163–6.

65. Mengiardi B, Pfirrmann CW, Vienne P, et al. Anterior tibial tendon abnormalities: MR imaging findings. Radiology 2005;235(3):977–84.

66. Na JB, Bergman AG, Oloff LM, et al. The flexor hallucis longus: tenographic technique and correlation of imaging findings with surgery in 39 ankles. Radiology 2005;236(3):974–82.

67. De Maeseneer M, Madani H, Lenchik L, et al. Normal anatomy and compression areas of nerves of the foot and ankle. Radiographics 2015;35(5):1469–82.

68. Farooki S, Theodorou DJ, Sokoloff RM, et al. MRI of the medial and lateral plantar nerves. J Comput Assist Tomogr 2001;25(3):412–6.

MR Imaging of the Plantar Plate

Normal Anatomy, Turf Toe, and Other Injuries

Caio Nery, MD[a,b,*], Daniel Baumfeld, MD[c],
Hilary Umans, MD[d], André F. Yamada, MD[e,f]

KEYWORDS

- Metatarsophalangeal joints • Turf toe • Sand toe • Plantar plate tears
- Magnetic resonance imaging • Instability • Forefoot

KEY POINTS

- Acute and traumatic injuries are more common at the first MTP joint and degenerative injuries are the main cause of lesser MTP plantar plate tears.
- MR imaging is the most powerful imaging tool to evaluate soft tissue and cartilaginous damage related to the turf toe and plantar plate injuries.
- Familiarity with typical patterns and classifications of plantar plate tears of the lesser MTP joints enhances detection and characterization of the lesions by the interpreting radiologist.
- Lesser metatarsal supination and second metatarsal protrusion may correlate with plantar plate tears.

INTRODUCTION

Forefoot pathology is a most challenging orthopedic subject owing to the anatomic complexity, the sophistication of its biomechanics, and the range of pathology, stressors, and injury that may occur over the course of a lifetime. The fine-tuned balance of the human forefoot can be disturbed by subtle forces, repetitive trauma, and degenerative conditions that set off a deleterious chain of events that lead to pain, overload, and, finally, permanent deformities.

Recognition that injuries to the greater and lesser metatarsophalangeal (MTP) joints can be terribly disabling has inspired increased interest in research and treatment of MTP joint pathology. The onset of new and efficient diagnostic and therapeutic alternatives for forefoot pathology must be based on robust knowledge of the regional anatomy, clinical observation, and an understanding of the range of conditions that affect the MTP joints.

Disclosures: Dr C. Nery is consultant of Arthrex, USA. Drs D. Baumfeld, H. Umans, and A.F. Yamada have nothing to disclose.
[a] Department of Orthopedics and Traumatology, UNIFESP - Federal University of São Paulo, São Paulo, São Paulo, Brazil; [b] Albert Einstein Jewish Hospital, São Paulo, São Paulo, Brazil; [c] Department of Surgery, Orthopedics and Traumatology, UFMG - Federal University of Minas Gerais, Belo Horizonte, Minas Gerais, Brazil; [d] Albert Einstein College of Medicine, Lenox Hill Radiology, Imaging and Associates, Bronx, NY, USA; [e] Department of Diagnostic Imaging, UNIFESP - Federal University of São Paulo, São Paulo, São Paulo, Brazil; [f] Department of Radiology, Hospital do Coração – Hcor, São Paulo, São Paulo, Brazil
* Corresponding author. Department of Orthopedics and Traumatology, UNIFESP - Federal University of São Paulo, São Paulo, São Paulo, Brazil.
E-mail address: caionerymd@gmail.com

Magn Reson Imaging Clin N Am 25 (2017) 127–144
http://dx.doi.org/10.1016/j.mric.2016.08.007
1064-9689/17/© 2016 Elsevier Inc. All rights reserved.

ANATOMY OF THE METATARSOPHALANGEAL JOINTS

Although the general structure of MTP joints of the great and lesser toes follows a similar pattern, important anatomic differences exist between the first and the second through fifth rays. All 5 metatarsal heads are rounded and convex in the sagittal plane, but the head of the first metatarsal has a larger transverse than vertical dimension, which results in a slightly flattened appearance. Conversely, the heads of the lesser metatarsals (second to fifth) are larger in the vertical than the transverse dimension, resulting in a more slender appearance in the coronal plane.[1]

The first metatarsal head has 2 different articular surfaces. The superior surface, which articulates with the proximal phalanx, is convex and wide, extending to the dorsal aspect of the metaphysis. A sagittal plane crest (the "crista") divides the plantar articular surface into 2 grooves, one for each hallucal sesamoid. The medial groove is deeper and wider than the lateral groove to accommodate the larger tibial sesamoid (Fig. 1).

Sagittal plane stability of the first ray MTP joint is provided by the glenosesamoid apparatus, a gliding and pressure-absorbing mechanism formed by the 2 sesamoids embedded in a thick fibrous tissue (Gillette, 1872)[1]—in combination with the intrinsic and extrinsic muscles of the hallux. The medial plantar tubercle at the base of the proximal phalanx of the hallux is the insertion site for the medial head of the flexor hallucis brevis (medial) and abductor hallucis tendons. The plantar plate anchors to the adjacent inferior margin of the proximal phalanx. The lateral head of the flexor hallucis brevis (lateral) and conjoint tendon of the adductor hallucis muscle (adductor hallucis oblique and transverse bellies) all insert onto the lateral plantar tubercle of the proximal phalanx. Both sesamoids are embedded in the plantar plate, which receives fibers from flexor hallucis brevis tendons, lateral deep intermetatarsal ligament, plantar fascia, and suspensory ligaments (Table 1).

Of the hallucal sesamoids, the medial one is slightly larger. A strong intersesamoid ligament binds the tibial and fibular sesamoids and forms the roof of a fibrous tunnel for the flexor hallucis longus tendon (Figs. 2 and 3).

At the dorsal aspect of the first MTP joint, the extensor system includes the extensor hallucis longus and extensor hallucis brevis tendons and the extensor hood that is composed of oblique and transverse aponeurotic fibers that extend around the capsule and blend on the plantar aspect with the plantar plate and deep transverse intermetatarsal ligament.

The lesser metatarsal distal articular surfaces are bicondylar, with 2 plantar articular segments separated by a central concavity; typically, the lateral condyle is larger. In rare instances (1.8%),[1] there are sesamoids of the lesser MTP joints.

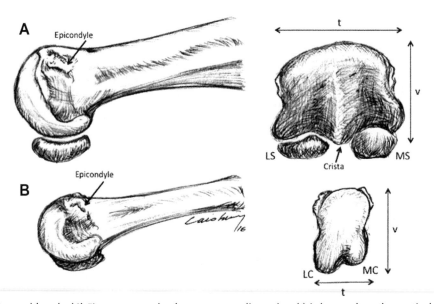

Fig. 1. Metatarsal heads. (*A*) First metatarsal—the transverse dimension (*t*) is larger than the vertical dimension (*v*). (*B*) Lesser metatarsals—the vertical dimension (*v*) is larger than the transverse dimension (*t*). LC, lateral condyle; LS, lateral sesamoid; MC, medial condyle; MS, medial sesamoid.

Table 1
Anatomy of the first MTP joint plantar plate ligaments and tendons

Anatomic Structure	Special Characteristics
FHB tendon (medial head)	Inserts on medial plantar tubercle at base of proximal phalanx of the hallux
Abductor hallucis tendon	Inserts on medial plantar tubercle at base of proximal phalanx of the hallux (together with FHB)
Plantar plate	Formed by fibers from the FHB tendon, lateral deep intermetatarsal ligament, plantar fascia, and suspensory ligaments, with contribution from aponeurotic fibers of extensor hood Extends from distal margin of the intersesamoidal ligament Inserts on inferior plantar margin of the proximal phalanx Often difficult to visualize as distinct structure unless thickened or surrounded by edema
FHB tendon (lateral head)	Inserts on lateral plantar tubercle of the proximal phalanx of the hallux
Adductor hallucis tendon (conjoint tendon from oblique and transverse muscle bellies)	Inserts on lateral plantar tubercle of the proximal phalanx of the hallux (together with FHB)
Proper collateral ligaments (medial and lateral)	Course obliquely to insert on medial and lateral phalangeal tubercles
Accessory collateral ligaments (medial and lateral)	Insert broadly along medial and lateral borders of the MTP joint plantar plates
Hallucal sesamoids (tibial and fibular)	The medial sesamoid is slightly wider and larger than the lateral
Intersesamoid ligament	Transverse ligament that runs between the tibial and fibular sesamoids
Metatarsal–sesamoid ligaments (medial and lateral)	Thickened portions of the plantar capsule that may be hard to distinguish from capsule Originate with joint capsule from plantar aspect of first metatarsal and attach to proximal margin of respective sesamoid
Sesamoidal–phalangeal ligaments (medial and lateral)	Extend from distal margin of sesamoids to plantar base of the proximal phalanx

Abbreviations: FHB, flexor hallucis brevis; MTP, metatarsophalangeal.

On each side of the lesser metatarsal heads, there are bony tubercles (epicondyles) that provide insertion sites for the MTP collateral ligaments (proper collateral ligaments) and for the fan-shaped suspensory metatarsoglenoid ligaments (accessory collateral ligaments).[2,3] The MTP joint proper collateral ligaments, which course obliquely to insert onto the medial and lateral

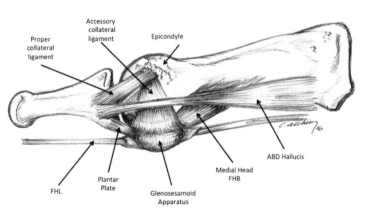

Fig. 2. Anatomy of the first metatarsophalangeal joint, medial view. ABD, abductor; FHB, flexor hallucis brevis; FHL, flexor hallucis longus.

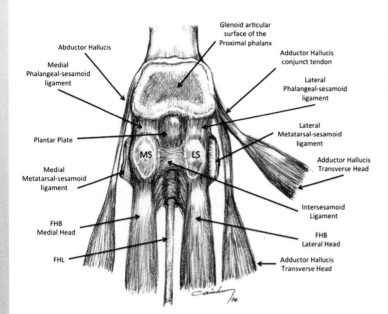

Fig. 3. Anatomy of the first metatarsophalangeal joint, dorsal view (the first metatarsal was removed). FHB, flexor hallucis brevis; FHL, flexor hallucis longus; LS, lateral sesamoid; MS, medial sesamoid.

phalangeal tubercles, play an important role in stabilization of the joint in the transverse plane. The suspensory (accessory collateral) ligaments broadly insert along the medial and lateral borders of the MTP joint plantar plates, which they stabilize.

The rounded metatarsal heads articulate with shallow, ovoid, concave bases of the proximal phalanges. These "glenoid" cavities are smaller than the articular surfaces of the metatarsal heads, conferring a degree of inherent instability to the MTP joints.

The anatomy of the lesser MTP joints is somewhat simpler than that of the first ray. The fibrocartilaginous plantar plate is now recognized as the primary stabilizer of the lesser MTP joints, especially in the dorsal–plantar direction.[2,4–6] The plantar plate firmly inserts onto the plantar bases of the lesser toe proximal phalanges. Along with its connections from the distal plantar fascia, accessory collateral ligaments (suspensory ligaments) and deep transverse intermetatarsal ligament, it acts as a cradle for the metatarsal head.[2,7] Dorsal and plantar interossei and lumbrical tendons insert onto the bases of the proximal phalanges, helping to maintain balance and function of the lesser MTP joints. At the central plantar surface of the plantar plate, a fibrous tunnel accommodates the flexor digitorum longus and brevis tendons (**Table 2**).

Both the extensor digitorum longus and brevis tendons cross the dorsal surface of the lesser MTP joint inside a fibroaponeurotic sling—the extensor hood—that helps to maintain joint balance (**Figs. 4** and **5**).

TURF TOE (FIRST METATARSOPHALANGEAL JOINT)

Hyperextension injury of the first MTP joint was first reported by Ryan and colleagues in 1975. The following year, Bowers and Martin coined the term "turf toe" owing its prevalence in American football players injured while wearing flexible shoes on artificial turf.[8–10]

Unfortunately, varied pathologies of the first MTP joint have been incorrectly bundled along with the diagnosis of turf toe, creating some confusion in the literature.[10] The classic "turf toe" lesion occurs when an axial force is applied to the foot while the great toe is fixed to the ground with hyperextension of the MTP joint (**Fig. 6**). The glenosesamoid apparatus and the plantar ligaments are the most frequently injured structures.[8,9,11] Depending on the intensity of the force applied to the foot, injuries can range in severity from mild sprain to complete disruption of the plantar structures (**Table 3**).

In contradistinction to turf toe, "sand toe" was described as an injury resulting from hyperplantarflexion of any of the MTP joints. This most commonly occurs in barefoot beach volleyball players. The most frequently affected structures in sand toe are the extensor tendons, the extensor hood and the articular capsule.[12]

Diagnosis

The diagnosis of the first MTP joint injuries is based not only on an accurate history, but also thorough physical examination and imaging studies. It is important to identify the points of

Table 2
Intrinsic muscles acting in the dynamic stabilization and function of the metatarsophalangeal joints

	Proximal	Phalanx
	Medial Plantar Tubercle (1) **Medial Metatarsophalangeal Joint** **Capsule (2)**	**Lateral Plantar Tubercle**
Great toe	Abductor hallucis + medial head of flexor hallucis brevis (1)	Adductor hallucis + lateral head of flexor hallucis brevis
Second toe	First dorsal interosseous (1) First lumbrical (2)	Second dorsal interosseous
Third toe	First plantar interosseous (1) Second lumbrical (2)	Third dorsal interosseous
Fourth toe	Second plantar interosseous (1) Third lumbrical (2)	Fourth dorsal interosseous
Fifth toe	Third plantar interosseous (1) Fourth lumbrical (2)	Abductor digitus V + digitus V short flexor

tenderness, ecchymosis, and swelling to correlate them with the deep anatomic structures potentially involved in the lesion.

The MTP joint drawer test is very useful to establish and grade joint instability. It is important to test the joint stability in different directions—varus stress/valgus stress/hyperflexion—because of the possibility of coexisting lesions in multiple planes. Comparison with the asymptomatic contralateral foot is extremely helpful.

Weight-bearing anteroposterior and lateral radiographs may show avulsion fractures of the proximal phalanx and sesamoids as well as proximal migration of the sesamoids, which may accompany complete rupture of the distal insertion of the glenosesamoid apparatus.[13] Waldrop and colleagues[10] showed that, when the distance between the sesamoids and the proximal phalanx differed by 3 mm or more between the right and left feet, then that was a significant and predictive of severe injury to the hallucal plantar plate (**Fig. 7**).

A dorsiflexed lateral radiograph of the hallux or fluoroscopic imaging can easily assess proximal migration of the glenosesamoid apparatus, diastasis of sesamoids, fractures or other coexisting lesions.

MR imaging is the most powerful diagnostic tool for assessment of soft tissue and cartilaginous injuries related to turf toe. By comparison, radiography, arthrography, and computed tomography have limited tissue contrast resolution, which is necessary to delineate the fine anatomic structures of the MTP joint of the great toe.[14] Although high-resolution ultrasonography can delineate soft

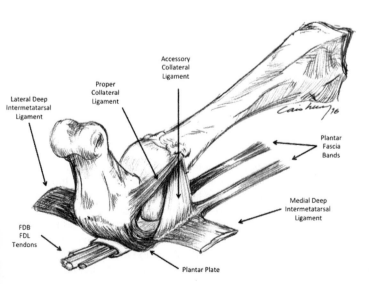

Fig. 4. Anatomy of the lesser metatarsophalangeal joints, dorsomedial view. FDB, flexor digitorum brevis; FDL, flexor digitorum longus.

Accessory Collateral Ligament

Proper Collateral Ligament

Lateral Deep Intermetatarsal Ligament

Plantar Fascia Bands

Medial Deep Intermetatarsal Ligament

FDB FDL Tendons

Plantar Plate

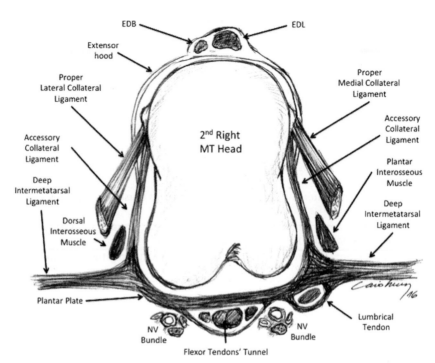

Fig. 5. Anatomy of the lesser metatarsophalangeal joints, coronal cut. EDB, extensor digitorus brevis; EDL, extensor digitorus longus; NV, neurovascular.

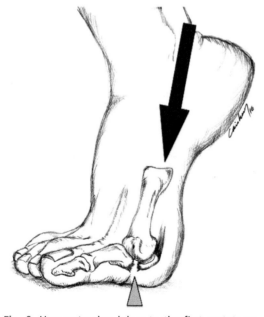

Fig. 6. Hyperextension injury to the first metatarso-phalangeal (MTP) joint. "Turf toe" injury occurs when an axial force (*black arrow*) is applied to the foot while the great toe is fixed on the ground, with hyperextension of the MTP joint and rupture of the glenosesamoid apparatus (*gray arrow head*).

tissue structures about the first MTP joint, it is not useful for the evaluation of the associated osseous and cartilaginous injuries.[15]

The MR imaging protocol should include at least 1 non–fat-suppressed T1-weighted or proton density-weighted sequence to delineate the anatomy (**Figs. 8** and **9**).[16] Some authors prefer proton density weighted sequences because of the superior detail of the ligaments and tendons and the improved delineation of the chondral surfaces.[17] In addition, fat-suppressed proton density-weighted sequences or short tau inversion recovery sequences in the coronal, axial, and sagittal planes are recommended for optimal evaluation of fluid and edema associated with acute pathology.[16]

The plantar plate and hallucal sesamoids are analyzed best in sagittal and coronal short axis planes. MR imaging can show variable patterns related to heterogeneous signal intensity resulting from a partial or complete tear of the plantar plate.[18] The lateral deep intermetatarsal ligament is visualized only in the coronal short axis plane.[14] Main collateral ligaments and sesamoid ligaments are analyzed best in the axial long axis and coronal short axis plane. Although it is not commonly performed, and unnecessary in the context of acute

Table 3
Classification and grading system for turf toe injury according to Anderson and Shawen

Injury	Grade	Description
Hyperextension (turf toe)	I	Attenuation of the glenosesamoid complex
		Local tenderness, minimal swelling and ecchymosis
	II	Partial tear of the glenosesamoid complex
		Diffuse tenderness, moderate swelling and ecchymosis
		Restricted painful movement
	III	Complete disruption of the glenosesamoid complex
		Severe tenderness, marked swelling and ecchymosis
		Limited painful movement + positive MTP drawer test
Hyperflexion (sand toe)		Hyperflexion injury of MTP or interphalangeal joint
		Lesser MTP joints may be involved
Dislocation	I	Dislocation of the hallux with the sesamoids
		No lesion of the intersesamoid ligament
	IIA	Associate disruption of the intersesamoid ligament
	IIB	Associate transverse fracture of one of both sesamoids
	IIC	Complete disruption of the intersesamoid ligament with fracture of one of the sesamoids

Abbreviation: MTP, metatarsophalangeal.

Data from Anderson RB, Shawen SB. Great-toe disorders. In: Porter DA, Schon LC, editors. Baxter's the foot and ankle in sport. 2nd edition. Philadelphia: Elsevier Health Sciences; 2007. p. 411–33.

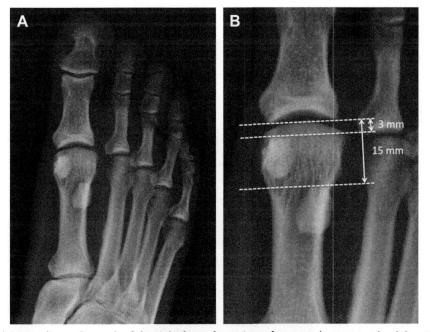

Fig. 7. (*A*) Plain standing radiograph of the right foot of a patient after acute hyperextension injury to the great toe or "turf toe." The lateral sesamoid is grossly displaced proximally suggesting a partial tear of the glenosesamoid apparatus. (*B*) Magnified view of the first metatarsal. The tibial sesamoid is in its normal position 3 mm proximal to the phalangeal border and the fibular sesamoid lies 15 mm proximal in relation to the phalangeal border indicating a significant injury.

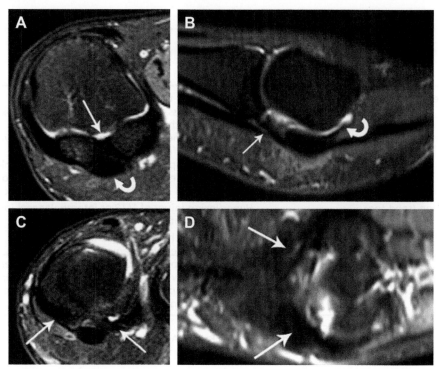

Fig. 8. MR images of a normal metatarsophalangeal hallucal complex. Coronal T2-weighted fat-suppressed image (*A*) demonstrate intersesamoid ligament with low signal intensity (*straight arrow*), deep to the normal flexor hallucis longus tendon (*curved arrow*). Sagittal T2-weighted fat suppressed image (*B*): normal anatomy of the sesamoid phalangeal ligament (*straight arrow*) and metatarsosesamoid ligament (*curved arrow*). Sesamoid phalangeal ligament (*straight arrow*) can also be identified on coronal (*C*) and axial (*D*) planes.

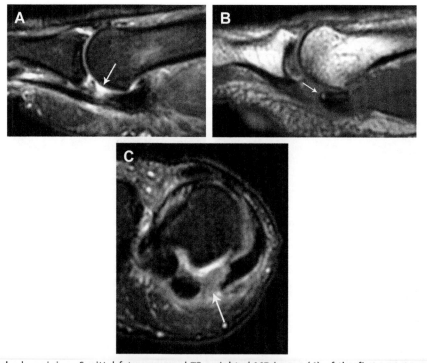

Fig. 9. Squash player injury. Sagittal fat-suppressed T2-weighted MR image (*A*) of the first metatarsophalangeal (MTP) illustrates a complete tear of the proximal medial sesamoid phalangeal ligament (*arrow*). Sagittal T1-weighted MR image (*B*) of the first MTP. Note the proximal retraction of the medial sesamoid (*arrow*). Coronal short axis fat-suppressed T2-weighted (*C*), demonstrates sesamoid-phalangeal ligament tear with adjacent edema (*arrow*).

injury with posttraumatic fluid signal distention of the joint, MR arthrography has been reported to enhance visualization of many of these structures.[14]

Treatment

First-line treatment of turf toe is conservative based on "RICE" (rest, ice, compression, and elevation). Non–weight-bearing protection or immobilization of the joint is essential to control pain and prevent additional tissue damage in the acute posttraumatic period. After a few days, as pain subsides, careful rehabilitation commences. The challenge lies in finding the balance between the restoring the physiologic range of motion and protecting the healing tissues. Taping and rigid insoles are often used to protect the great toe MTP joint, until recovery is complete.

All grades of turf toe can be treated conservatively; however, higher grade injuries take longer to heal, with greater delay in return to full activity. Fortunately, few cases of turf toe require surgical treatment. According to McCormick and Anderson,[8,9] there are strict indications for surgical treatment of turf toe that include (**Box 1**): (1) large capsular avulsion with unstable joint (coronal, sagittal or transverse planes), (2) diastasis and/or retraction of the sesamoids (fracture or bipartite), (3) traumatic hallux valgus/varus deformity, (4) osteochondral injury (including loose bodies), and (5) failed conservative treatment.[8]

Box 1

Indications for turf toe surgical treatment

Strict indications for surgical treatment of the turf toe lesions

1. Large capsular avulsion with unstable metatarsophalangeal joint (coronal, sagittal or transverse planes)

2. Diastasis and/or retraction of the sesamoids (fracture or bipartite)

3. Traumatic hallux valgus/varus deformity

4. Osteochondral injury (first metatarsal head), including loose bodies

5. Failed conservative treatment (unstable and painful joint)

Data from McCormick JJ, Anderson RB. The great toe: failed turf toe, chronic turf toe, and complicated sesamoid injuries. Foot Ankle Clin 2009;14:135–50; and McCormick JJ, Anderson RB. Turf toe: anatomy, diagnosis, and treatment. Sports Health 2010;2:487–94.

LESSER METATARSOPHALANGEAL JOINT INSTABILITY

Although acute trauma can lead to lesser MTP joint instability (16%), instability of the lesser MTP joints is more commonly a chronic, degenerative condition.[5] Compressive and tensile forces chronically applied to the hyperextended MTP joint contribute to attenuation and insufficiency of the stabilizing structures, which ultimately results in a painful, deformed, and dysfunctional toe.[19] The "crossover toe" is the end-stage disabling deformity, which was first described by Coughlin in 1987[20] (**Fig. 10**). Although the normal function of the lesser MTP joints depends on an intricate balance between bones, articular ligaments, and tendons, the deterioration and rupture of the plantar plate seems to be the most important fact in the genesis of lesser MTP joint instability.[4]

Acute pain under the affected metatarsal head and the sensation of plantar swelling are the very first clinical signs. A few days later, widening of the interdigital space can be seen. Clinical distinction of acute metatarsalgia owing to plantar plate tear, intermetatarsal bursitis, interdigital (Morton) neuroma, and stress fracture may be very challenging.

The affected toe progressively loses "ground touch" and "toe purchase" (the dynamic ability of the toe to push against the ground, which connotes normal muscle balance and function), that can be detected and measured using the "paper pull out test."[21] The most predictive and reliable test to identify and quantify MTP joint instability is the Hamilton-Thompson MTP drawer test, which measures the degree of subluxation or dislocation at the MTP joint (**Fig. 11**).[5]

Coughlin and colleagues[6] proposed a Clinical Staging System for MTP joint instability that correlates toe alignment with the most important

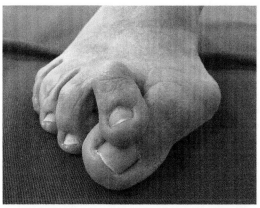

Fig. 10. The classic crossover toe deformity. This represents end-stage deformity resulting from plantar plate injury of the second metatarsophalangeal joint.

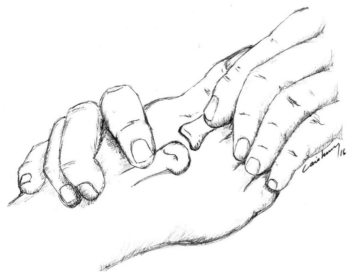

Fig. 11. Hamilton-Thompson MTP drawer test is a predictive and reliable clinical test for MTP joint instability, assessing the degree of subluxation or dislocation under stress. *P*<.0001. MTP, metatarsophalangeal.

Correlation	Grade 0 (%)	Grade 1 (%)	Grade 2 (%)	Grade 3 (%)	Grade 4 (%)
MTP drawer test: grade I (<50%)	100	72	60	35	0
MTP drawer test: grade 2 (>50%)	0	8	40	42	35
MTP drawer test: grade 3 (dislocatable)	0	0	0	13	29
MTP drawer test: grade 4 (dislocated)	0	0	0	0	35

(*From* Nery C, Coughlin MJ, Baumfeld D, et al. Classification of metatarsophalangeal joint plantar plate injuries: history and physical examination variables. J Surg Orthop Adv 2014;23:218; with permission.)

physical findings (**Table 4**). Based on cadaveric studies and a surgical series, an Anatomic Grading System for the plantar plate lesions was proposed[6,22,23] (**Figs. 12** and **13**, **Table 5**). This anatomic grading has been shown to correlate strongly with the clinical staging system. The comparison of the ability to identify and describe lesser toes plantar plate tears by 2 groups of radiologists (one who were knowledgeable of the anatomic pattern of plantar plate tears and another that had no notion of the anatomic patterns of the tears) showed that familiarity with the anatomic grading system improved radiologists' diagnostic accuracy in characterizing plantar plate tears, which is an important help to the surgeons in preoperative planning.[5,24]

Diagnosis

The primary evaluation of plantar plate injury is based on the clinical examination with adjunctive diagnostic imaging. Radiographs, ultrasound imaging, and MR imaging have been the primary diagnostic imaging tools used by clinicians to assist in their evaluation.[25] There has even been reported utility of dual-energy computed tomography in a recent case report.[26]

At initial presentation, foot standing radiographs are obtained to rule out other osseous pathology, including fracture, dislocation, and advanced osteonecrosis,[27] keeping in mind that both fracture and early stage osteonecrosis are commonly radiographically occult. Radiography is helpful for assessment of MTP joint arthritis, hallucal sesamoid position, metatarsal length, phalangeal deviation, subluxation, and hyperextension.

There are both developmental anatomic factors that might predispose to, and acquired deformities that may result from, plantar plate tears. Three measurements based on anteroposterior weight-bearing radiographs (an increased first metatarsal declination angle, and increased second metatarsal declination angle, and a second metatarsal protrusion distance of >2 mm) were shown to correlate with plantar plate tear in greater than 75% of cases in a series reported by Klein and colleagues.[27] This indicates that a long second metatarsal likely predisposes to plantar plate tear. In a

Table 4
MTP joint instability: Clinical staging system

Grade	Alignment	Physical Examination
0	MTP joint alignment; pain with no deformity	Plantar pain, thickening or swelling under MTP joint, reduced toe purchase, negative drawer test
1	Mild misalignment, widening of web space, medial toe deviation	MTP joint pain and swelling, loss of toe purchase, mild positive drawer test (<50% subluxable)
2	Moderate misalignment, medial, lateral, dorsal or dorsomedial deformity, hyperextension of toe	MTP joint pain, reduced swelling, no toe purchase, moderate positive drawer test (>50% subluxable)
3	Severe misalignment, dorsal or dorsomedial deformity, crossover toe or flexible hammertoe	MTP joint and toe pain, little swelling, no toe purchase, very positive drawer test (dislocatable MTP joint) and flexible hammertoe
4	Dorsomedial or dorsal dislocation, severe deformity, fixed hammertoe	MTP joint and toe pain, little or no swelling, no toe purchase, dislocated MTP joint, fixed hammertoe

Abbreviation: MTP, metatarsophalangeal.

recent publication by Umans and colleagues[28] based on MR imaging, second metatarsal protrusion of greater than 4 mm was also found to trend toward correlation with plantar plate tear (**Fig. 14**).

Related predisposing morphology includes subtle cavus foot structure, mildly increased metatarsus adductus, a supinated foot, or a forefoot varus deformity, all of which result in a plantar-flexed "shortened" position of the first ray. With relative shortening of the first ray, the second metatarsal is relatively "lengthened." Resultant overload of the second metatarsal head and plantar structures, including the plantar plate, predisposes to tissue deterioration. As the supporting soft tissue structures deteriorate, toe deformity ensues and manifests radiographically as transverse plane splaying of the digits (tibial deviation of the second toe and fibular deviation of the third

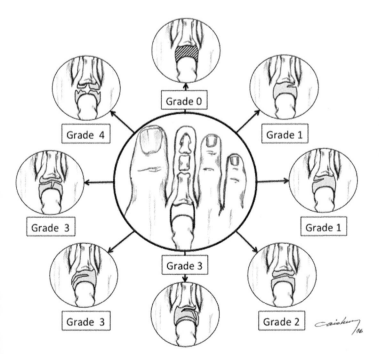

Fig. 12. Anatomic grading system of lesser metatarsophalangeal joint plantar plate tears: grade 0 = attenuation; grade 1 = partial transverse distal tear (<50%)—lateral or medial; grade 2 = complete transverse distal tear (>50%–100%); grade 3 = combination of transverse and longitudinal tears – "7," "T," or "inverted 7" shapes; grade 4 = extensive tear with buttonhole.

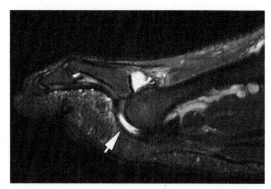

Fig. 13. Sagittal MR image of the second metatarsophalangeal joint, showing an extensive plantar plate tear with the characteristic buttonhole appearance (*arrow*).

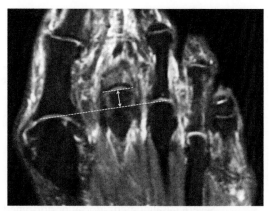

Fig. 14. Second metatarsal protrusion. A line tangent to the most distal points of the first and third metatarsals heads is drawn. The "second metatarsal protrusion" is the perpendicular distance (in millimeters) from this baseline to the distal tip of the second metatarsal head. Note that the landmarks of the distal borders of the metatarsal heads may lie on adjacent images and may be necessary to scroll between them to determine exactly your references.

toe), sagittal plane instability (varus angulation of the second MTP joint angle >6°), or both.

The metatarsal parabola is an old, but useful, concept that aims to understand the physiologic relationship between the lengths of the metatarsals in a normal subject. According to Maestro, "in the normal parabola the metatarsal heads were positioned according to a geometric progression by a factor of 2."[27] This concept defines forefoot radiologic images where one can see the second metatarsal 3 mm longer than the third that is 6 mm longer than the fourth that is 12 mm longer than the fifth metatarsal (the harmonic morphotype).[27,29] It can be assessed according to 3 methods: (1) the arc method described by Hardy and Clapham, (2) the second metatarsal protrusion

distance, and (3) the harmonious morphotype method described by Maestro and colleagues. All methods were found to be of equal usefulness by Klein and colleagues.[27] This description is useful for assessing disharmonious morphotypes that are associated with pathology, and for surgical planning to correct the metatarsal parabola. In radiologic evaluation, weight-bearing anteroposterior and lateral views suffice, without the need for special forefoot or toe views.[29]

MR imaging and ultrasound examination provide further details in the diagnostic evaluation of plantar plate pathology. The plantar plate is a superficial fibrocartilaginous structure which is easily accessible and visible in its entirety by ultrasound[30,31] (**Figs. 15** and **16**). Gregg and colleagues[30] compared ultrasound and MR imaging detection of plantar plate pathology in both symptomatic and asymptomatic feet and found only fair correlation between MR imaging and intraoperative findings, whereas longitudinal and transverse plane sonographic images showed moderate to high correlation, respectively.[30] It should be noted, however, that operative correlation was available in only 10 of the 160 symptomatic joints.[32] Klein and colleagues[32] also compared plantar plate ultrasound and MR imaging with a surgical gold standard and showed that MR imaging and ultrasound examination were both highly sensitive (73.9% and 91.5%, respectively), but MR imaging offered 100% specificity, whereas ultrasound examination was poorly specific. In all series, sonography is extremely sensitive for detection of plantar

Table 5
Anatomic grading system of plantar plate tears

Grade	Patterns of Soft Tissue Evolvement
0	Plantar plate and capsular attenuation and/or discoloration
1	Transverse distal tear adjacent to insertion to the proximal phalanx (<50%, more frequently at the lateral area)
2	Transverse distal tear (>50%, almost 100%)
3	Transverse distal tear (>50%, frequently 100%) combined with a longitudinal extensive tear: Medial (inverted "7" shape), Central ("T" shape) or Lateral ("7" shape)
4	Extensive tear with buttonhole (dislocation) resulting from the combination of transverse and longitudinal tears. Little or no plantar plate tissue to repair

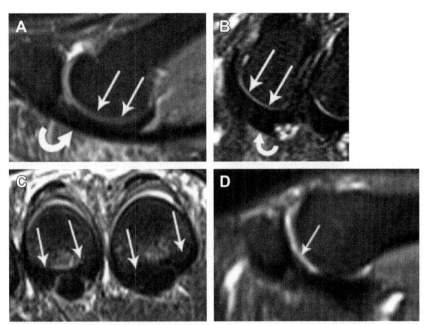

Fig. 15. MR images of a normal lesser metatarsophalangeal joint. Sagittal T2-weighted fat-suppressed image (*A*): normal appearance of the plantar plate (PP; *straight arrow*) with low signal intensity, deep to the normal flexor tendons (*curved arrow*). Coronal T2-weighted fat-suppressed image (*B*) of the central portion of a normal PP (*straight arrow*) at the level of the metatarsal head. In the same image, one can see the normal flexor tendons (*curved arrow*). Distally it is possible to see normal insertion of PP (*straight arrow*) at the base of proximal phalanx (*C*). This insertion can also be seen in the sagittal plane (*straight arrow*) (*D*).

plate pathology, but is relatively nonspecific in distinguishing between degeneration and tear.

Although MR imaging and ultrasound examination are appropriate modalities for the evaluation of plantar plate, ultrasound performance is strongly user dependent, and reproducible only in the hands of highly skilled professionals. Based on our experience, MR imaging is affords a greater degree of reproducibility between different institutions.

Different MR imaging protocols for evaluation of the plantar plate have been reported in the literature. Podiatrists Klein and colleagues[32] and Sung and colleagues[25] reported good diagnostic performance using 0.3 T MR imaging, imaging in 3 orthogonal planes using T1, T2 and short T1 inversion recovery sequences. Most radiologists, however, favor imaging of small parts using high field strength MR imaging, given the inherent superiority in spatial resolution and practical advantage of more rapid imaging time. Gregg and colleagues[33] and Umans and colleagues[34] used 1.5 T and 3.0 T MR imaging. Gregg and colleagues[33] performed proton density fast-spin echo sequences and T2-weighted fat-suppressed fast-spin echo sequences in the coronal, axial, and sagittal

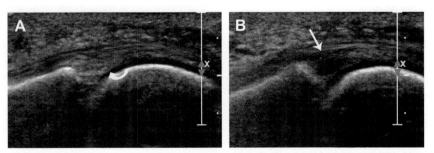

Fig. 16. Plantar plate (PP) ultrasound image of the second metatarsophalangeal, sagittal plane. (*A*) Normal appearance of PP as a labral-like, slightly echogenic and homogeneous structure (*curved arrow*). (*B*) Hypoechoic area of discontinuity (*arrow*) in the distal attachment of the PP, adjacent to the base of the proximal phalanx, compatible with PP tear.

planes using a 10 cm field of view and 2-mm slices with no gap. Umans and colleagues[34] performed axial long axis and coronal short axis T1-weighted and fat-suppressed proton-density, T2-weighted and sagittal fat-suppressed proton-density, or T2-weighted images using 10- to 12-cm of view and 2- to 3-mm slice thickness in the short axis and sagittal plane and 2- to 2.5-mm slice thickness in the long axis images.

Although arthrography is not widely used in the evaluation of plantar plate tears, it has been reported as a useful adjunct to MR imaging. Yao and colleagues[18] first reported pathologic communication of MTP intraarticular contrast with the flexor tendon sheath as diagnostic of plantar plate tear using conventional arthrography. Subsequently, using a cadaveric model, Mohana-Borges and colleagues[35] showed MR arthrography to be superior to standard MR imaging for depiction of the articular surface of plantar plate, proximal and distal attachments, and the connections of plantar plate with collateral ligaments. Kier and colleagues[36] later described the use of MR arthrography for the evaluation of painful conditions of second and third MTP joints, but did not compare the relative diagnostic performance of conventional MR imaging to MR arthrography. Recently, Lepage-Saucier and colleagues[36] reported the combination of toe traction and MR arthrography to be superior to conventional MR imaging in assessment of articular cartilage and plantar plate pathology in a small cadaveric series.

In our experience, MR imaging of the plantar plate is ideally performed using high field units, typically without intraarticular contrast using a small field of view and small surface coil. Axial long axis and coronal short axis T1-weighted, sagittal, axial long axis, and coronal short axis fat-suppressed T2-weighted or proton-density images should be obtained, with contiguous thin slices no thicker than 3 mm in the sagittal and coronal short axis. It is important to achieve high spatial resolution, because tears can be quite small and the plantar plate measures only 12 mm in the transverse plane.

MR IMAGING OF THE NORMAL PLANTAR PLATE

In the sagittal plane, proton-density and T2-weighted sequences depict the normal plantar plate as a uniform dark signal. The plantar plate cradles and articulates with the metatarsal head. The hypointense flexor tendon courses beneath the plantar plate and seems to blend with it, with a typically nondiscernable intervening cleavage plane. The origin of the plantar plate at the level of the metatarsal shaft, just proximal to the flare

of the metatarsal head, is poorly delineated from the flexor tendon. The insertional fibers are well-delineated against the articular cortex of the proximal phalanx.[31]

Umans and Elsinger reported a normal, discretely marginated, high signal intensity zone at the midsagittal phalangeal insertion of the plantar plate that measures up to 2.5 mm.[34] Mohana-Borges and colleagues[35] subsequently clarified that this represents an anatomic recess, which they identified in the midsagittal plane in 47% of imaged MTP joints. This normal capsular recess must not be mistaken for a plantar plate tear (**Fig. 17**).

In coronal short axis proton density and T2-weighted fat-suppressed images, the plantar plate appears as a C-shaped low signal intensity band centered under the metatarsal head. On the plantar surface a central groove accommodates the flexor tendons. The plantar plate is of low signal intensity, similar to the flexor tendons. The proper collateral ligaments blend with the plantar plate at their insertion bilaterally onto the base of proximal phalanx. The insertional fibers are also hypointense adjacent to the articular cortex of the proximal phalanx.[31] Collateral ligaments have a close relationship with the interosseous, abductor digiti minimi, and flexor digiti minimi brevis tendons. Distally, these complexes are attached both to the base of the proximal phalanges and the plantar plate. Axial long axis images are best for evaluating the attachment of collateral ligaments onto the bilateral base of the proximal phalanges, but coronal short axis and sagittal images are necessary for evaluating the integrity of the plantar plate.[35]

MR IMAGING OF PLANTAR PLATE TEARS

Yao and colleagues[18] first described the utility of MR imaging in evaluating plantar plate tear.[34,38] Using a surgical gold standard, they found that

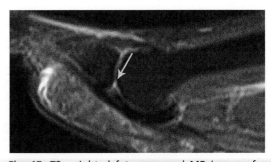

Fig. 17. T2-weighted fat-suppressed MR image of a normal plantar plate (PP), sagittal plane. Poorly defined area of moderately increased signal intensity, compatible with normal PP recess (*arrow*).

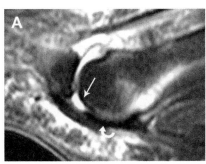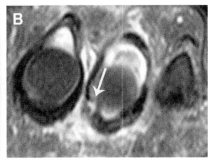

Fig. 18. T2-weighted fat-suppressed MR image of direct sign of plantar plate (PP) tear, sagittal (*A*) and coronal (*B*) planes of the third metatarsophalangeal. Replacement of normal low signal PP fibers with a hyperintense focus (*arrow*), compatible with PP tear. The intact proximal portion of the plantar plate is seen on the sagittal image (*curved arrow*).

focal high signal intensity of the plantar plate identified on fluid-sensitive sequences correlated with plantar plate tear.[39] A bright T2 signal defect at the insertion of the plantar plate is accepted as a direct sign of a plantar plate tear[28,39] (**Fig. 18**). Tears appear hyperintense on both proton density-weighted and T2-weighted fat-suppressed images. Retraction of a torn plantar plate is best assessed in the sagittal plane. Coronal short axis images best delineate the location of tear in relation to the collateral ligaments and flexor tendon. Although the distinction can be difficult, partial versus full-thickness tears can be assessed in both the sagittal and coronal planes.

Umans and colleagues[34] reported intermetatarsal space nonneuromatous lesions in association with plantar plate tear. Pericapsular fibrosis accompanies most cases of plantar plate tear and, like some Morton neuromas, it is intermediate signal on T1- and T2-weighted images[34] (**Fig. 19**). The key difference is that pericapsular fibrosis is eccentrically located within the interspace and broadly abuts the plantar lateral and lateral aspect of the MTP joint, whereas Morton neuroma is centrally located within the interspace, typically extending plantar to the level of the deep transverse intermetatarsal ligament. The importance of this finding is 2-fold. Eccentric pericapsular fibrosis is now recognized as a useful correlate, which may be more readily apparent than a small defect, for the diagnosis of plantar plate tear. It has also been recognized that many cases of plantar plate tear with associated pericapsular fibrosis have been misdiagnosed and mistreated as neuroma. Misdiagnosis of plantar plate tear and pericapsular fibrosis and mistreatment; neuroma can prolong pain and dysfunction, permit development of progressive deformity, and possibly adversely affect outcomes of definitive surgery.

Although the classic direct sign of plantar plate tear on MR imaging is widely accepted, represented by partial or complete discontinuity of the plantar plate on fluid-sensitive sequences with fluid interposition, there is no consensus regarding other morphologic changes of the plantar plate seen on MR imaging studies. In our experience, other changes include thinning or nonvisualization of the plantar plate, pericapsular fibrosis, increased distance between the distal margin of plantar plate and the base of the proximal phalanx, and distortion of the interosseous tendon and collateral ligament complex, all of which might help in the diagnosis of plantar plate tear. In our unpublished data (André F. Yamada and colleagues, 2016), pericapsular fibrosis was strongly associated with plantar plate tears, with an odds ratio of 103.3 (95% confidence interval, 9.6–1108.5; $P<.001$). In addition, these data indicated that the distance between the distal margin of plantar plate and the base of the proximal phalanx, with a cutoff value of 0.28 cm, showed a significant association with plantar plate tears (odds ratio, 18.3; 95% confidence interval, 2.9–161.0; $P = .009$).

TREATMENT

The acute posttraumatic form and early stages of chronic, degenerative lesser MTP joint instability can be treated conservatively. The main purpose of noninvasive treatment is pain control, combined with protection and stabilization of the forefoot. This is achieved with taping of the central lesser toes in slight flexion, temporary suspension of weight bearing and reduction of the range of motion of the affected joints. Corticosteroid injections must be avoided because of the potential damage to the soft tissues of the region.

Successful treatment lies in the balance between joint rehabilitation and the protection of

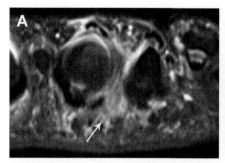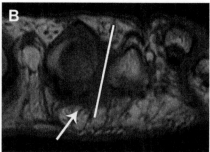

Fig. 19. Coronal short axis fat-suppressed T2-weighted (*A*) and T1-weighted (*B*) images. Pericapsular fibrosis accompanies most cases of plantar plate tear and, like some Morton neuromas, it is intermediate signal on T1 and T2 weighted images (*arrow*). Unlike neuromas, pericapsular fibrosis is positioned eccentrically within the intermetatarsal space (*line*), abutting the second metatarsophalangeal lateral capsule and PP.

the healing tissues. Unfortunately, outcome studies suggest that although conservative therapy may reduce or eliminate pain, deformity and MTP instability tend to worsen over time. When conservative therapy fails to reduce discomfort and deformities worsen, surgery is indicated.

Older surgical techniques focused on restoration of joint function through soft tissue transfers and reconstruction, but did not attempt to repair the main anatomic structures. Based on unpublished research by Dr Garry P. Jolly, Ford and colleagues[37] in 1998, demonstrated that direct plantar plate repair was a viable alternative for stabilization of the lesser MTP joints. Ever since, repair and reinsertion of the plantar plate onto the base of the phalanx has been considered the surgical treatment of choice. Controversy remains as to whether or not there is a need to combine plantar plate repair with Weil osteotomy and how to address grade 4 lesions in which there is no salvageable soft tissue.

New treatment alternatives must focus on the early stages of MTP joint instability to achieve better patient outcomes. Based on the literature[19,20,33,39–41] and our own experience,[5,42,43] our goals in the treatment of patients with plantar plate tear are to:

1. Correct the metatarsal parabola (to correct lesser metatarsal head protrusion);
2. Reduce pressure under the metatarsal head (to alleviate metatarsalgia);
3. Create room to permit access to the plantar plate (to reinsert it and repair it); and
4. Repair the original anatomic structures and tissues.
5. Consider the impact on the whole forefoot (pay attention to PIP and DIP joints)

In our service, we are using a treatment algorithm[43] for the lesser MTP joint instability based on the Anatomic Grading System that can be summarized as follows:

- Grade 0 and 1 tears—arthroscopic radiofrequency shrinkage plus Weil osteotomy.
- Grades 2 and 3 (all variants)—plantar plate repair and reinsertion through the dorsal approach plus capsular and ligament reefing plus Weil osteotomy.
- Grade 4—flexor digitorus longus tendon transfer to the extensor hood plus Weil osteotomy.

In our practice, all joints are first evaluated by MTP joint arthroscopy. This enables us to grade the tear and treat according to the algorithm as described. The direct repair and reinsertion of the plantar plate in the proximal phalanx can be performed via dorsal or plantar approaches. The dorsal approach is greatly preferred because it permits evaluation and correction of the dynamic and static anatomic structures. Lengthening of the extensor tendons, repairing and balancing the proper and accessory collateral ligaments and joint capsule, and shortening an elongated metatarsal is almost impossible through a plantar approach. Repair of the plantar plate via a dorsal approach has only been made possible by innovations in surgical instruments and techniques, which have only been available in the last 5 years.

Generally, the transverse component of the tear is debrided and reinserted onto the base of the proximal phalanx. Once sutures secure the plantar plate at its phalangeal insertion, they are passed through bone holes and tied in the dorsal aspect the proximal phalanx. Longitudinal tears are repaired using two or three 4-0 or 5-0 nonabsorbable sutures. Lateral soft tissue reefing may be performed as needed to improve toe alignment and stability.

The most common postoperative complications are arthrofibrosis and joint stiffness. This is likely owing to the extent of dissection and soft tissue release in a small anatomic area. It is essential, therefore, to perform all the surgical steps as gently as possible to minimize scarring and retraction of the transected structures. Reefing and balancing the joint and careful hemostasis in all dissected planes at the end of the procedure helps prevent these complications.

POSTOPERATIVE

Healing occurs within 6 weeks but requires another 4 to 6 months for complete maturation. It is important to protect the toes during this period. We recommend keeping the toes in 20° of flexion in a postoperative shoe for 6 weeks. An aggressive rehabilitation program starts at the end of the first week to reduce scarring at the incision site, strengthen the flexor tendons, and maintain joint mobility. It is crucial to prevent passive and active dorsiflexion of the toes for 6 weeks to avoid damaging the plantar plate sutures. Low-heeled shoes with wide toe boxes are advised for 6 months after the surgery, during which time high-impact sports activities should be avoided. Return to play should occur gradually and carefully, to protect the surgical repair and prevent reinjury.

EXPECTATIONS

Direct plantar plate repair using a dorsal approach are promising. Some studies reported excellent pain relief with improved digital strength and realignment at an average follow-up of 1.5 years.[42] Recently, authors have reported favorable results in the treatment of early stages of plantar plate injuries with better postoperative results when compared with correction of later stages with gross instability. These results suggest that surgical treatment of MTP joint instability in the early stages might yield better outcomes.

SUMMARY

The complex anatomy of the MTP joints is critical for proper balance and biomechanics. Imaging studies, particularly MR imaging, play a crucial role in diagnosing plantar plate tear and turf toe injury and for the heterogeneous group of disorders affecting the first and the lesser MTP joint. Equipped with knowledge of local anatomy and the diverse pathologies that can affect this complex, the radiologist can help the referring clinician or surgeon to determine the appropriate treatment plan to minimize morbidity and facilitate faster recovery and rehabilitation.

REFERENCES

1. Sarrafian SK, Kelikian AS. Syndesmology. Sarrafian's anatomy of the foot and ankle: descriptive, topographic, functional. 3rd edition. Philadelphia: Wolters Kluwer/Lippincott Williams & Wilkins; 2011.
2. Deland JT, Lee KT, Sobel M, et al. Anatomy of the plantar plate and its attachments in the lesser metatarsal phalangeal joint. Foot Ankle Int 1995;16: 480–6.
3. Deland JT, Sung IH. The medial crossover toe: a cadaveric dissection. Foot Ankle Int 2000;21:375–8.
4. Chalayon O, Chertman C, Guss AD, et al. Role of plantar plate and surgical reconstruction techniques on static stability of lesser metatarsophalangeal joints: a biomechanical study. Foot Ankle Int 2013; 34:1436–42.
5. Nery C, Coughlin MJ, Baumfeld D, et al. Classification of metatarsophalangeal joint plantar plate injuries: history and physical examination variables. J Surg Orthop Adv 2014;23:214–23.
6. Coughlin MJ, Baumfeld DS, Nery C. Second MTP joint instability: grading of the deformity and description of surgical repair of capsular insufficiency. Phys Sportsmed 2011;39:132–41.
7. Deland JT, Sobel M, Arnoczky SP, et al. Collateral ligament reconstruction of the unstable metatarsophalangeal joint: an in vitro study. Foot Ankle 1992; 13:391–5.
8. McCormick JJ, Anderson RB. The great toe: failed turf toe, chronic turf toe, and complicated sesamoid injuries. Foot Ankle Clin 2009;14:135–50.
9. McCormick JJ, Anderson RB. Turf toe: anatomy, diagnosis, and treatment. Sports Health 2010;2: 487–94.
10. Waldrop NE 3rd, Zirker CA, Wijdicks CA, et al. Radiographic evaluation of plantar plate injury: an in vitro biomechanical study. Foot Ankle Int 2013; 34:403–8.
11. McCormick JJ, Anderson RB. Rehabilitation following turf toe injury and plantar plate repair. Clin Sports Med 2010;29:313–23, ix.
12. Frey C, Andersen GD, Feder KS. Plantarflexion injury to the metatarsophalangeal joint ("sand toe"). Foot Ankle Int 1996;17:576–81.
13. Prieskorn D, Graves SC, Smith RA. Morphometric analysis of the plantar plate apparatus of the first metatarsophalangeal joint. Foot Ankle 1993;14: 204–7.
14. Theumann NH, Pfirrmann CWA, Mohana Borges AVR, et al. Metatarsophalangeal joint of the great toe: normal MR, MR arthrographic, and MR bursographic findings in cadavers. J Comput Assist Tomogr 2002;26:829–38.

15. Luukkainen R, Ekman P, Luukkainen P, et al. Ultrasonographic findings in metatarsophalangeal and talocrural joints in healthy persons. Clin Rheumatol 2008;28:311–3.

16. Crain JM, Phancao JP, Stidham K. MR imaging of turf toe. Magn Reson Imaging Clin N Am 2008;16:93–103, vi.

17. Shindle MK, Foo LF, Kelly BT, et al. Magnetic resonance imaging of cartilage in the athlete: current techniques and spectrum of disease. J Bone Joint Surg Am 2006;88(Suppl 4):27–46.

18. Yao L, Do HM, Cracchiolo A, et al. Plantar plate of the foot: findings on conventional arthrography and MR imaging. AJR Am J Roentgenol 1994;163:641–4.

19. Doty JF, Coughlin MJ, Weil L Jr, et al. Etiology and management of lesser toe metatarsophalangeal joint instability. Foot Ankle Clin 2014;19:385–405.

20. Coughlin MJ. Crossover second toe deformity. Foot Ankle 1987;8:29–39.

21. Bouche RT, Heit EJ. Combined plantar plate and hammertoe repair with flexor digitorum longus tendon transfer for chronic, severe sagittal plane instability of the lesser metatarsophalangeal joints: preliminary observations. J Foot Ankle Surg 2008;47:125–37.

22. Cooper MT, Coughlin MJ. Sequential dissection for exposure of the second metatarsophalangeal joint. Foot Ankle Int 2011;32:294–9.

23. Coughlin MJ, Schutt SA, Hirose CB, et al. Metatarsophalangeal joint pathology in crossover second toe deformity: a cadaveric study. Foot Ankle Int 2012;33:133–40.

24. Nery C, Coughlin MJ, Baumfeld D, et al. MRI evaluation of the MTP plantar plates compared with arthroscopic findings: a prospective study. Foot Ankle Int 2013;34:315–22.

25. Sung W, Weil L Jr, Weil LS Sr, et al. Diagnosis of plantar plate injury by magnetic resonance imaging with reference to intraoperative findings. J Foot Ankle Surg 2012;51:570–4.

26. Stevens CJ, Murphy DT, Korzan JR, et al. Plantar plate tear diagnosis using dual-energy computed tomography collagen material decomposition application. J Comput Assist Tomogr 2013;37:478–80.

27. Klein EE, Weil L Jr, Weil LS Sr, et al. The underlying osseous deformity in plantar plate tears: a radiographic analysis. Foot Ankle Spec 2013;6:108–18.

28. Umans R, Umans B, Umans, H, et al. Predictive MRI correlates of lesser Metatarsophalangeal Joint (MPJ) Plantar Plate (PP) tear. Radiological Society of North America 2014 Scientific Assembly and Annual Meeting. Chicago, IL, November 30-December 5, 2014.

29. Doty JF, Coughlin MJ. Metatarsophalangeal joint instability of the lesser toes and plantar plate deficiency. J Am Acad Orthop Surg 2014;22:235–45.

30. Gregg J, Silberstein M, Schneider T, et al. Sonographic and MRI evaluation of the plantar plate: a prospective study. Eur Radiol 2006;16:2661–9.

31. Gregg JM, Silberstein M, Schneider T, et al. Sonography of plantar plates in cadavers: correlation with MRI and histology. AJR Am J Roentgenol 2006;186:948–55.

32. Klein EE, Weil L Jr, Weil LS Sr, et al. Magnetic resonance imaging versus musculoskeletal ultrasound for identification and localization of plantar plate tears. Foot Ankle Spec 2012;5:359–65.

33. Gregg J, Silberstein M, Clark C, et al. Plantar plate repair and Weil osteotomy for metatarsophalangeal joint instability. J Foot Ankle Surg 2007;13:116–21.

34. Umans H, Srinivasan R, Elsinger E, et al. MRI of lesser metatarsophalangeal joint plantar plate tears and associated adjacent interspace lesions. Skeletal Radiol 2014;43:1361–8.

35. Mohana-Borges AVR, Theumann NH, Pfirrmann CWA, et al. Lesser metatarsophalangeal joints: standard MR imaging, MR arthrography, and MR bursography—initial results in 48 cadaveric joints. Radiology 2003;227:175–82.

36. Lepage-Saucier M, Linda DD, Chang EY, et al. MRI of the metatarsophalangeal joints: improved assessment with toe traction and MR arthrography. AJR Am J Roentgenol 2013;200:868–71.

37. Ford LA, Collins KB, Christensen JC. Stabilization of the subluxed second metatarsophalangeal joint: flexor tendon transfer versus primary repair of the plantar plate. J Foot Ankle Surg 1998;37:217–22.

38. Yao L, Cracchiolo A, Farahani K, et al. Magnetic resonance imaging of plantar plate rupture. Foot Ankle Int 1996;17:33–6.

39. Doty JF, Coughlin MJ. Metatarsophalangeal joint instability of the lesser toes. J Foot Ankle Surg 2014;53:440–5.

40. Weil L Jr, Sung W, Weil LS Sr, et al. Anatomic plantar plate repair using the Weil metatarsal osteotomy approach. Foot Ankle spec 2011;4:145–50.

41. Klein EE, Weil L Jr, Weil LS Sr, et al. Clinical examination of plantar plate abnormality: a diagnostic perspective. Foot Ankle Int 2013;34:800–4.

42. Nery C, Coughlin MJ, Baumfeld D, et al. Lesser metatarsophalangeal joint instability: prospective evaluation and repair of plantar plate and capsular insufficiency. Foot Ankle Int 2012;33:301–11.

43. Nery C, Coughlin MJ, Baumfeld D, et al. Prospective evaluation of protocol for surgical treatment of lesser MTP joint plantar plate tears. Foot Ankle Int 2014;35:876–85.

MR Imaging of Impingement and Entrapment Syndromes of the Foot and Ankle

Edward Sellon, MBBS, MRCS, FRCR,
Philip Robinson, MBChB, MRCP, FRCR*

KEYWORDS

• Ankle • Impingement • Entrapment • MR imaging • Athletic injuries

KEY POINTS

- Impingement is a clinical syndrome of chronic pain and restricted range of movement caused by compression of abnormal bone or soft tissue within the ankle joint.
- Common sites of impingement in the ankle include posterior, posteromedial, anteromedial, anterolateral, and, less commonly, direct anterior; these often coexist and occur in conjunction with other ankle pathologies.
- The presence of synovitis, pericapsular oedema and bone marrow oedema on MR imaging support a diagnosis of impingement in the right clinical context.
- In most cases ankle impingement is managed conservatively, with arthroscopic or open debridement of the abnormal bone or soft tissue reserved for refractory cases.

INTRODUCTION

Impingement syndromes of the ankle are a common cause of chronic pain, instability, and limited range of movement in athletes and the active population. They most commonly occur after a sprain injury or repetitive microtrauma at the extreme ranges of movement. The resultant hemorrhage, reactive synovial hyperplasia, and scarring can lead to abnormal soft tissue interposition within the joint. Developmental or acquired bony spurs or prominences also may impede the normal range of movement. It is painful soft tissue or osseous entrapment within the joint that characterises impingement. The diagnosis is largely clinical but may be supported with a range of imaging techniques. MR imaging is particularly valuable in being able to detect not only the soft tissue and osseous abnormalities involved in these syndromes but also a wide variety of concomitant injuries and other potential causes of ankle pain that also may need to be addressed clinically. It is important to remember that although MR imaging findings help direct surgery and have a high concordance with surgical findings, subclinical asymptomatic disease is often present in athletes, and close correlation with the clinical picture is required.

This heterogenous group of pathologies is categorized according to the anatomic relation to the tibiotalar joint. Broadly speaking there are 3 main types[1]:

1. Anterior impingement, which can be subdivided into anterolateral, anteromedial, and purely anterior impingement.

The authors have nothing to disclose.
Musculoskeletal Centre X-Ray Department, Chapel Allerton Hospital, Chapeltown Road, Leeds LS7 4SA, UK
* Corresponding author.
E-mail address: philip.robinson10@nhs.net

Magn Reson Imaging Clin N Am 25 (2017) 145–158
http://dx.doi.org/10.1016/j.mric.2016.08.004
1064-9689/17/© 2016 Elsevier Inc. All rights reserved.

2. Posterior impingement, subdivided into posterior and posteromedial impingement.
3. Extra-articular lateral hindfoot impingement, which encompasses talocalcaneal and subfibular impingement secondary to a planovalgus foot deformity.

In most cases, ankle impingement is managed conservatively, with arthroscopic or open debridement of the joint reserved for refractory cases. In this review, we describe the anatomy, pathophysiology, clinical presentation, imaging features, and treatment approach of each of ankle impingement syndrome, with a focus on the MR imaging findings.

ANTERIOR IMPINGEMENT SYNDROME

Anterior ankle impingement is a well-established and relatively common cause of chronic ankle pain, particularly in soccer players, runners, and ballet dancers, who sustain repetitive ankle dorsiflexion. Symptoms are generally progressive and relate to impingement of hypertrophied synovial scar tissue and bony spurs within the anterior ankle joint.

Anatomy and Pathophysiology

Ankle instability or repetitive forceful dorsiflexion can result in microtrauma to the anterior joint cartilage and deeper bone layers. Over time, attempted repair, including fibrosis and fibrocartilage proliferation, leads to the formation of bony spurs on the anterior rim of the tibia and sulcus of the talus.[2] These bony spurs or osteophytes can cause anterior joint space narrowing, limiting ankle dorsiflexion (Fig. 1).[3] The term osteophyte does not imply conventional osteoarthritis, rather a proliferative effect of focal premature degeneration. Like any other osteophyte, however, they may break off into the joint, forming a loose body.

Repetitive supination injuries are also known to cause osteophyte formation secondary to damage to the anterior and medial margin of the articular cartilage. Another proposed aetiological factor is direct microtrauma caused by ball striking in soccer with direct impact of the ball typically over the anteromedial tibiotalar joint, where the cartilage is covered only by thin subcutaneous fat.[4] Both mechanisms described occur frequently in soccer players, and it is therefore unsurprising that this population of athletes is so commonly afflicted.[5] Indeed, the condition was first described in European soccer players as "footballer's ankle."[5,6] The theory hypothesised at the time, however, was one of repetitive traction injury of the anterior joint capsule in extreme plantarflexion causing

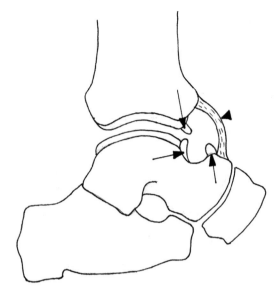

Fig. 1. Diagrammatic representation of the anterior ankle (sagittal) with intra-articular tibiotalar spurs (*arrows*) and hypertrophied anterior capsular thickening (*arrowhead*). (*Courtesy of* Jenna Fielding, MBChB, MRCP, Sheffield, United Kingdom.)

anterior exostoses. This is certainly not the case in the anteromedial ankle, where cadaveric analysis has shown that the bony spurs are intra-articular, consistent with osteophyte formation.[7] The traction hypothesis, however, may still hold true laterally, where growth is sometimes extra-articular and may represent enthesophyte formation.[7]

It is important to remember that the finding of anterior bone spurs does not necessarily mean that the patient is symptomatic. Studies of asymptomatic athletes have found that a significant proportion (45%–59%) have anterior tibiotalar spurs on plain radiograph.[8] It is thought that the associated anterior synovial thickening and scarring, rather than the spurs alone, are responsible for producing the clinical symptoms.[9] Indeed, postexcision recurrence of the bony spurs is not necessarily accompanied by recurrence of symptoms.[9,10] Recent attention has been given to congenital anatomic variants as predisposing factors for the formation of anterior joint space spurs and soft tissue hypertrophy. A cam-type deformity of the talar dome has been described, whereby contact between a noncircular arc morphology of the dome with the anterior tibial plafond during dorsiflexion causes abnormal loading of the talar dome cartilage.[3] In these patients, a cavo-varus foot type is more commonly observed, and the associated external rotation of the tibia is thought to further reduce the tibiotalar joint space.[3] In addition, the orthopaedic literature describes several cases of soft tissue anterior impingement treated successfully by arthroscopic resection of a congenital intra-articular plicae or fibrous bands.[11,12]

Clinical Presentation

The typical symptoms are of chronic anterior ankle pain with subjective feeling of blocking on dorsiflexion. On examination, there is restricted and painful dorsiflexion. There may also be a palpable soft tissue swelling or a spur over the anterior joint. The palpable bone spurs are commonly felt over the anteromedial aspect, whereas the symptoms of soft tissue impingement are on the anterolateral aspect of the ankle.[11,13]

Imaging Features

Diagnosis of anterior impingement is primarily clinical, but conventional, preferably weight-bearing, radiographs are useful for the evaluation of bony spurs and the tibiotalar joint space (**Fig. 2**). Anteromedial osteophytes are best demonstrated on the oblique anteromedial impingement (AMI) view.[14] The plié view (lateral weight-bearing view with the ankle in maximal dorsiflexion) can demonstrate joint space loss and osseous impingement.[15] Radiographic assessment of the tibiotalar joint for secondary signs of degeneration, particularly joint space loss, has prognostic importance. The Van Dijk radiographic classification system, based on osteophyte appearance and degree of joint space narrowing, demonstrated the importance of osteoarthritis as a postoperative prognostic factor.[16] Several more recent studies have agreed that secondary osteoarthritis confers a poorer postoperative prognosis.[9,10]

Further imaging is usually unnecessary. Conventional MR imaging can be used, however, to further characterise the location of the spurs within the joint space and to review the degree of synovitis and joint capsule thickening (**Fig. 3**). It is also useful to check for concomitant pathology, such as osteochondral lesions that may not have been detected on radiography.

Treatment

- Most patients recover with conservative measures, including rest, activity modification, and physical therapy. Particularly in ballet dancers this should be performed in conjunction with correction of technique to correct overpronation where appropriate. Ultrasound can be used to direct intra-articular injection of cortisone and local anaesthetic (**Fig. 4**).
- In resistant cases, however, surgery has been shown to have a long-term benefit. In athletes, arthroscopic resection of the osseous spurs and soft tissue abnormality has shown excellent functional and symptomatic results.[9] The overall prognosis after surgery does depend on the degree of degenerative change evident in the rest of the tibiotalar joint at the time of the surgery.[9,10,17]

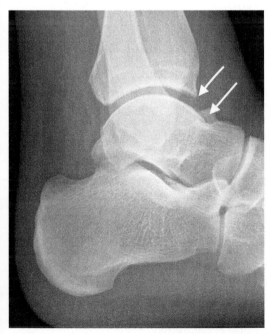

Fig. 2. Soccer player with clinical anterior impingement. Lateral radiograph shows tibiotalar bony spurs (*arrows*).

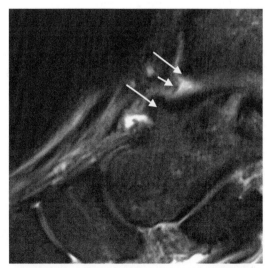

Fig. 3. Sagittal short TI inversion recovery MR image of the ankle of a cricket player shows irregular capsular thickening (*short arrow*) and anterior tibial and talar spurs (*long arrows*).

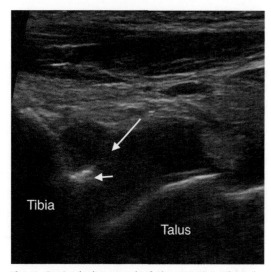

Fig. 4. Sagittal ultrasound of the anterior tibiotalar joint in a rugby player shows hypoechoic synovitis in the anterior joint space (*long arrow*), and an anterior tibial spur (*short arrow*). Ultrasound was used to direct intra-articular injection of corticosteroid and local anaesthetic.

ANTEROLATERAL IMPINGEMENT SYNDROME

Anterolateral impingement is well described in the orthopedic and radiology literature and describes soft tissue hypertrophy and entrapment within the anterolateral recess of the ankle. It is classically described in young athletic patients following an inversion sprain injury with subsequent chronic anterolateral pain and swelling.[2]

Anatomy and Pathophysiology

The anterolateral recess is a triangular structure bordered posteromedially by the anterolateral tibia and talus and posterolaterally by the anterior fibula. Anteriorly it is bordered by the anterolateral joint capsule and capsular ligaments. These include the anterior talofibular, anterior inferior tibiofibular and calcaneofibular ligaments (**Fig. 5**). Ligamentous and capsular tearing and the resultant microinstability and haemorrhage following an ankle sprain may lead to reactive synovial hyperplasia and scarring in the anterolateral gutter.[18,19] Compression of the abnormal soft tissue in the anterolateral gutter during dorsiflexion or eversion can cause severe morbidity and pain, particularly amongst athletes and the younger population. It is estimated that the incidence of anterolateral impingement syndrome is 3% following ankle sprains.[4,17] In advanced cases, the soft tissue can become molded to the triangular shape of the anterolateral gutter. This connective tissue mass was originally described as a

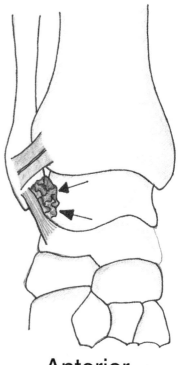

Anterior

Fig. 5. Diagrammatic representation of the anterior ankle (coronal) indicating the typical location of synovitis (*arrows*) within the anterolateral recess involving the capsule between the tibiofibular and tibiotalar ligaments in anterolateral impingement syndrome. (*Courtesy of* Jenna Fielding, MBChB, MRCP, Sheffield, United Kingdom.)

"meniscoid lesion" based on its macroscopic meniscuslike appearance.[20]

Anterolateral impingement also has been described in a subset of patients with an accessory fascicle of the anteroinferior tibiofibular ligament. The ligament is invariably multifascicular, but a discreet inferior fascicle separated from the main body by a fibrofatty septum is variably present (identified in 21%–97% of ankles depending on the exact definition) and considered a normal variant.[18,21] The accessory fascicle of the anteroinferior tibiofibular ligament (Bassett ligament) may normally contact the anterolateral corner of the talus but it is thought that increased contact in dorsiflexion may lead to synovial hypertrophy and impingement within the anterolateral joint space. Ligamentous abrasion of the exposed anterolateral talar cartilage also can sometimes be seen.

Clinical Presentation

The clinical diagnosis of anterolateral impingement is reasonably accurate and based on the anterolateral tenderness, swelling, and pain exacerbated by single-leg squatting, ankle eversion, or dorsiflexion. A provocative physical examination test can be performed in which pressure is applied over the anterolateral ankle while the ankle is brought from the plantar flexed position to full dorsiflexion. A 94.8% sensitivity and 88.0% specificity was reported in a prospective study.[13]

Imaging Features

Anterolateral impingement is predominantly a soft tissue abnormality and therefore radiography and conventional computed tomography (CT) have limited specific utility. Ultrasound and MR imaging can potentially detect abnormal nodular soft tissue extruding anteriorly from the anterolateral gutter. In a retrospective evaluation of ultrasound in a small group of elite soccer players with resistant anterolateral impingement awaiting arthroscopy, synovitic lesions were detected using ultrasound with 100% sensitivity[22] (Fig. 6).

MR imaging has the advantage over ultrasound in being able to assess for whole ankle pathology, including coexisting or alternative causes of prolonged ankle pain, such as marrow contusions, chondral lesions, intra-articular bodies, and sinus tarsi syndrome. MR imaging can show synovial hypertrophy in the anterolateral recess.

The most reliable sign is the obscuration of the anterolateral recess with scar tissue (Fig. 7). It must be remembered that an abnormal nodular or irregular contour of the recess is commonly found in the asymptomatic population and can merely reflect previous anterolateral trauma or surgery. The diagnostic ability of MR imaging in the absence of joint distention with either contrast material or a native effusion remains controversial, with some investigators previously preferring MR

arthrography, as it has a reported sensitivity of 97% and specificity of 100%.[23]

However, with advances in MR imaging hardware technology, MR arthrography is now largely redundant and, with sufficient experience, the diagnosis can be made on conventional MR imaging with relative confidence (75%–83% sensitivity and 75%–100% specificity, depending on the experience of the reporter).[24] Axial T1-weighted images were deemed the most useful for detecting the intermediate to low signal hypertrophy and scarring in the anterolateral gutter.[25] Sagittal T1-weighted images are a useful adjunct, demonstrating anterior displacement of the normal hyperintense fat anterior to the fibula by the hypointense scar tissue. Specificity, however, for all these findings on ultrasound or MR imaging is poor, particularly with regard to the detection of thickened nonenhancing scar tissue.

Treatment

- The initial treatment is conservative, with immobilization, physiotherapy, and nonsteroidal anti-inflammatory medication. Dry needling of the abnormal soft tissue with an intra-articular injection of cortisone and local anaesthetic may be performed under ultrasound guidance, allowing a return to previous levels of activity, even in elite athletes, but this technique has not been evaluated in the literature.
- If these measures fail, arthroscopic evaluation and resection of hypertrophied synovium and scar tissue, including the distal fascicle of the anterior tibiofibular ligament when that is the underlying etiology, has yielded good to excellent symptomatic and functional results.[24,26]

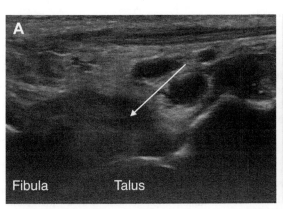
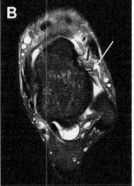

Fig. 6. Rugby league player with previous ankle injuries and persistent anterolateral joint line tenderness. Ultrasound (A) and (B) axial T2-weighted fat-suppressed MR image of the ankle showing a synovitic mass in the anterolateral recess (arrow).

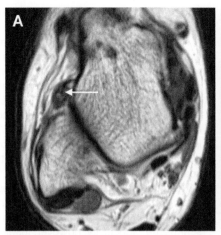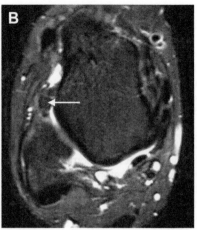

Fig. 7. Rugby league player with a previous lateral ligament injury now presenting with clinical signs of antero-lateral impingement. Axial PD-weighted (*A*) and T2-weighted fat-suppressed (*B*) MR images of the ankle showing a synovitic mass in the anterolateral recess (*arrows*).

ANTEROMEDIAL IMPINGEMENT SYNDROME

AMI is an uncommon cause of chronic ankle pain and usually occurs alongside other pathology, including anterior or anterolateral impingement and chondral lesions. Classic findings include hypertrophic spurs, reactive fibrosis and synovial proliferation along the anteromedial gutter of the tibiotalar joint.

Anatomy and Pathophysiology

Although originally thought to result from a pronation (eversion) injury with traction on the anterior tibiotalar ligament of the deltoid complex, it is now believed to be a rare consequence of a supination (inversion) injury, probably with a rotational component, causing microtrauma and tearing of the anteromedial capsule and tibiotalar ligament[16,25] (**Fig. 8**). The resulting capsular, ligamentous, and synovial hypertrophy and thickening can become compressed during dorsiflexion and inversion.

Clinical Presentation

The diagnosis is usually a clinical one, characterised by anteromedial ankle pain on dorsiflexion and inversion. There is tenderness and swelling along the anteromedial joint line and sometimes restriction of movement and palpable marginal osteophytes on examination.

Imaging Features

If bone spurs are suspected, the AMI view radiograph can be useful.[14] MR imaging features include posttraumatic synovitis, synovial hyperplasia, capsular thickening, and scarring of the anterior tibiotalar ligament (**Fig. 9**).[27] There are,

however, no large imaging studies of AMI. The largest surgical series involved 22 female patients actively involved in competitive gymnastics and demonstrated that 86% had concomitant ankle

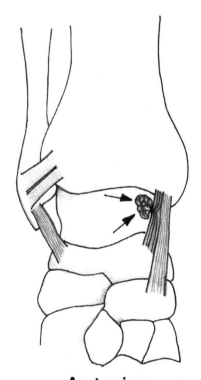

Anterior

Fig. 8. Diagrammatic representation of anteromedial ankle impingement with a "meniscoid" lesion (*arrows*), and a thickened anterior tibiotalar ligament. (*Courtesy of* Jenna Fielding, MBChB, MRCP, Sheffield, United Kingdom.)

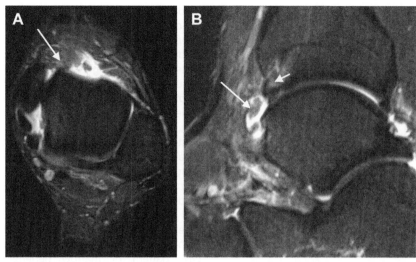

Fig. 9. Rugby league player with AMI. Axial (*A*) and sagittal (*B*) T2-weighted fat-suppressed MR images with irregular soft tissue thickening within the anteromedial ankle joint (*arrow*). The sagittal view (*B*) shows abnormal capsular thickening (*long arrow*) and bone marrow oedema in the anteromedial spur on the distal tibia (*short arrow*).

lesions found at arthroscopy.[28] MR imaging therefore has added value in assessing for related concomitant pathologies.

Treatment

- There are no accounts in the literature of management with purely conservative measures, but these typically involve physiotherapy and heel lifts to improve ankle joint biomechanics.[10,29] One group uses an anaesthetic-only injection at the area of presumed impingement with the patient reassessed clinically a few hours later.[28] Those with a favourable response in terms of pain and mobility return for a localised ultrasound-guided soft tissue steroid injection (**Fig. 10**).
- Surgical osteophyte and soft tissue debridement may give symptomatic relief and functional improvement. In a group of 22 female gymnasts with refractory AMI pain, 64% returned to competitive gymnastics following surgery.[28] Murawski and Kennedy[30] reported good or excellent functional outcomes in 91% of their series of 100 arthroscopic debridements (age range 13–60) with a 5% complication rate and mean return to play in the athletic subpopulation of 7 weeks.

POSTEROMEDIAL IMPINGEMENT

Posteromedial ankle impingement is thought to occur as a consequence of a severe inversion injury. Although there are few reported series in the literature, the identified soft tissue imaging findings on ultrasound and MR imaging are relatively characteristic.[31–33]

Anatomy and Pathophysiology

First described in a surgical case report in 1993, posteromedial impingement has become recognised as an uncommon consequence of severe ankle inversion injury in which the deep fibres of the posterior tibiotalar ligament and the posteromedial capsule become compressed between the medial wall of the talus and posterior margin of the medial malleolus (**Fig. 11**).[31,33,34]

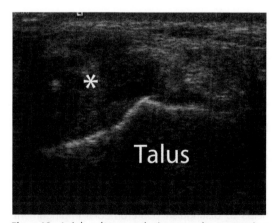

Fig. 10. Axial ultrasound image demonstrating nodular hypoechoic synovitis (*asterisk*) in the anteromedial ankle in a patient with clinical signs of anteromedial impingement. Ultrasound was used to direct intra-articular injection of corticosteroid and local anaesthetic.

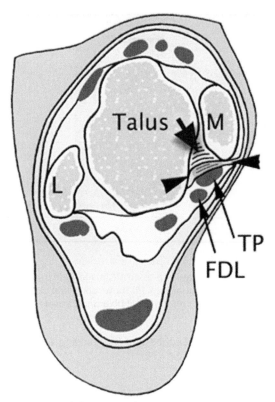

Fig. 11. Axial illustration shows structures involved in posteromedial impingement. FDL, flexor digitorum longus tendon; L, lateral malleolus; M, medial malleolus; TP, tibialis posterior tendon. Arrowheads donate posterior fibres of tibiotalar ligament; short arrow indicates deep fibers of tibiotalar ligament. (*From* Messiou C, Robinson P, O'Connor PJ, et al. Sub-acute posteromedial impingement of the ankle in athletes: MR imaging evaluation and ultrasound guided therapy. Skeletal Radiol 2006;35:89; with permission.)

Inadequate healing and fibrosis can cause painful chronic posteromedial joint impingement. The abnormal hypertrophic soft tissue may displace or encase the surrounding tendons, particular the posterior tibialis tendon.[32,33]

Clinical Presentation

Patients usually present with posteromedial pain, which may occur gradually once the precipitating anterolateral inversion injury signs have resolved. The pain is exacerbated by provocative testing, by palpating the site while moving the ankle into plantarflexion and inversion. This clinical sign helps to distinguish posteromedial impingement from pure posterior tibialis tendon dysfunction.

Imaging Features

Ultrasound and MR imaging have been described in 3 case series, but MR imaging is the imaging modality of choice, as it permits identification of coexisting anterolateral and posteromedial capsule-ligament lesions and particularly associated osteochondral lesions.[1,31–33] Axial proton-density (PD)-weighted and T2-weighted sequences show loss of striation of the posterior tibiotalar ligament, capsular thickening, and oedema around the posteromedial tendons (Fig. 12A, B). Messiou and colleagues[33] demonstrated that, of 9 elite athletes with clinical posteromedial impingement, there was signal abnormality in the posterior tibiotalar ligament in all cases, displacement of the posterior tibialis tendon and flexor digitorum tendon in 7 cases, and disruption of the posterior tibiotalar ligament fibres in 4 cases. Posteromedial tendon encasement was more common in chronic cases. No specific pattern of marrow oedema has been described. As with other impingement syndromes, MR imaging findings are nonspecific, with mild synovitis and thickening sometimes found in asymptomatic cases.

Symptomatic patients with isolated posteromedial synovitis and no associated chondral or ligamentous instability may benefit from ultrasound-guided therapeutic injection. Ultrasound findings include hypoechoic posteromedial capsular thickening deep to and sometimes displacing the tibialis posterior tendon, obscuring the striated detail of the posterior tibiotalar ligament (Fig. 12C).[33]

Treatment

- If conservative measures have failed, ultrasound can be used to identify the capsular abnormality and guide percutaneous dry needling and injection of steroid and local anaesthetic. This approach allows a return to previous levels of activity in elite athletes. In the study by Messiou and colleagues,[33] all athletes returned to preinjury activity within 3 weeks.
- For resistant cases, successful outcome has been reported following surgical resection of abnormal posteromedial soft tissue without ligamentous repair.[31,32]

POSTERIOR IMPINGEMENT

Posterior ankle impingement is a common cause of posterior ankle pain in sports that involve repetitive hyperplantar flexion. It has been extensively described in ballet dancers (due to the "en pointe" or "demi-pointe" positions), in football players (when kicking the ball), cricket players and javelin throwers (front foot planting while throwing or bowling), and horizontal jump athletes (lead foot on toe-off).[35,36] Albisetti and colleagues[37] identified a prevalence of 6.5% during a 1-year

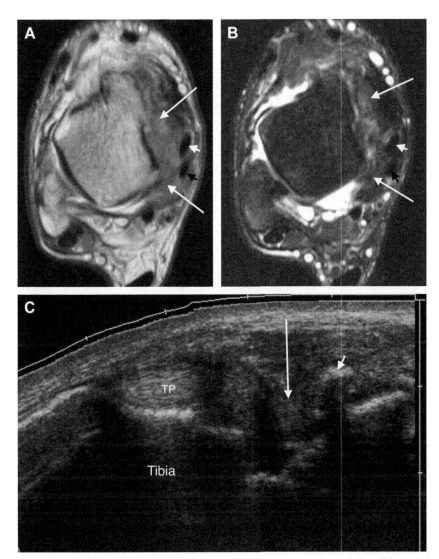

Fig. 12. Volleyball player with posteromedial impingement. Axial PD-weighted (*A*) and T2-weighted fat-suppressed (*B*) MR images show disorganisation of the deltoid and posteromedial tissues with scarring and soft tissue thickening (*long arrows*) displacing the tibialis posterior (*white short arrow*) and flexor digitorum longus (*black short arrow*) tendons. Axial oblique ultrasound (*C*) of the posteromedial ankle showing hypoechoic soft tissue thickening (*long arrow*) within the posteromedial recess and around tibialis posterior (TP) tendon with dystrophic calcification (*short arrow*).

observation of 186 ballet dance trainees.[38] Injury audit data from the English Cricket Board revealed that posterior ankle impingement was the most common cause for players deemed unfit to train or play secondary to foot and ankle problems over the 2001–2002 season. It principally affects the front foot of fast bowlers and represented more days lost for injury to foot and ankle pathology that season than to lateral ankle ligament and Achilles tendon pathologies combined.[38]

Other names, such as "os trigonum syndrome," "talar compression syndrome," and "posterior block" have also been attributed to this collective syndrome of pathologies, all of which are characterised by forced or repeated ankle plantar flexion with subsequent compression of bone or soft tissues between the posterior articular lip of the tibia and the calcaneus.[4,17]

Anatomy and Pathophysiology

There are many causes of posterior impingement, including bone lesions, soft tissue lesions, and anomalous and accessory muscles. The posterior talar process has 2 posterior projections or tubercles. These form a fibro-osseous groove through which the flexor hallucis longus tendon runs. The lateral tubercle (or posterolateral process) is larger than the medial one and contains a secondary ossification centre. This usually mineralises between 7 and 13 years of age and fuses by 1 year. In 7% to 14% of adults it remains as a separate accessory bone, the os trigonum, and is bilateral in 1.4% of cases (**Fig. 13A**).[39] This structure is usually asymptomatic but may become painful if there is disruption of the synchondrosis leading to a cycle of inflammation and soft tissue hypertrophy. Alternatively, chronic stress may lead to a fracture. An elongated posterolateral process of the talus (Stieda or trigonal process), can also be important in posterior impingement (**Fig. 13B**).

Another anatomic consideration is the morphology of the posterior articular surface of the tibia (posterior malleolus) and the calcaneal tuberosity. A more down-sloping configuration of the posterior malleolus or a prominent posterior process of the calcaneus may be contributory.[40]

Soft tissue impingement between the posterior tibial plafond and the superior aspect of the calcaneus typically involves scarring and oedematous thickening of the posterior capsule. The supporting posterior talofibular, tibiofibular, and intermalleolar ligaments also can get compressed but are rarely primarily abnormal. It is hypothesised that subclinical thickening exists in many athletes and any acute injury to the ankle that produces haemarthrosis can cause further thickening that may explain why many athletes present during rehabilitation for a seemingly previous remote acute injury.[41] The flexor hallucis longus tendon can also become secondarily involved with tendinopathy and tenosynovitis with symptoms that can mimic impingement.

The posterior intermalleolar ligament is an anatomic variant of the posterior ligaments of the ankle. First described by Rosenberg and colleagues[42] in 1995, it was identified in 56% of cadaveric specimens. The ligament extends obliquely from the posterior margin of the medial malleolus to the superior margin of the fibular malleolar fossa. It lies between the inferior tibiofibular ligament and the posterior talofibular ligament. When the foot is in plantarflexion, the posterior intermalleolar ligament can protrude into the joint and become entrapped and torn. Bucket handle tears and entrapment of the ligament have been described as a cause of posterior impingement in ballet dancers.[43] Although the presence of a posterior intermalleolar ligament is common, posterolateral impingement related to it is rare. In addition, generalized hypermobility or talocrural laxity relating to previous anterior talofibular ligament disruption also can put stress on the posterior capsule-ligament complex and predispose to posterior impingement.[35]

Clinical Presentation

Presentation is usually with progressive posterior ankle pain, but diagnosis can be difficult as it may mimic other pathologies such as Achilles, flexor hallucis, or peroneal tendon pathology. Like other ankle impingement symptoms, it can present subacutely after a seemingly remote acute ankle injury as the athlete rehabilitates. The pain is aggravated by running, kicking, jumping, or cutting maneuvers, and with either plantar or dorsiflexion due to either compression or stretching of the abnormal posterior soft tissue. Pain relating to an os trigonum or Stieda process is more often posterolateral, whereas flexor hallucis issues are more commonly posteromedial.[44] It is often difficult, however, to clinically localise the pain to a side.

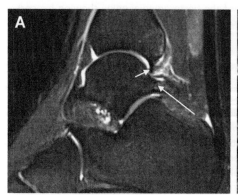
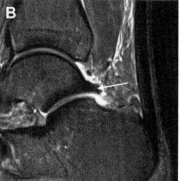

Fig. 13. Osseous anatomic structures of the talus associated with posterior impingement. Sagittal T2-weighted fat-suppressed MR images show (*A*) os trigonum with patchy increased signal around the synchondrosis due to normal intrinsic vascularity (*long arrow*) and down-sloping posterior tibia (*short arrow*). (*B*) Stieda process (*arrow*).

On examination, impingement testing by applying passive plantar flexion to the ankle with the patient lying in the prone position and the knee flexed is invariably positive. Involvement of the flexor hallucis longus tendon is suspected if resisted isometric plantar flexion of the first metatarsal phalangeal joint results in posterior ankle pain.

Imaging Features

Plain radiography is the first step in identifying the os trigonum or Stieda process osseous variants. It should be remembered, however, that symptom severity is not related to the size or even the presence of these 2 structures.[45] The shape of the posterior malleolus and the calcaneal tuberosity also can be assessed.

Sagittal T1-weighted and fat-suppressed fluid-sensitive sequences allow optimal visualisation of an os trigonum, a Stieda process, a down-sloping posterior malleolus, or prominent calcaneal tubercle. Bone marrow oedema may be seen in all these osseous structures and fluid signal may be seen at the synchondrosis within a nonunited synchondral fracture. However, this latter feature must be carefully evaluated, as a normal synchondrosis will show patchy increased T2-weighted signal due to normal intrinsic vascularity (see **Fig. 13**A). Axial and sagittal fat-suppressed fluid-sensitive images allow visualisation of soft tissue abnormalities, such as posterior capsular thickening, ligament disruption, flexor hallucis tenosynovitis, and soft tissue oedema and synovitis.[46,47] The combined presence of bone marrow oedema and posterior ankle synovitis suggests a diagnosis of posterior ankle impingement (**Fig. 14**).[48,49]

As with other ankle impingement syndromes, MR imaging is used to look for other related pathologies or unrelated mimics, such as Achilles tendinopathy, subtalar arthritis, flexor hallucis tenosynovitis, Haglund deformity, retrocalcaneal bursitis, and osteochondral lesion.

Ultrasound is increasingly being used to demonstrate the hypoechoic nodularity of capsular thickening around the lateral aspect of the posterolateral process or os trigonum. The main role, however, is to target percutaneous therapy.

Treatment

- Initial management is conservative with taping and bracing to limit plantar flexion, followed by manual mobilisation and anti-inflammatory medication. An injection of local anaesthetic into an os trigonum synchondrosis under fluoroscopic guidance can be a useful diagnostic adjunct and can help therapeutically where there is a flare-up during a performance season.[44] If symptoms persist, an ultrasound-guided injection of corticosteroid and local anaesthetic into the abnormal area of soft tissue with dry needling can be useful, particularly in the absence of an os trigonum.[41]
- If symptomatic osseous impingement fails to resolve, operative management is advised. Surgical excision of osseous and soft tissue elements have a high success rate in returning athletes back to their sport of choice.[44]

EXTRA-ARTICULAR LATERAL HINDFOOT IMPINGEMENT

Severe pes planus and hindfoot valgus deformity can lead to extra-articular lateral hindfoot impingement, including talocalcaneal and subfibular

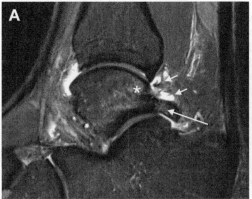
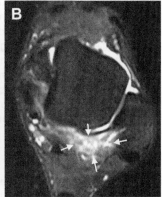

Fig. 14. Posterior impingement. Sagittal (*A*) and axial (*B*) T2-weighted fat-suppressed MR images of posterior ankle impingement with posterior capsular synovitis (*short arrows*). There is low-grade oedema in the os trigonum (*long arrow*), and posterior body of the talus (*asterisk*).

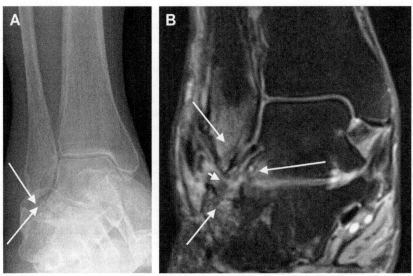

Fig. 15. Patient with pes planus, hindfoot valgus following a calcaneal fracture who presented with lateral hindfoot tenderness. Frontal radiograph (*A*) shows close approximation of the fibular tip with the calcaneus (*arrows*). Coronal PD-weighted MR image (*B*) shows extra-articular subfibular impingement with bone marrow oedema in the fibular tip and lateral margins of the talus and calcaneus (*long arrows*). There is associated soft tissue oedema and synovial thickening (*short arrow*).

impingement. This can present with progressive lateral ankle pain and deformity.

Anatomy and Pathophysiology

Valgus deformity of the ankle is associated with a shift of weight-bearing force from the talar dome to the lateral talus and fibula. Subsequent talocalcaneal impingement may follow, with or without subfibular impingement. This may occur secondary to malunion after calcaneus fracture, posterior tibialis tendon dysfunction, neuropathic arthropathy, or inflammatory athritides.[50]

Clinical Presentation

Regardless of the initial cause of flatfoot, patients with rigid flatfoot deformity experience decreased range of motion at the midfoot and hindfoot and decreased ankle dorsiflexion.[50,51] Although the pain may initially locate to the medial ankle in cases of posterior tibialis tendon dysfunction, lateral ankle pain predominates in chronic severe dysfunction.[52] Further midfoot and hindfoot pain is associated with secondary degeneration and progressive deformity.

Imaging Features

Weight-bearing radiographs are useful to assess the plantar arch and hindfoot valgus. Although there are no definite radiographic criteria for lateral hindfoot impingement, subfibular osseous impingement should be suspected if the distance

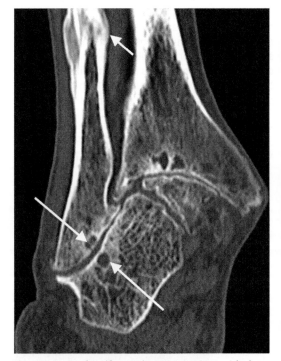

Fig. 16. Severe hindfoot valgus in a patient with rheumatoid arthritis. There is pseudoarticulation between the fibula and calcaneus with sclerosis, articular irregularity, and extensive cystic change (*long arrows*). Also note previous associated chronic diaphysial fracture of the distal fibula (*short arrow*).

between the fibula and the lateral process of the talus on the anteroposterior view measures 1 mm or less (**Fig. 15**).[53] CT also can be used (**Fig. 16**) and is similarly suspicious if there is a bony protrusion of 2 mm or more at the lateral surface of the talus on axial view or if bone spurs are seen on the lateral process of the talus and on adjacent fibula on coronal view.[53] MR imaging may show marrow oedema or sclerosis at the posterior subtalar joint, fibular tip, lateral process of the talus, and lateral calcaneus. There also may be thickening of the subfibular soft tissues with calcaneofibular ligament entrapment and subluxation of the peroneal tendons.[50] MR imaging is also used to check for posterior tibialis tendinopathy and other associated sources of pain, such as lateral bursitis and distal fibular stress fractures (see **Fig. 16**).

Treatment

- Conservative early measures are directed at preventing further osseous deformity with physiotherapy and orthotics.
- Surgical correction of hindfoot deformity is, however, usually required and consists of either calcaneal osteotomy or, in the most severe cases, arthrodesis.

SUMMARY

Ankle impingement syndromes are an established cause of persistent ankle pain in young and athletic populations, particularly presenting during rehabilitation after a sprain injury. MR imaging is used to help support the clinical diagnosis, to evaluate the rest of the joint for associated injury and to plan treatment. Although we have described the different syndromes as distinct entities, they often coexist and commonly occur together with other pathologies. MR imaging features of impingement may be found in asymptomatic patients and the diagnosis therefore requires careful clinical correlation. Most patients, including elite athletes, are managed successfully with conservative measures with percutaneous injection techniques used in selected patients. Surgical treatment for resistant cases are effective in allowing a prompt return to play.

REFERENCES

1. Pesquer L, Guillo S, Meyer P. US in ankle impingement syndrome. J Ultrasound 2014;17:89–97.
2. Hopper MA, Robinson P. Ankle impingement syndromes. Radiol Clin North Am 2008;46:6.
3. Amendola N, Newhoff D, Vaseenon T, et al. CAM-type impingement in the ankle. Iowa Orthop J 2012;32:1–8.
4. Cerezal L, Abascal F, Canga A, et al. MR imaging of ankle impingement syndromes. AJR Am J Roentgenol 2003;181(2):551–9.
5. McMurray TP. Footballer's ankle. J Bone Joint Surg Br 1950;32B:68–9.
6. Morris LH. Athlete's ankle. J Bone Joint Surg 1943; 25:220.
7. Hayeri MR, Trudell DJ, Resnick D. Anterior ankle impingement and talar bony outgrowths: osteophyte or enthesophyte? Paleopathologic and cadaveric study with imaging correlation. Am J Roentgenol 2009;193(4):W334–8.
8. Cheng JC, Ferkel RD. The role of arthroscopy in ankle and subtalar degenerative joint disease. Clin Orthop Relat Res 1998;(349):65–72.
9. Tol JL, Verheyen CPPM, Van Dijk CN. Arthroscopic treatment of anterior impingement in the ankle: a prospective study with a five-to-eight year follow-up. J Bone Joint Surg Br 2001;83:9–13.
10. Coull R, Raffiq T, James LE, et al. Open treatment of anterior impingement of the ankle. J Bone Joint Surg Br 2003;85:550–3.
11. Valkering KP, Golanó P, van Dijk CN, et al. "Web impingement" of the ankle: a case report. Knee Surg Sports Traumatol Arthrosc 2013;21(6):1289–92.
12. Hess GW. Ankle impingement syndromes: a review of etiology and related implications. Foot Ankle Spec 2011;4(5):290–7.
13. Malloy S, Solan S, Bendall SP. Synovial impingement in the ankle. A new physical sign. J Bone Joint Surg Br 2003;85(3):330–3.
14. Tol JL, Verhagen RA, Krips R, et al. The anterior ankle impingement syndrome: diagnostic value of oblique radiographs. Foot Ankle Int 2004;25:63–8.
15. O'Kane JW, Kadel N. Anterior impingement syndrome in dancers. Curr Rev Musculoskelet Med 2008;1:12–6.
16. Van Dijk CN, Tol JL, Verheyen C. A prospective study of prognostic factors concerning the outcome of arthroscopic surgery for anterior ankle impingement. Am J Sports Med 1997;25:737–45.
17. Robinson P, White LM. Soft-tissue and osseous impingement syndromes of the ankle: role of imaging in diagnosis and management. Radiographics 2002;22:1457–69.
18. Bassett FH 3rd, Gates HS 3rd, Billys JB, et al. Talar impingement of the anteroinferior tibiofibular ligament. A cause of chronic pain in the ankle after inversion sprain. J Bone Joint Surg Am 1990;72:55–9.
19. Ferkel RD, Karzel RP, Del Pizzo W. Arthroscopic treatment of anterolateral impingement of the ankle. Am J Sports Med 1991;19:440–6.
20. Wolin I, Glassman F, Sideman S, et al. Internal derangement of the talofibular component of the ankle. Surg Gynecol Obstet 1950;91:193–200.

21. Nikolopoulos CE, Tsirikos AI, Sourmelis S, et al. The accessory anteroinferior tibiofibular ligament as a cause of talar impingement: a cadaveric study. Am J Sports Med 2004;32:389–95.

22. McCarthy CL, Wilson DJ, Coltman TP. Anterolateral ankle impingement: findings and diagnostic accuracy with ultrasound imaging. Skeletal Radiol 2008; 37(3):209–16.

23. Robinson P, White LM, Salonen DC, et al. Anterolateral impingement of the ankle: MR arthrographic assessment of the anterolateral recess. Radiology 2001;221:186–90.

24. Meislin RJ. Arthroscopic treatment of synovial impingement of the ankle. Am J Sports Med 1993; 21:186–9.

25. Duncan D, Mologne T, Hildebrand H, et al. The usefulness of magnetic resonance imaging in the diagnosis of anterolateral impingement of the ankle. J Foot Ankle Surg 2006;45(5):304–7.

26. Lui HI, Raskin A, Osti I, et al. Arthroscopic treatment of anterolateral ankle impingement. Arthroscopy 1994;10:215–8.

27. Jose J, Mirpuri T, Lesniak B, et al. Sonographically guided therapeutic injections in the meniscoid lesion in patients with anteromedial ankle impingement syndrome. Foot Ankle Spec 2014;7:409–13.

28. Vann MA, Manoli A. Medial ankle impingement syndrome in female gymnastics. Oper Tech Sports Med 2010;18(1):50–2.

29. Van Dijk C, van Bergen C. Advancements in ankle arthroscopy. J Am Acad Orthop Surg 2008;16: 635–46.

30. Murawski C, Kennedy JG. Anteromedial impingement in the ankle joint: outcomes following arthroscopy in the first one hundred cases. Arthroscopy 2011;27(5):e58–9.

31. Paterson RS, Brown JN. The posteromedial impingement lesion of the ankle: a series of six cases. Am J Sports Med 2001;29:550–7.

32. Koulouris G, Connell D, Schneider T, et al. Posterior tibitotalar ligament injury resulting in posteromedial impingement. Foot Ankle Int 2003;24(8):575–83.

33. Messiou C, Robinson P, O'Connor PJ, et al. Subacute posteromedial impingement of the ankle in athletes: MR imaging evaluation and ultrasound guided therapy. Skeletal Radiol 2006;35:88–94.

34. Liu S, Mirzayan R. Posteromedial ankle impingement. Arthroscopy 1993;9(6):709–11.

35. Rogers J, Dukstra P, McCourt P, et al. Posterior ankle impingement syndrome: a clinical review with reference to horizontal jump athletes. Acta Orthop Belg 2010;76:572–9.

36. Giannini S, Buda R, Mosca M, et al. Posterior ankle impingement. Foot Ankle Int 2013;34(3):459–65.

37. Albisetti WJ, Ometti M, Pascale V, et al. Clinical evaluation and treatment of posterior impingement in dancers. Am J Phys Med Rehabil 2009;88(5): 349–54.

38. Ribbans WJ, Ribbans HA, Cruickshank JA, et al. The management of posterior ankle impingement syndrome in sport: a review. Foot Ankle Surg 2015; 21(1):1–10.

39. Lawson JP. Symptomatic radiographic variants in extremities. Radiology 1985;157(3):625–31.

40. Peace KAL, Hillier JC, Hulme A, et al. Features of posterior ankle impingement syndrome in ballet dancers: a review of 25 cases. Clin Radiol 2004; 59:1025–33.

41. Robinson P, Bollen SR. Posterior ankle impingement in professional soccer players: effectiveness of sonographically guided therapy. AJR Am J Roentengol 2006;187:W53–8.

42. Rosenberg ZS, Cheung YY, Beltran J, et al. Posterior intermalleolar ligament of the ankle: normal anatomy and MR imaging features. Am J Roentgenol 1995; 165:387–90.

43. Hamilton WG. Foot and ankle injuries in dancers. Clin Sports Med 1988;7(1):143–73.

44. Coetzee JC, Seybold JD, Moser BR, et al. Management of posterior impingement in the ankle in athletes and dancers. Foot Ankle Int 2015;36(8): 988–94.

45. Hamilton WG, Geppert MJ, Thompson FM. Pain in the posterior aspect of the ankle in dancers: differential diagnosis and operative treatment. J Bone Joint Surg Am 1996;78:1491–500.

46. Karasick D, Schweitzer ME. The os trigonum syndrome: imaging features. Am J Roentgenol 1996; 166:125–9.

47. Bureau NJ, Cardinal E, Hobden R, et al. Posterior ankle impingement syndrome: MR imaging findings in seven patients. Radiology 2000;215:497–503.

48. Umans H. Ankle impingement syndromes. Semin Musculoskelet Radiol 2002;6:133–40.

49. Fiorella D, Helms CA, Nuley JA. The MR imaging features of the posterior intermalleolar ligament in patients with posterior impingement syndrome of the ankle. Skeletal Radiol 1999;28:573–6.

50. Donovan A, Rosenberg ZS. MRI of ankle and lateral hindfoot impingement syndromes. Am J Roentgenol 2010;195:595–604.

51. Pedowitz WJ, Kovatis P. Flatfoot in the adult. J Am Acad Orthop Surg 1995;3:293–302.

52. Bluman EM, Myerson MS. Stage IV posterior tibial tendon rupture. Foot Ankle Clin 2007;12:341–62.

53. Ahn JY, Choi HJ, Lee WC. Talofibular bony impingement in the ankle. Foot Ankle Int 2015; 36(10):1150–5.

MR Imaging of Common Soft Tissue Masses in the Foot and Ankle

 CrossMark

Mary G. Hochman, MD, MBA*, Jim S. Wu, MD

KEYWORDS

- Foot • Ankle • Soft tissue mass • MR imaging • Plantar fibroma • Giant cell tumor of tendon sheath
- Ganglion cyst • Synovial sarcoma

KEY POINTS

- Soft tissue masses in the foot and ankle may represent true neoplasms or other, nonneoplastic entities that mimic musculoskeletal tumors. Malignant tumors can occur, but are rare.
- Although a definitive diagnosis may not be possible, imaging characteristics can help narrow the diagnosis for a soft tissue mass and, occasionally, provide a specific diagnosis.
- On reviewing MR imaging, consider signal intensity, contrast enhancement, lesion location, association with anatomic structures, findings on radiographs, patient history, examination, and demographics.
- Some solid masses have high T2 signal intensity and can be mistaken for cysts. Intravenous contrast helps in making the distinction.
- Malignant sarcomas can be nonaggressive in appearance and can demonstrate indolent growth.

Soft tissue masses may be encountered in the foot and ankle as incidental findings or as part of the workup of a palpable mass or other abnormality. These lesions may represent true neoplasms, either malignant or benign, or may represent other, nonneoplastic entities that mimic musculoskeletal tumors. The goal of this article is to review common soft tissue masses that can be encountered in the foot or ankle, highlight their MR imaging appearance, and outline common pitfalls. Technical considerations for imaging of soft tissue masses in the foot and ankle are also discussed.

BACKGROUND

The incidence of different lesions in the foot and ankle is difficult to quantify, because reported series differ in terms of anatomy covered, patient age, and the kinds of masses included.[1,2] Overall, true soft tissue neoplasms of the foot and ankle are uncommon.[3] However, soft tissue masses encountered in the foot include not only true neoplasms, as classified by the World Health Organization,[4] but also a variety of cystic and solid benign masses—and even some normal anatomic structures—that are relatively common and that can be mistaken for tumors. Kirby and colleagues[5] reviewed a series of 83 consecutive biopsied soft tissue masses in the foot and ankle and found 87% were benign and 13% were malignant. Berquist and Kransdorf presented a compilation of soft tissue masses from a several different studies.[3,5–9] In their compilation, the most common benign lesions were ganglion cyst, plantar fibroma, giant cell tumor of the tendon sheath, hemangioma, lipoma, soft tissue chondroma, and benign nerve

Disclosure Statement: The authors have nothing to disclose.
Musculoskeletal Imaging and Intervention, Department of Radiology, Beth Israel Deaconess Medical Center, Harvard Medical School, 330 Brookline Avenue, Boston, MA 02215, USA
* Corresponding author.
E-mail address: mhochman@bidmc.harvard.edu

Magn Reson Imaging Clin N Am 25 (2017) 159–181
http://dx.doi.org/10.1016/j.mric.2016.08.013
1064-9689/17/© 2016 Elsevier Inc. All rights reserved.

mri.theclinics.com

sheath tumors. The most common malignant lesions were malignant vascular tumors, synovial sarcoma, fibrosarcoma, melanotic clear cell tumor, and undifferentiated pleomorphic sarcoma.

IMAGING EVALUATION OF SOFT TISSUE MASSES

MR imaging is the preferred method for evaluation of soft tissue tumors because of the high intrinsic soft tissue contrast, demonstration of features that can aid in tissue characterization, and accuracy for demonstrating extent of bone and soft tissue involvement.[10] Nonetheless, radiographs remain an important adjunct modality for evaluation of soft tissue tumors, in particular because radiographs are superior to MR imaging in demonstrating soft tissue calcifications and reactive changes in bone.[10] Radiographs may also demonstrate large fatty masses or effacement of usual fat planes. Gartner and colleagues[11] found that 62% of radiographs (n = 454) in patients with proven soft tissue tumors had positive radiographic findings.

Ultrasound imaging can differentiate between cystic and solid masses, can help in characterization of some masses such as lipomas, vascular lesions, and nerve sheath tumors,[12] and can be used for image guidance of lesion aspiration and biopsy.[10] In general, ultrasound imaging requires sufficient operator and radiologist expertise to be most useful.

Computed tomography (CT) scans can also be useful in evaluation of soft tissue masses about the foot and ankle, although they lack the level of intrinsic soft tissue contrast inherent in MR images and require ionizing radiation.[10] However, CT images can demonstrate soft tissue calcifications such as phleboliths, lesion matrix mineralization, and reactive changes in bone, and can be useful in evaluation of fatty lesions. Intravenous (IV) contrast-enhanced CT images can help to demonstrate masses that might otherwise not be distinguishable from surrounding soft tissue and CT angiographic techniques can reveal features of vascular malformations and information about lesion vascularity. The use of dual energy CT techniques to demonstrate monosodium urate content for characterization of gouty tophi has also been described.[13,14]

MR IMAGING TECHNIQUES

Effective MR imaging depends on producing images of high spatial resolution. Images should be obtained using a local coil and, whenever possible, a small field of view, targeted to the area of interest. In the workup of soft tissue masses, however, this must be balanced against the need to include the entire extent of the lesion and its surrounding soft tissues. Imaging planes should be optimized to best demonstrate the relationship between the lesion and surrounding anatomic structures.[15]

Imaging protocols vary, but should include T1-weighted (T1W) images and fluid-sensitive sequences. T2-weighted (T2W) images without fat saturation are useful, because classic early descriptions of mass lesions described their T2 signal intensity characteristics and because T2 images without fat saturation are more sensitive for detection of signal heterogeneity within lesions. However, practically speaking, many protocols eschew T2W images in favor of fat-saturated T2-weighted, short tau inversion recovery (STIR), and fat-saturated proton density-weighted images.

Administration of IV contrast allows for distinction between cystic and solid lesions, with cysts demonstrating only a thin rim of peripheral enhancement and no internal enhancement. To assess for the presence of contrast enhancement, it is important to compare sequences that are identical in imaging parameters. Although precontrast and postcontrast images are generally performed using frequency selective fat saturated T1W sequences, it can be difficult to achieve homogeneous fat saturation in the foot and ankle. In those cases, preconstrast and postcontrast imaging on T1W images without fat saturation can serve as an alternative, either by direct comparison, or based on subtraction of the precontrast and postcontrast images. The use of Dixon techniques has also been described as a means to provide more robust fat saturation.[16] Stabilization of the foot within the coil is important to minimize motion and to facilitate the use of subtraction images.

Some supplementary MR imaging sequences can be considered. Production of diagnostic images can be particularly challenging in the setting of hardware or postoperative changes. The use of various metal artifact reduction techniques has been described.[17,18] T2*-weighted gradient echo sequences can be used to demonstrate blooming owing to the presence of hemosiderin, which can be seen in giant cell tumor of the tendon sheath (GCT-TS) and pigmented villonodular synovitis, and which can also be caused by dense calcification. Hemosiderin can also occasionally be seen surrounding vascular tumors that have leaked or at sites of previous hematoma.[19,20] The use of diffusion weighted MR images and MR spectroscopy to help characterize musculoskeletal soft tissue masses has been described, but these techniques are not yet in common clinical use in the musculoskeletal system.[21–25]

SYSTEMATIC APPROACH TO ANALYSIS

Although it may not be possible to arrive at a definitive diagnosis for every soft tissue tumor encountered in the foot and ankle, imaging characteristics can help to narrow the differential diagnosis for a soft tissue mass and in some cases can help to arrive at a specific diagnosis.[19,26] Characteristics such as signal intensity on T1W images, signal intensity on T2W images, contrast enhancement characteristics, lesion location, and association with other anatomic structures, as well as findings on correlative radiographs, can be useful in this regard (**Box 1**).[27,28]

Many mass lesions are isointense to muscle on T1W images and relatively hyperintense on T2W images. However, substances that seem to be high signal on T1W images include fat, proteinaceous fluid (of specific concentration range), hemorrhage (methemoglobin phase), melanin, and, of course, gadolinium (**Box 2**). Substances that seem to be low signal on T2W images include calcification, fibrous material (scar tissue, fibrous neoplasm), and hemosiderin (**Box 3**). IV contrast can help to distinguish cystic lesions, which demonstrate peripheral rim enhancement, from solid lesions, which have high T2 signal intensity on fluid-sensitive images, but demonstrate internal enhancement. Dynamic contrast enhancement can be used to assess the degree of lesion vascularity.[19] Various forms of "tail signs" can be seen in nerve sheath tumors, ganglia, and, after contrast administration, in plantar fibromas, whereas a "target sign" is highly suggestive of a nerve sheath tumors. Bursae occur in characteristic anatomic locations, whereas other lesions characteristically arise in association with other anatomic structures, for example, giant cells tumors of tendon sheath (tendons), nerve sheath tumors (nerves), plantar fibromas (plantar fascia), and synovial cysts (joints). In addition, radiographs may provide findings that can aid in diagnosis, such as phleboliths (hemangiomas), foreign bodies (foreign body granulomas), pleomorphic calcifications (synovial sarcomas), calcified masses (gout), and well-defined erosions (gout, giant cell tumor of tendon sheath).

With this in mind, a systematic approach can be applied to aid in decision making when a mass is encountered in the foot or ankle (**Boxes 4–6**).[26]

BENIGN SOFT TISSUE TUMORS
Plantar Fibroma

Plantar fibromas are the most common solid soft tissue neoplasm encountered in the foot and ankle in Berquist and Kransdorf's compilation, and the second most common mass after ganglion cysts.[3] A plantar fibroma is a nodular mass composed of spindle cells and variable amounts of collagen that arises in the plantar aponeurosis of the foot.[4] Plantar fibromas are related to palmar fibromas seen in Dupuytren disease, as well as other forms

---

Box 2
High signal on T1-weighted images

- Fat
- Proteinaceous fluid
- Methemoglobin
- Melanin
- Gadolinium

Box 1
MR imaging features for systematic analysis

T1-weighted signal

T2-weighted signal

Contrast enhancement

- Peripheral/central
  - Peripheral: thin/smooth versus thick/irregular
- Homogeneous/heterogeneous
- Dynamic enhancement: early or late

Special imaging features

- Tail sign
- Target sign

Characteristic location

- Bursae

Associated anatomy

- Tendon
- Nerve
- Vessel
- Plantar fascia
- Joint

Box 3
Low signal on T2-weighted images

- Calcification
- Fibrous tissue—scar
- Fibrous tissue—fibrous neoplasms
- Hemosiderin

Box 4
For lesions that are high signal on T1-weighted images

1. Does the lesion suppress using chemically specific (frequency-selective) fat saturation? If so, it is composed of fat and the differential would include entities such as lipoma, well-differentiated liposarcoma (rare in the foot or ankle), or hemangioma.

2. Does the radiograph show a focal collection of phleboliths, suggesting an hemangioma?

3. Does the enhancement pattern indicate a cystic structure, such as a hemorrhagic or proteinaceous ganglion cyst?

Box 6
For lesions that are high signal and cyst-like on T2-weighted images

1. If there is a thin rim of peripheral enhancement, this suggests a cystic structure, such as a ganglion cyst. Be aware that soft tissue chondromas can also demonstrate thin peripheral enhancement. It also important to confirm that the cystic structure is not a smaller component of a larger mixed cystic and solid structure.

2. If the peripheral enhancement is thick, rather than thin, this could indicate and inflamed or infected cyst or bursa or an abscess or, alternatively, a solid lesion with central necrosis. Nerve sheath tumors that display a "target sign" on T2-weighted images may also show predominantly peripheral enhancement on postcontrast images.

3. Is there central enhancement? If so, a solid high T2 signal mass should be considered. This can be seen with a variety of benign and malignant lesions and the differential includes a synovial or other myxoid sarcomas, other myxomatous soft tissue masses, and hemangiomas.

---

of fibromatosis. They typically occur in patients older than 30 years of age, and more commonly in men. The etiology is uncertain, but likely multifactorial, with family history and trauma both implicated.[4]

Patients with plantar fibromas may present with a palpable nodule or area of focal thickening along the plantar aspect of the foot and may experience mild pain after standing or walking for long periods. Lesions may be bilateral in 20% to 50% of patients.[9]

On MR imaging, plantar fibromas are seen as nodular masses adherent to the plantar aponeurosis, typically medial rather than lateral.[29] They are well-defined with respect to the overlying plantar subcutaneous fat, but are often not well-demarcated with respect to the plantar aponeurosis and underlying muscle.[30] Most lesions are heterogeneous in signal intensity, isointense to slightly hyperintense to muscle on fluid-sensitive

sequences, and demonstrate heterogeneous, enhancement, which is variable in degree.[30] Contrast enhancement may extend along the plantar aponeurosis, creating a "fascial tail" sign.[29] Multiple lesions can be present at the same time (synchronous) and new lesions can arise after treatment (metachronous).[29] Lesions do not metastasize, but can recur locally (**Fig. 1**).[4]

Giant Cell Tumor of the Tendon Sheath

A GCT-TS is a benign neoplastic mass consisting of mononuclear and inflammatory cells, arising from the tendon sheath.[4,31] The lesion can be localized or diffuse. Histologically, GCT-TS resembles intraarticular pigmented villonodular synovitis. GCT-TS occurs most commonly in the hands and feet, with about 17% occurring in the foot and ankle.[3,32,33] In data compiled by Berquist and Kransdorf, GCT-TS was the third most common benign mass encountered in the foot and ankle.[3] Patients with GCT-TS present with a usually painless mass that develops gradually, often over several years. GCT-TS usually occurs in patients between 30 to 50 years of age and is more common in women (F:M 2:1).[34]

Lesions are typically occult on radiographs, but, on occasion, a focal soft tissue mass and/or nonaggressive erosion of the abutting bone may

---

Box 5
For lesions that are low signal on T2-weighted images

1. Does the radiograph show rounded or ovoid calcified mass, as might be seen in a gouty tophus?

2. Is there blooming on T2*-weighted images? If there are no calcifications on the radiographic to account for this, then giant cell tumor of the tendon sheath or residua from hemorrhage around a vascular lesion or old hematoma should be considered.

3. Does the lesion location suggest a diagnosis, such as a giant cell tumor of the tendon sheath arising from a tendon sheath or a plantar fibroma arising from the plantar fascia?

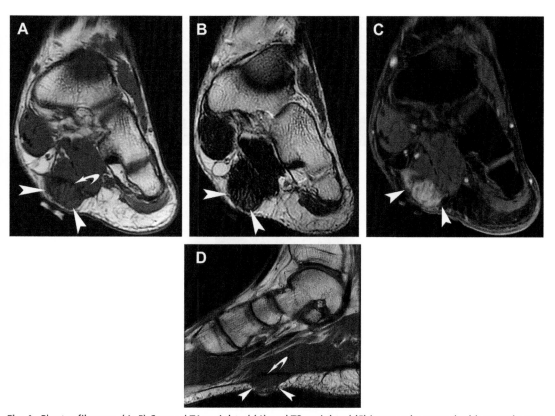

Fig. 1. Plantar fibroma. (*A, B*) Coronal T1-weighted (*A*) and T2-weighted (*B*) images show a palpable mass (*arrowheads*) that is isointense to muscle on both sequences. It arises from the plantar fascia (*curved arrow*) and projects into the overlying plantar subcutaneous fat. (*C*) Coronal postcontrast fat-saturated T1-weighted image shows diffuse, slightly heterogeneous enhancement of the plantar fibroma (*arrowheads*). (*D*) Sagittal T1-weighted image shows the mass (*arrowheads*) adhering to—and arising from—the plantar fascia (*curved arrow*).

be visible.[35] The MR imaging appearance of GCT-TS can be highly suggestive of the diagnosis. On MR imaging, the lesions appear as focal masses that are adherent to the surface of a tendon. Small lesions may be rounded, but large, lobulated lesions can also be seen. The lesions are classically low signal on both T1- and T2-weighted images. Low T2 signal is attributed to abundant collagen and hemosiderin.[36] When sufficient hemosiderin is present, these lesions may demonstrate blooming on T2* gradient echo images, that is, the lesion may demonstrate low signal that appears darker and/or more extensive on the T2*W gradient echo images. However, some lesions may not contain enough hemosiderin to be T1 and T2 hypointense or to cause blooming artifact on gradient echo images.[37] The gadolinium enhancement pattern is variable, but lesions often show pronounced homogeneous enhancement (**Fig. 2**).[36]

A fibroma of the tendon sheath can a similar MR appearance, but fibromas are less common in this location and are not characterized by hemosiderin or by blooming on T2*W gradient echo images.[38]

Hemangioma

Hemangiomas are benign vascular lesions that consist of hyperplastic endothelial cells, together with mast cells, and may be superficial (cutaneous or subcutaneous) or deep.[39] These lesions are often associated with fat (angiolipoma), fibrous tissue, and/or smooth muscle. Based on the vessels that comprise them, hemangiomas can be further classified histologically as capillary, cavernous, venous, or arteriovenous.[40]

Hemangiomas are common, accounting for 7% of all benign soft tissue lesions and 9% of benign lesions in the foot and ankle.[3,32] Hemangiomas are common in infancy and childhood, but can occur at any age. Most patients present by 30 years of age. The incidence is similar in men and women.[3] Patients may present with blue discoloration on the skin. Hemangiomas may

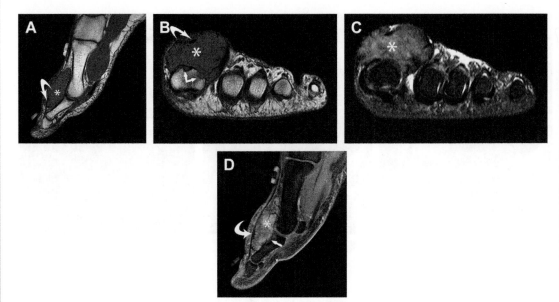

Fig. 2. Giant cell tumor of the tendon sheath (GCT-TS). (*A*) Sagittal T1-weighted image shows a large lobulated mass (*asterisk*), very slightly hyperintense to muscle, wrapping around the extensor hallucis tendon (*curved arrow*). (*B, C*) Coronal T1-weighted (*B*) and fat-saturated T2-weighted (*C*) images shows the mass (*asterisk*) and tendon (*curved arrow*) and demonstrates subtle nonaggressive erosions in the proximal phalanx (*arrowheads*), owing to the mass effect from the lesion. (*C*) The lesion (*asterisk*) is of a higher signal intensity on the fat saturated T2-weighted image than it would be expected to be on a T2-weighted image without fat saturation. (*D*) Heterogeneous, but still prominent, contrast enhancement of the GCT-TS (*asterisk*) is seen on the postcontrast fat saturated T1-weighted image. Encasement of the tendon (*curved arrow*) and bone erosion (*arrowhead*) are again noted.

fluctuate in size and can become painful after exercise, owing to shunting of blood away from the surrounding tissue.[29]

Radiographs play an important role in the imaging diagnosis of hemangioma, because they demonstrate phleboliths (focal dystrophic mineralization within thrombus) in up to 50% of cavernous hemangiomas (**Fig. 3**C). In up to 33% of patients, radiographs may demonstrate a soft tissue mass and bony reactive changes, such as cortical or periosteal thickening.[41]

On MR imaging, hemangiomas may be either well- or poorly circumscribed. Lesions may have high T1 signal owing to varying amounts of fatty

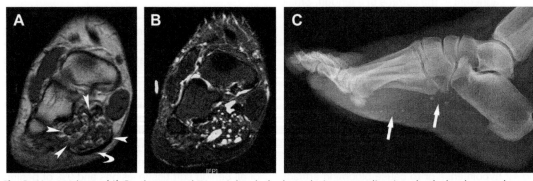

Fig. 3. Hemangioma. (*A*) On the coronal T1-weighted, the large lesion extending into both the deep and superficial plantar compartments of the midfoot is not readily visualized (*arrowheads*) or particularly well-demarcated. It includes slow-flowing venous channels that are isointense to muscle interspersed with areas of fat. Along its plantar border, the lesion bulges the plantar fascia (*curved arrow*). (*B*) On the coronal fat-saturated T2-weighted image, there is high signal owing to slow flow, and signal from the fatty components of the mass is suppressed. (*C*) Review of the patient's foot radiograph revealed clustered phleboliths (*arrows*) in the same location as the mass, highly suggestive of an hemangioma.

overgrowth or hemorrhage.[29] They are typically high signal on T2W images, owing to the presence of slow flow, and fluid–fluid levels may be visible. When high flow vessels are present, serpiginous signal voids ("flow voids") will be seen on nonflow sensitive sequences. Rounded foci of low signal within the lesions can indicate the presence of phleboliths and should be correlated with radiographs. Intramuscular lesions may be accompanied by a small amount of surrounding fatty atrophy owing to vascular steal phenomenon.[40] If perilesional hemorrhage has occurred, then low T2 signal hemosiderin may be seen at the periphery of the lesion and can cause blooming on T2*-weighted gradient echo images.[40] Hemangiomas typically show prominent contrast enhancement,[29] although delayed enhancement can also occur.[40] As on radiographs, reactive changes may be visible in adjoining segments of bone (**Fig. 3**A, B).

Because a focal hemangioma with slow flow can appear as a focal high T2 mass, care should be taken not to mistake an hemangioma for a cyst or for a myxoid soft tissue mass. IV contrast and ultrasound can be helpful in this regard.[29]

Lipoma

Lipomas are benign soft tissue tumors composed of mature white adipocytes, histologically identical to adipose fat.[4] Overall, lipomas are the most common soft tissue tumor in adults, with an incidence of up to 2.1 per 100 individuals.[42] In Berquist and Kransdorf's compilation, lipomas were the fifth most common soft tissue mass in the foot and ankle.[3]

A simple lipoma is composed entirely of fat. It may contain several thin septations, but thickened septations (>2 mm) and nodular soft tissue areas within the fatty tumor should raise concern for malignancy.[43] Other features concerning for malignancy include patient age, large lesion size (>10 cm), thickened septae, globular areas of nonfatty signal intensity, and lesions with less than 75% fat content.[43] It should be noted, however, that a substantial percentage of benign lipomas, as well as lipoma variants, contain nonfatty components.[4,43]

On radiographs, lipomas are often occult. When visible, they appear as a radiolucent mass, occasionally with thin septations or calcifications.[42] On MR imaging, lipomas follow the signal of subcutaneous or intramedullary fat on all sequences.[29] A simple lipoma is homogeneously high signal on T1W images and that high signal should suppress on T1W images obtained with chemically-specific ("frequency selective") fat saturation. As noted, although a lipoma may have thin septations, thickened septations (>2 mm) or nodular soft tissue components raise concern for malignancy. The lesion may have a thin surrounding capsule, although may be variably unencapsulated. Lipomas may occur in subcutaneous fat, deep fat, or between or within muscles.[42] When lipomas occur within muscle, longitudinal muscle fibers may traverse the lipoma and should not be mistaken for thickened septae (**Fig. 4**).

Liposarcomas in the foot and ankle are rare.[6,39] Well-differentiated liposarcomas contain large amounts of normal appearing fat and should be distinguished from lipoma using the criteria listed above.[43]

Soft Tissue Chondroma

Soft tissue chondromas are benign extraosseous and extrasynovial soft tissue tumors composed predominantly of mature hyaline cartilage.[4,39]

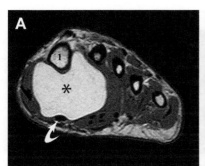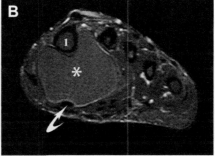

Fig. 4. Simple lipoma. (*A, B*) Coronal T1-weighted (*A*) and fat-saturated T2-weighted (*B*) images through the foot show a lobulated, well-circumscribed, homogeneous high T1 mass (*asterisk*) interposed between the first metatarsal (*1*) and the flexor hallucis tendon (*curved arrow*), displacing the tendon and the surrounding musculature. There is uniform loss of signal on the fat-saturated T2-weighted images, although loss of signal on a T1-weighted images obtained with frequency selective fat saturation is considered much more specific for fat. There was no internal enhancement.

Soft tissue chondromas occur over a broad age range (mean, 34.5 years) and demonstrate a slight male predominance (3:2).[4,44] The majority of soft tissue chondromas arise on the fingers and hands, followed by toes and feet.[4]

Most soft tissue chondromas are solitary and occur as a soft tissue mass near tendons and joints. On imaging, soft tissue chondromas are lobulated and well-demarcated, with central and peripheral calcifications that are arclike, punctate, spiculated, or coarsely geometric.[4,45] On MR imaging, soft tissue chondromas demonstrate the high T2 signal typical of chondroid lesions, but may have small signal voids owing to the matrix calcifications.[39] Large chondromas may be difficult to distinguish from chondrosarcoma (**Fig. 5**).[46]

Peripheral Nerve Sheath Tumors

Peripheral nerve sheath tumors (PNSTs) include benign and malignant PNSTs and are classified as nerve sheath tumors by the World Health Organization.[4] Benign PNSTs include both neurofibromas and the more common schwannomas (also known as neurilemmomas). Overall, these account for approximately 10.5% of benign soft tissue tumors.[1] In the Berquist and Kransdorf compilation, benign nerve sheath tumors represented the seventh most common benign soft tissue mass in the foot and ankle.[3] Schwannomas are composed of differentiated neoplastic Schwann cells, whereas neurofibromas consist of a mix of differentiated Schwann cells together with myelinated and unmyelinated axons in an extracellular matrix.[4] Both neurofibromas and schwannomas are typically seen in patients 20 to 40 years of age.[4] Clinically, patients may present with motor or sensory disturbances or both. Patients with neurofibromatosis may have multiple lesions. In the foot, most neurofibromas occur in the heel and great toe.[32] Neurofibromas are typically seen along cutaneous nerves.[4,33,47] Schwannomas typically occur along the flexor surface of the extremity.[4,29,47]

Although neurofibromas arise directly from the nerve and schwannomas arise from Schwann cells and lie eccentric to the nerve, the 2 lesions can be difficult to distinguish at imaging. In both cases, the lesion typically appears as a well-defined, smooth-bordered, fusiform mass aligned along the nerve. Signal intensity is often nonspecific, isointense to muscle on T1W and slightly hyperintense to fat on T2W images.[4] In some cases, the lesions may have a "target sign" appearance on T2W images, with higher signal peripherally and lower signal centrally, corresponding to myxoid and fibrocollagenous content, respectively.[48,49] The target appearance is seen in both neurofibromas and schwannomas, though more commonly in neurofibromas.[29] Contrast enhancement is variable. On occasion, the nerve from which the tumor arises becomes thickened immediately adjacent to the tumor, giving rise to a "tail sign."[50] When the PNST enlarges, a surrounding rim of fat is maintained—this becomes especially apparent on lesions that arise within muscle and is termed the "split fat sign" (**Fig. 6**).[26,29]

On imaging, it may be impossible to differentiate benign from malignant PNSTs, although malignant PNSTs are typically larger, have ill-defined margins, and central necrosis and demonstrate rapid growth.[48] Malignant neurofibromas are rare in the foot[32] and are associated with type I neurofibromatosis in 25% to 70% of cases.[29]

MALIGNANT SOFT TISSUE TUMORS

Malignant soft tissue tumors are very uncommon in the foot.[3] The most common sarcomas in the foot

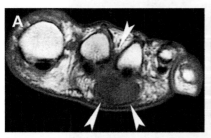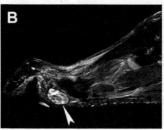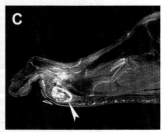

Fig. 5. Soft tissue chondroma. (*A*) Coronal T1-weighted image through the forefoot shows a nonspecific T1-weighted mass centered in the plantar subcutaneous fat, extending between the second and third toes (*arrowheads*). (*B*) Sagittal fat-saturated T2-weighted image shows a lobulated high signal mass, that contains several low signal foci, which seems to be relatively well-demarcated on this view (*arrowhead*). Although not specific in appearance, hyaline cartilage lesions tend to be high signal on T2-weighted images, often similar to fluid, and demonstrate a lobulated growth pattern. (*C*) The lesion (*arrowhead*) demonstrates heterogeneous contrast enhancement.

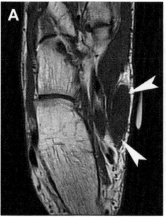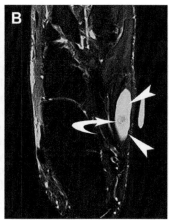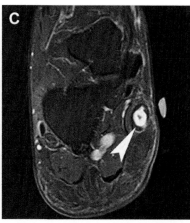

Fig. 6. Schwannoma. (*A, B*) Axial T1-weighted (*A*) and fat-saturated T2-weighted images through the midfoot show a well-circumscribed ovoid mass (*arrowheads*) within the substance of the abductor hallucis muscle. The lesion likely arises from a superficial nerve branch, although no thickened nerve is appreciated. There is a central focus of hyperintense T1/hypointense T2 signal within the lesion, compatible with a target sign, which is a feature that can be seen in nerve sheath tumors (both schwannomas and neurofibromas; *curved arrow*). (*C*) Contrast enhancement on the fat-saturated T1-weighted tracks with T2-weighted appearance, also showing a target sign, with more pronounced enhancement seen peripherally (*arrowhead*).

and ankle are malignant vascular tumors, accounting for nearly one-third of malignant soft tissue tumors in the foot and ankle[3,5,6] and synovial sarcoma, accounting for approximately one-fifth.[3,5,6] It is essential to be aware that soft tissue sarcomas can have a nonaggressive appearance on MR imaging and may present as a smooth bordered mass. Having said that, features that are more common in malignant than in benign lesions include large size (>5 cm), deep site, inhomogeneous signal intensity, hemorrhage and necrosis, early and inhomogeneous contrast enhancement, irregular margins, surrounding soft tissue edema, and invasion of adjacent structures, including bone and neurovascular structures.[3,15,19,51]

Although MR imaging may have limited utility for providing a specific histologic diagnosis, it is the method of choice for pretreatment and preoperative planning. Tumors should be assessed for their size and extent, for involvement of bone and neurovascular structures, and for extension into other surgical compartments, including intraarticular extension.[15]

Synovial Sarcoma

Synovial sarcoma is a malignant sarcoma classified by World Health Organization as a "tumor of uncertain differentiation."[4] It is a mesenchymal spindle cell tumor; biphasic synovial sarcomas contain both epithelial and spindle cell components.[4] Notwithstanding its name, synovial

sarcoma does not arise from existing synovium. Although it is often found near a joint or tendon sheath, fewer than 10% of lesions actually arise within a joint.[29] In Kransdorf's retrospective review, synovial sarcoma constituted the most common malignancy of the foot and ankle in patients 6 to 45 years of age.[2,29] Most synovial sarcomas are diagnosed between 10 and 40 years of age (mean, 32), with men and women affected equally.[52]

Patients with synovial sarcoma present with a mass that may or may not be painful. The lesion is often slow growing. As a result, diagnosis may be delayed, with 1 study showing a mean of 2.5 years between onset of symptoms and diagnosis.[52]

Radiographs show soft tissue calcification in up to 33% of cases. Calcifications are nonspecific in appearance, often eccentric or peripheral,[4,53] and may be difficult to appreciate by MR imaging. 11% to 20% of cases show extrinsic bone erosion, which can seem to be nonaggressive, or a periosteal reaction.[53]

Synovial sarcomas range in size from 3 to 10 cm. However, lesions in the extremities may be relatively small when they present.[52] On MR imaging, synovial sarcomas appear as lobulated soft tissue masses that may be heterogeneously isointense or slightly higher signal intensity than muscles and heterogeneously high signal on T2W images. Jones and colleagues[54] described a "triple" signal intensity appearance, referring to intermixed low, intermediate and high T2 signal within a synovial sarcoma, that reflected a combination of cystic (hemorrhage and necrosis) and solid components.[29,55] Fluid–fluid levels are seen in approximately 10% to 25% of cases.[29] Although not pathognomonic, the triple signal intensity together with fluid–fluid levels, deep location, and appropriate patient age should suggest the diagnosis.[29] Murphey and colleagues[53] described the combination of multilobulation, marked heterogeneous signal intensity, hemorrhage, fluid–fluid levels, and septae seen in synovial sarcomas as the "bowl of grapes" sign. Contrast enhancement is most often prominent and heterogeneous and may be peripheral and nodular.[54]

Because synovial sarcomas can present as small, high T2 signal lesions with smooth, well-defined, nonaggressive borders, and indolent growth,[4] care should be taken not to mistake these malignant neoplasms for a cystic lesion such as a ganglion cyst. When a cystlike lesion has atypical features or occurs in an atypical location, IV contrast should be administered to determine whether it is solid or truly cystic (**Fig. 7**).

CYSTIC TUMORLIKE LESIONS
Ganglion

Ganglia, or ganglion cysts, are benign fluid-filled masses that can arise from joint capsules, tendon sheaths, bursae, ligaments, and subchondral bone.[26,56] Ganglia are not true tumors. However, they are commonly encountered soft tissue masses about the foot and ankle.[39,57] In a series by Weishaupt and colleagues[57] (n = 167), ganglion cysts represented 42% of clinically suspected soft tissue masses in the foot and were found most commonly in tarsal tunnel, sinus tarsi and Lis-Franc joint.

Ganglia are lined by a capsule composed of flat spindle cells and, unlike synovial cysts, do not have a synovial lining.[58] Ganglia often contain viscous, gelatinous fluid. They may be composed of a simple unilocular cyst, although not infrequently, they are lobulated and contain thin septations.[3] Their origin is debated.[3,26,29] They have been theorized to develop owing to synovial herniation from a joint or tendon sheath, synovial rests, mesenchymal metaplasia, repetitive trauma, or ligamentous injury.[3,26,29,59] Lesions typically occur in adults, more commonly in women.[9]

Radiographs of patients with ganglion cysts are typically negative, but nonaggressive bony remodeling can occur.[60] On MR imaging, ganglia are well-defined rounded or multilobulated lesions, with high T2 signal and smooth borders.[29] Lesions vary in size and a given lesion can fluctuate in size, but they often measure 1.5 to 2.5 cm.[9] Lesions may be uniloculated or multiloculated.[60] They are isointense to muscle on T1W images when they contain simple fluid, but can be hyperintense on T1W images when they contain proteinaceous fluid or hemorrhage. After contrast administration, they demonstrate a thin, smooth rim of peripheral enhancement. They should have no internal enhancement, except for similarly thin, smooth septae. Ganglia that are inflamed or infected will show a thicker rim of peripheral enhancement. Lesions typically arise close to a joint or tendon, although they can extend far away from a joint.[61] A high T2 curvilinear channel or "tail" may extend between the ganglion cyst and its site of origin and, when visible, should be reported, to help guide surgical resection.[60] Some ganglia are associated with surrounding pericystic edema (**Fig. 8**).[60]

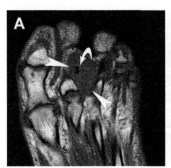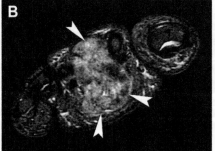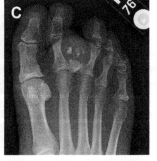

Fig. 7. Synovial sarcoma. (*A*) An axial T1-weighted image shows a lesion that is predominantly isointense to muscle (*arrowheads*) and contains a small low signal focus (*curved arrow*). (*B*) The lesion is heterogeneously high signal on the fat-saturated T2-weighted images (*arrowheads*) and splays the toes. Note the lobulated, well-circumscribed borders and relatively nonaggressive appearance of the mass. (*C*) The corresponding radiograph shows demonstrates calcifications within the mass, which account for the areas of internal low signal on the MR images. The calcifications are irregular and nonspecific in appearance. Radiographs show calcifications in up to 33% of cases of synovial sarcoma.

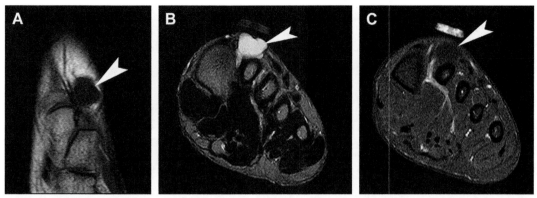

Fig. 8. Ganglion. (*A–C*) A lobulated well-circumscribed lesion (*arrowhead*) arising along the dorsum of them midfoot, just distal to the Lis-Franc ligament, is isointense to muscle on T1-weighted images and, to yield (*A*) hyperintense on T2-weighted images (*B*), reflecting simple fluid content. (*C*) On postcontrast fat-saturated T1-weighted images, there is no central enhancement and only trace peripheral enhancement is seen, confirming its cystic nature. Ganglion cysts are common in the foot, where they are often found in the tarsal tunnel, sinus, and about the Lis-franc joint.

Synovial Cyst

Synovial cysts are juxtaarticular fluid collections that arise from a joint and that possess a synovial lining. A synovial cyst is seen as a well-circumscribed fluidlike focus that communicates with the joint, isointense to muscle on T1W images and hyperintense on T2W images, with a thin rim of peripheral enhancement.[29] They can appear more complex, with higher T1 signal and thicker peripheral enhancement, when hemorrhage, inflammation, or infection is present. In practice, synovial cysts may be difficult to distinguish from ganglia at imaging unless a clear connection to the joint can be demonstrated. Unlike (some) ganglia, synovial cysts should not be multiloculated.

Bursae

Bursae occur in several characteristic locations in the foot and ankle. Congenital bursae include the intermetatarsal bursae (between the intermetatarsal heads) and retrocalcaneal bursa (posterior to the postero-superior tubercle of the calcaneus, deep to the distal Achilles tendon).[62,63] These are present at birth and represent normal anatomy. In contrast, adventitial bursae can develop sporadically, owing to increased friction, and include the retro-Achilles bursae (in the subcutaneous fat posterior to the calcaneus; also known as the superficial calcaneal or tendo-Achilles bursa),[64] the forefoot bursae (in the fat planter to the first metatarsal and in the fat plantar and lateral to the fifth metatarsal head),[65] and malleolar bursae (overlying the malleoli, medial more often

than lateral, typically seen in skaters owing to friction from the skate).[66]

Some fluid-containing bursae may be asymptomatic, but, when inflamed, they can present as a painful mass. Intermetatarsal bursae with fluid content measuring 3 mm or less in transverse diameter are considered physiologic.[67] Studler and colleagues[65] found that 84% of asymptomatic volunteers had signal changes related to adventitial bursae in the plantar fat pad of the forefoot.

Bursae may become inflamed owing to mechanical irritation or owing to involvement in inflammatory arthritides.[63] When inflamed, bursae may fill with fluid and/or thickened synovium. The distended bursa is typically isointense or slightly hyperintense to muscle on T1W images and hypertintense on T2W images. If fluid filled, they demonstrate a thin rim of enhancement. If the bursal synovium is thickened and inflamed, then that will also enhance, creating a thickened, enhancing rim peripherally and a more complex pattern of internal enhancement. In lesions in the forefoot, fibrosis sometimes predominates, leading to low T2 signal (**Fig. 9**).[65]

NONCYSTIC TUMORLIKE MASSES
Morton Neuroma

Morton neuromas are benign nonneoplastic masses that occur owing to fibrosis and neural degeneration surrounding the plantar digital nerve.[68] The majority of lesions occur in the second or third intermetatarsal space, along the plantar aspect of the transverse intermetatarsal

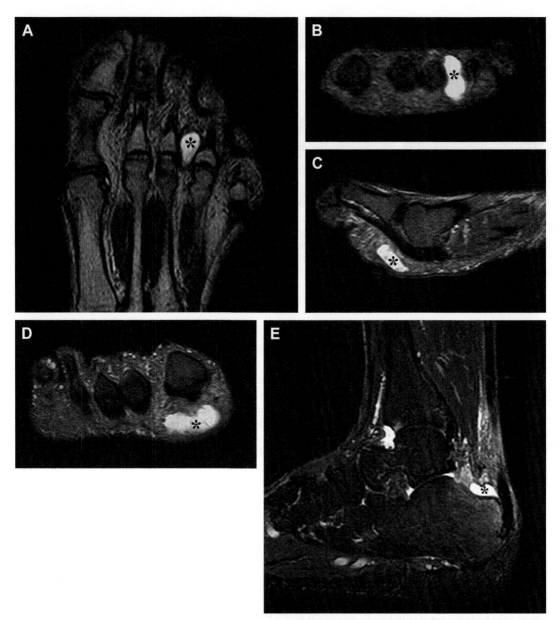

Fig. 9. Bursae. Both congenital and adventitial bursae can be recognized based on their characteristic locations and shapes. They demonstrate high T2 signal owing to fluid content and/or hyperemic synovium. Fluid-filled bursae show a thin peripheral rim of contrast enhancement, but, when the bursal synovium is thickened, the peripheral rim of enhancement can become thickened and irregular. (*A, B*) A distended intermetatarsal bursa has an hourglass shape, extending both dorsal and plantar within the intermetatarsal space (*asterisk*). (*C, D*) Adventitial bursae can form in the subcutaneous fat along the plantar and lateral aspects of the first and fifth metatarsophalangeal joints owing to chronic friction, and tend to have a pliable, discoid shape (*asterisk*). (*E*) The comma-shaped retrocalcaneal bursa lies between the posterior calcaneus and distal Achilles tendon and, when distended, extends into Hoffa's fat pad (*asterisk*).

ligament. Morton neuromas are thought to occur secondary to chronic repetitive microtrauma, with compression of the plantar digital nerve against the transverse ligament. Lesions are seen more commonly in women.[68]

Patients with Morton neuroma may be asymptomatic, but may also present with pain radiating to the toes and with forefoot numbness, often exacerbated by standing or walking.[69] On physical examination, there may be a positive Tinel sign and a positive Mulder sign (a "click" when metatarsal bones are squeezed together).

Radiographs are often negative, but large Morton neuromas may be associated with splaying of the metatarsal heads. MR imaging with the patient in the prone position can be helpful in demonstrating a Morton neuroma.[70] On MR imaging, Morton neuromas are best visualized in the coronal plane (coronal to the body). A Morton neuroma appears as a focal, rounded, or teardrop-shaped mass that is isointense to muscle on T1W images and hypointense to fat on T2W images, owing to its fibrosis.[67] Lesions may be relatively inconspicuous on T2W images obtained without fat saturation.[29,67] Enhancement of Morton neuromas is variable.[29,68] Small lesions may not be visualized on MR imaging and large lesions may be asymptomatic.[69] Asymptomatic lesions that are visible on MR imaging are often smaller than their symptomatic counterparts (**Fig. 10**).[67,69]

The differential diagnosis for a mass in the intermetatarsal space includes the intermetatarsal bursa, which demonstrates high signal on T2W images and which, unlike Morton neuroma, extends above (dorsal) to the level of intermetatarsal ligament.[67]

Soft Tissue Callus

In response to chronic mechanical pressure, a benign fibroblastic response can occur and give rise to focal soft tissue thickening in the superficial plantar subcutaneous fat, typically in the forefoot and heel. This soft tissue "callus" appears lower signal compared with surrounding fat on T1W and T2W MR images.[71] In diabetic patients, this lesion can be come ulcerated and infected, and can become a conduit for deep infection (**Fig. 11**).[72]

Foreign Body Granuloma

The foot is a common site for foreign bodies. Depending on circumstances, a foreign body may elicit a fibrohistiocytic and giant cell granulomatous reaction within the soft tissues and thereby mimic a neoplastic mass. The MR imaging appearance of a foreign body granuloma may vary

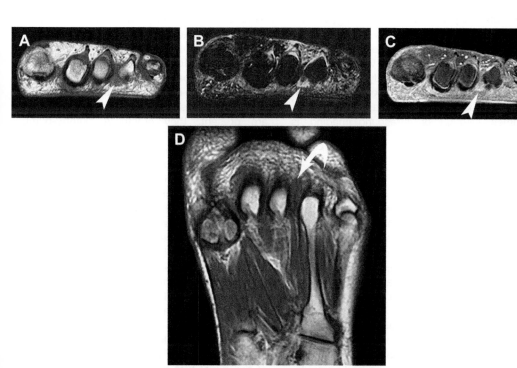

Fig. 10. Morton neuroma. (*A*) T1-weighted and (*B*) fat-saturated T2-weighted images of the forefoot show a well-circumscribed, tear-drop shaped mass (*arrowheads*) in the third intermetatarsal interspace that is isointense to muscle on proton density-weighted and heterogeneously hyperintense on fat-saturated T2-weighted images. (*C*) It demonstrates heterogeneous enhancement on the fat-saturated T1-weighted images (*arrowhead*). (*D*) An axial T1-weighted images shows the mass interposed between the 2 metatarsal heads (*curved arrow*). It represents fibrosis surrounding the plantar digital nerve and characteristically arises along the plantar surface, below the level of the transverse metatarsal ligament.

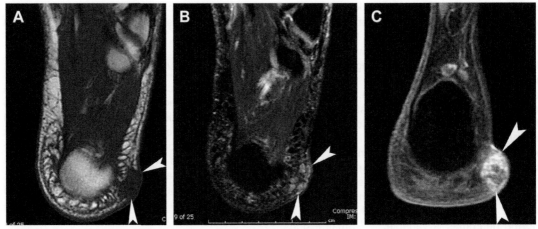

Fig. 11. Soft tissue callus. Soft tissue callus is a benign fibroblastic response that can occur in the superficial plantar subcutaneous in fat response to chronic mechanical pressure, typically seen in the heel and forefoot. (*A, B*) A focal, moderately well-defined mass (*arrowheads*) is seen in the superficial subcutaneous fat of the lateral heel. The lesion (*arrowheads*) is nonspecific in appearance, isointense to muscle on T1-weighted images and heterogeneous on the fat-saturated T2-weighted images. (*C*) Enhancement is heterogeneous (*arrowheads*).

depending on the composition of the foreign body itself and on the nature of the soft tissue response, but foreign body granulomas are often low-to-intermediate signal on T1W images and intermediate-to-high signal on T2W images.[29,73,74] The presence of contrast enhancement is likely to vary based on composition, vascularity and inflammation.[29] The foreign body itself may or may not be apparent on MR imaging. Correlation with clinical history and with radiographs and, sometimes, with CT or ultrasound imaging, is important to help identify the foreign body and aid in diagnosis (**Fig. 12**).

Gout

Gout is a common disorder related to hyperuricemia and is increasing in prevalence in the United States.[75,76] Soft tissue masses owing to gouty tophi are typically encountered in patients with chronic gout, but, on occasion, tophi may be present at the time of the initial attack of gout.[77] Tophi can occur within bone, about joints, within tendons, and in the soft tissues. Paraarticular tophi can give rise to characteristic erosions. Gouty tophi form owing to deposition of monosodium urate crystals, which may be accompanied by intercrystalline matrix, and foreign body granulomatous reaction.[78]

Radiographic changes typically develop only after repeated attacks of gout and are seen in approximately 40% of patients.[39] On radiographs, gouty tophi composed of monosodium urate will be radiolucent, often slightly more

dense than surrounding soft tissues, although they may be apparent owing to mass effect and owing to their characteristic well-circumscribed paraarticular erosions, demarcated by sclerotic rims and overhanging edges of bone. Calcification of the tophus is unusual.[78] However, when calcium coprecipitates with sodium urate, mineralization may be radiographically visible as an irregular or cloudlike calcification, often peripheral in distribution.[78] When multiple tophi are present, they create a "lumpy-bumpy" appearance.

A gouty tophus could be mistaken for a soft tissue neoplasm on MR imaging, so it is important to review the clinical history and to obtain correlative radiographs and serum uric acid studies. On MR imaging, gouty tophi have a nonspecific appearance. The tophi are variable in appearance, generally isointense or hypointense to muscle on TW and variable, but often intermediate to low signal, on T2W images, which may influenced by variable amounts of calcium.[29,75] Contrast enhancement may be uniform or heterogeneous, often with a nonenhancing center.[39,75] Bone erosions and variable amounts of marrow edema may be present. Clues to the diagnosis are site and distribution of findings. The medial aspect of the distal first metatarsal is a characteristic site for gout; gout also can be seen in the midfoot. However, when there is a skin ulcer adjacent to the mass, even in characteristic locations, osteomyelitis should be considered, because concomitant infection of gouty tophi can also occur (**Fig. 13**).[79]

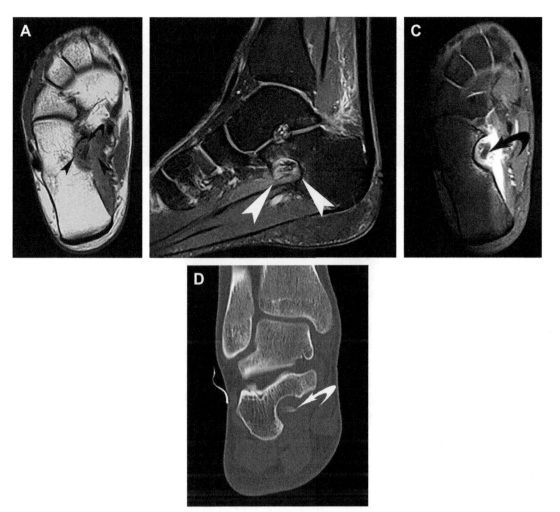

Fig. 12. Foreign body granuloma. (*A*) An axial T1-weighted image shows a mass that is predominantly slightly hyperintense intense to T1 (*arrowheads*) with a central linear focus of lower T1 signal (*curved arrow*). The mass has caused nonaggressive bony remodeling of the adjoining medial wall of the calcaneus (*arrowheads*). The mass is not well-demarcated form the overlying muscle. (*B*) On a sagittal fat-saturated T2-weighted image, the mass (*arrows*) is heterogeneously low signal. (*C*) Postcontrast axial fat-saturated T1-weighted image shows intense enhancement of the lesion, with a small amount of enhancement in the adjoining calcaneus. The central low signal focus does not enhance and remains visible (*curved arrow*). (*D*) Computed tomography scan obtained after the MR image demonstrated a radiopaque foreign body (*curved arrow*), corresponding to the nonenhancing focus on MRI. The enhancing mass was a foreign body granuloma that formed around a fragment of horseshoe crab spine and that had created a pressure erosion in the adjoining calcaneus.

Rheumatoid Nodule

Rheumatoid nodules are benign granulomatous foci with central necrosis that are relatively common in advanced cases of rheumatoid arthritis. They occur in 20% to 30% of individuals with rheumatoid arthritis, often over bony prominences, and are more common in women.[63] Occurrence in the feet is uncommon.[3]

There are few descriptions of rheumatoid nodules in the literature, but the MR imaging appearance has been presented as a nonspecific, ill-defined mass that is isointense to muscle on T1W images and heterogeneously hyperintense on T2W images, with intense, heterogeneous enhancement.[39,80] In our experience, the T2 signal intensity and contrast enhancement characteristics vary based on the lesion's degree of fibrosis (low T2 signal), central necrosis (high T2 signal), and hyperemia (high T2 signal), and with overall disease activity. Correlation with a history of rheumatoid arthritis is important in making the diagnosis (**Fig. 14**).

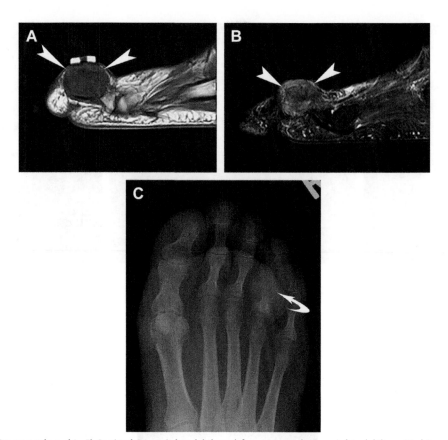

Fig. 13. Gouty tophus. (*A, B*) Sagittal T1-weighted (*A*) and fat-saturated T2-weighted (*B*) sagittal images of the forefoot, show a large, well-defined ovoid mass (*arrowheads*) that is isointense to muscle on T1-weighted and heterogeneously low signal on fluid sensitive images. (*C*) On the radiograph, the mass seems to be aggressive, destroying portions of the phalanges (*curved arrow*). The mass is nonspecific in appearance, although relative low signal on the fluid-sensitive images suggests calcification and/or fibrous material. The patient had a history of gout, making a gouty tophus a likely etiology. The diagnosis of a tophus was confirmed by aspiration.

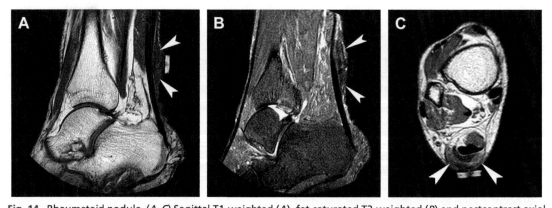

Fig. 14. Rheumatoid nodule. (*A–C*) Sagittal T1-weighted (*A*), fat-saturated T2-weighted (*B*) and postcontrast axial T1-weighted images through the hindfoot show an elongated, relatively well-circumscribed mass centered in the subcutaneous fat along the posterior surface of the Achilles tendon (*arrowheads*). The lesion is predominantly isointense to muscle on T1, heterogeneously low signal on the fluid-sensitive image, and demonstrates heterogeneous enhancement. In the literature, however, rheumatoid nodules are described as heterogeneously hyperintense on fluid sensitive images. In our experience, T21W single intensity and enhancement characteristics of rheumatoid nodules vary with the nodule composition and overall disease activity.

Table 1
Imaging characteristics of common masses about the foot and ankle

	Margins	T1	T2	Contrast	Features	Location	Radiographs
Benign soft tissue tumors							
Plantar fibroma[30]	Nodular mass, well-defined superficially, ill-defined along deep surface	Isointense to slightly hyperintense to muscle	Isointense to slightly hyperintense to muscle (on STIR), heterogeneous	Variable; heterogeneous	Tail sign of enhancement along plantar fascia	Adherent to plantar fascia; Can be multiple	Typically negative
Giant cell tumor of the tendon sheath[35–37]	Rounded or large, lobulated; well-defined	Isointense to hypointense to muscle	Isointense or hypointense to fat, can be somewhat heterogeneous	Variable; often intense homogeneous enhancement	May show blooming on T2*W gradient echo images	Adherent to tendon sheath	Occasional nonaggressive bony remodeling
Hemangioma[40,41]	Well or poorly circumscribed	May be high T1 owing to varying amounts of fatty overgrowth and/or hemorrhage	Typically high signal, owing to slow flow	Prominent contrast enhancement; can be delayed or heterogeneous	Fluid–fluid levels; Signal voids owing to high flow vessels (serpiginous) or phleboliths (rounded); Fatty atrophy in surrounding muscle Perilesional blooming on T2*W owing to hemosiderin, if has bled	Nonspecific	Phleboliths in ≤50% Bony reactive changes (cortical or periosteal thickening) in ≤33%
Lipoma[42,43]	Often, but not always, encapsulated	High signal, isointense to fat	Isointense to fat	Thin rim of enhancement, no internal enhancement except for thin septae (<2 mm)	Uniformly loses signal with frequency selective fat saturation	Nonspecific	Occasionally visible as a lucent mass; thin septations and calcifications sometimes visible

(continued on next page)

Table 1
(continued)

	Margins	T1	T2	Contrast	Features	Location	Radiographs
Soft tissue chondroma[44–46]	Well defined	Intermediate signal intensity, with matrix calcifications seen as low signal foci	High T2 signal with matrix calcifications seen as low signal foci	Not well-described	Lobulated pattern reflects growth pattern of hyaline cartilage	Near tendons and joints	Peripheral and central calcifications, including "chondroid" calcifications
Peripheral nerve sheath tumor[48,49]	Well-defined smooth bordered fusiform mass aligned along the nerve; (exception: plexiform neurofibromas)	Isointense to muscle	Slightly hyperintense to fat	Variable; heterogeneous	Target sign Tail sign Split fat sign	Along nerve	Typically negative
Malignant soft tissue tumors (selected)							
Synovial sarcoma[52–55]	Often rounded, and lobulated well-defined	Isointense to muscle	Hyperintense to fat on T2, often very heterogeneous unless small	Intense, usually heterogeneous, often nodular foci	Triple signal appearance (intermixed low, intermediate, and high T2 signal); Fluid–fluid levels in 10%–25% Septations "Bowl of grapes" appearance	Almost always extra-articular, though often near a joint	Lesion mineralization, often peripheral, seen in as many as one-third of patients Bone involvement (periosteal reaction, osseous remodeling, frank bony invasion) in 11%–20%
Cystic tumor like masses							
Ganglion[58–61]	Rounded, well-circumscribed; Uniloculated or multiloculated	Isointense or hyperintense to muscle	Fluidlike; hyperintense to fat and muscle	Thin rim of peripheral enhancement (thicker if inflamed)	Tail sign—thin fluidlike channel points to site of origin	Usually near joint or tendon, but can extend far away	Typically negative, can see nonaggressive bone remodeling

Mass	Shape	T1 signal	T2 signal	Enhancement		Location	Radiographs
Synovial cyst[58-61]	Well-circumscribed, rounded, tear-drop shaped	Isointense or slightly hyperintense to muscle	Fluidlike; hyperintense	Thin or thick rim of enhancement, depending on degree of synovial thickening	N/A	Extends from joint	Negative
Bursa[62-67]	Well-circumscribed; fibrous lesions in forefoot can be less well-circumscribed Shape varies with type of bursa	Isointense or slightly hyperintense to muscle	Fluidlike; hyperintense	Thin or thick rim of enhancement, depending on degree of synovial thickening	N/A	Characteristic locations	Typically negative
Noncystic tumorlike masses							
Morton neuroma[67,69]	Focal, rounded or teardrop shape	Isointense to muscle	Hypointense to fat	Variable in degree and pattern	N/A	Arises around plantar digital nerve, typically plantar to transverse intermetatarsal ligament	Typically negative, splaying of metatarsal heads when large
Soft tissue callus[71,72]	Focal, but not well-defined	Hypointense to fat	Hypointense to fat	Not well-described, likely variable	N/A	Subcutaneous fat, at sites of mechanical pressure, typically forefoot and heel	Typically negative, may see nonspecific increased density in subcutaneous fat
Foreign body granuloma[73,74]	Focal	Varies, often low-to-intermediate signal	Varies, often intermediate to high signal	Varies	N/A	Nonspecific	Can see foreign body, if radiopaque

(continued on next page)

Table 1
(continued)

	Margins	T1	T2	Contrast	Features	Location	Radiographs
Gouty tophus[75,76,78]	Focal	Isointense or hypointense to muscle	Variable, but often intermediate to low signal	Uniform or heterogeneous, often with a nonenhancing center	N/A	Medial aspect of distal first metatarsal is characteristic, though can occur elsewhere	Well-defined periarticular erosions with sclerotic rims and overhanging edges; "lumpy bumpy appearance"; mass may have irregular or cloudlike calcification
Rheumatoid nodule[6,80]	Focal, variable degree of definition	Isointense to muscle	Heterogeneously hyperintense, may be lower when fibrotic	Intense heterogeneous enhancement, may be lower when fibrotic	N/A	Nonspecific	May see other findings of rheumatoid arthritis, such as marginal erosions

Abbreviation: STIR, short T1 inversion recovery.

Variable = Degree of enhancement.

Homogeneous or heterogeneous = Pattern of enhancement.

Based on original study, signal intensity of some lesions were described in relation to fat, others in relation to muscle. Some lesions were originally characterized on T2-weighted images, others on fat saturated T2-weighted or STIR images.

SUMMARY

Soft tissue masses in the foot and ankle may represent true neoplasms, either malignant or benign, or may represent other, nonneoplastic entities that mimic musculoskeletal tumors. The most common benign lesions include ganglion cyst, plantar fibromatosis, GCT-TS, hemangioma, lipoma, soft tissue chondroma, and benign nerve sheath tumors. The most common malignant lesions include malignant vascular tumors, synovial sarcoma, fibrosarcoma, melanotic clear cell tumor, and undifferentiated pleomorphic sarcoma. Although a definitive diagnosis may not be possible in many cases, imaging characteristics can help to narrow the differential diagnosis for a soft tissue mass and, occasionally, provide a specific diagnosis. Patient demographics, clinical history and physical examination remain relevant. Radiographs can provide important information regarding soft tissue calcifications, foreign bodies, bone erosions, and periostitis. On MR imaging, consider signal intensity on T1W andT2W images, contrast enhancement characteristics, lesion location, and lesion association with other anatomic structures (**Table 1**). Some solid masses have high T2 signal intensity and can be mistaken for cysts. IV contrast helps in making the distinction. Malignant sarcomas can be nonaggressive in appearance and can demonstrate indolent growth.

REFERENCES

1. Kransdorf MJ. Benign soft-tissue tumors in a large referral population: distribution of specific diagnoses by age, sex, and location. AJR Am J Roentgenol 1995;164:395–402.

2. Kransdorf MJ. Malignant soft-tissue tumors in a large referral population: distribution of diagnoses by age, sex, and location. AJR Am J Roentgenol 1995;164:129–34.

3. Berquist TH, Kransdorf MJ. Bone and soft tissue tumors and tumor-like conditions. Chapter 6. In: Berquist TH, editor. Imaging of the foot and ankle. Philadelphia: Wolters Kluwer/Lippincott Williams & Wilkins; 2011. p. 375–435.

4. Fletcher CD, Bridge JA, Hogendoorn PC, et al, editors. WHO classification of tumours of soft tissue and bone. Lyon (France): IARC Press; 2013.

5. Kirby EJ, Shereff MJ, Lewis MM. Soft-tissue tumors and tumor-like lesions of the foot. An analysis of eighty-three cases. J Bone Joint Surg Am 1989;71: 621–6.

6. Bakotic BW, Borkowski P. Primary soft-tissue neoplasms of the foot: the clinicopathologic features of 401 cases. J Foot Ankle Surg 2001;40:28–35.

7. Blume PA, Niemi WJ, Courtright DJ, et al. Fibrosarcoma of the foot: a case presentation and review of the literature. J Foot Ankle Surg 1997; 36:51–4.

8. Gibbons CL, Khwaja HA, Cole AS, et al. Giant-cell tumour of the tendon sheath in the foot and ankle. J Bone Joint Surg Br 2002;84:1000–3.

9. Weiss SW, Goldblum JR. Enziger and Weiss' soft tissue tumors. St Louis (MO): Mosby; 2001.

10. Zoga AC, Weissman BN, Kransdorf MJ, et al. ACR appropriateness criteria® soft-tissue masses. American College Radiology; 2012. Available at https://acsearch.acr.org/docs/70546/Narrative/. Accessed September 29, 2016.

11. Gartner L, Pearce CJ, Saifuddin A. The role of the plain radiograph in the characterisation of soft tissue tumours. Skeletal Radiol 2009;38:549–58.

12. Pham H, Fessell DP, Femino JE, et al. Sonography and MR imaging of selected benign masses in the ankle and foot. AJR Am J Roentgenol 2003;180: 99–107.

13. Fritz J, Henes JC, Fuld MK, et al. Dual-energy computed tomography of the knee, ankle, and foot: noninvasive diagnosis of gout and quantification of monosodium urate in tendons and ligaments. Semin Musculoskelet Radiol 2016;20:130–6.

14. Desai MA, Peterson JJ, Garner HW, et al. Clinical utility of dual-energy CT for evaluation of tophaceous gout. Radiographics 2011;13:1365–75.

15. Manaster BJ. Soft-tissue masses: optimal imaging protocol and reporting. AJR Am J Roentgenol 2013;201:505–14.

16. Maas M, Dijkstra PF, Akkerman EM. Uniform fat suppression in hands and feet through the use of two-point Dixon chemical shift MR imaging. Radiology 1999;210:189–93.

17. Talbot BS, Weinberg EP. MR Imaging with metal-suppression sequences for evaluation of total joint arthroplasty. Radiographics 2016;36:209–25.

18. Ariyanayagam T, Malcolm PN, Toms AP. Advances in metal artifact reduction techniques for periprosthetic soft tissue imaging. Semin Musculoskelet Radiol 2015;19:328–34.

19. Chhabra A, Soldatos T. Soft-tissue lesions: when can we exclude sarcoma? AJR Am J Roentgenol 2012; 199:1345–57.

20. Papp DF, Khanna AJ, McCarthy EF, et al. Magnetic resonance imaging of soft-tissue tumors: determinate and indeterminate lesions. J Bone Joint Surg Am 2007;89(Suppl 3):103–15.

21. van Rijswijk CS, Kunz P, Hogendoorn PC, et al. Diffusion-weighted MRI in the characterization of soft-tissue tumors. J Magn Reson Imaging 2002;15: 302–7.

22. Jeon JY, Chung HW, Lee MH, et al. Usefulness of diffusion-weighted MR imaging for differentiating between benign and malignant superficial soft

tissue tumours and tumour-like lesions. Br J Radiol 2016;89:20150929.

23. Lee SY, Jee WH, Jung JY, et al. Differentiation of malignant from benign soft tissue tumours: use of additive qualitative and quantitative diffusion-weighted MR imaging to standard MR imaging at 3.0 T. Eur Radiol 2016;26:743–54.

24. Fisher SM, Joodi R, Madhuranthakam AJ, et al. Current utilities of imaging in grading musculoskeletal soft tissue sarcomas. Eur J Radiol 2016;85:1336–44.

25. Fayad LM, Jacobs MA, Wang X, et al. Musculoskeletal tumors: how to use anatomic, functional, and metabolic MR techniques. Radiology 2012;265: 340–56.

26. Wu JS, Hochman MG. Soft-tissue tumors and tumor-like lesions: a systematic imaging approach. Radiology 2009;253:297–316.

27. Sundaram M, McGuire MH, Herbold DR, et al. High signal intensity soft tissue masses on T1 weighted pulsing sequences. Skeletal Radiol 1987;16:30–6.

28. Sundaram M, McGuire MH, Schajowicz F. Soft-tissue masses: histologic basis for decreased signal (short T2) on T2-weighted MR images. AJR Am J Roentgenol 1987;148:1247–50.

29. Kransdorf MJ, Murphey MD. Imaging of soft tissue tumors. Philadelphia: Lippincott, William & Wilkins; 2006.

30. Morrison WB, Schweitzer ME, Wapner KL, et al. Plantar fibromatosis: a benign aggressive neoplasm with a characteristic appearance on MR images. Radiology 1994;193:841–5.

31. van der Heijden L, Gibbons CL, Hassan AB, et al. A multidisciplinary approach to giant cell tumors of tendon sheath and synovium–a critical appraisal of literature and treatment proposal. J Surg Oncol 2013;107:433–45.

32. Johnston MR. Epidemiology of soft-tissue and bone tumors of the foot. Clin Podiatr Med Surg 1993;10: 581–607.

33. Walling AK, Gasser SI. Soft-tissue and bone tumors about the foot and ankle. Clin Sports Med 1994;13: 909–38.

34. Ushijima M, Hashimoto H, Tsuneyoshi M, et al. Giant cell tumor of the tendon sheath (nodular tenosynovitis). A study of 207 cases to compare the large joint group with the common digit group. Cancer 1986;57:875–84.

35. Karasick D, Karasick S. Giant cell tumor of tendon sheath: spectrum of radiologic findings. Skeletal Radiol 1992;21:219–24.

36. De Beuckeleer L, De Schepper A, De Belder F, et al. Magnetic resonance imaging of localized giant cell tumour of the tendon sheath (MRI of localized GCTTS). Eur Radiol 1997;7:198–201.

37. Narvaez JA, Narvaez J, Aguilera C, et al. MR imaging of synovial tumors and tumor-like lesions. Eur Radiol 2001;11:2549–60.

38. Fox MG, Kransdorf MJ, Bancroft LW, et al. MR imaging of fibroma of the tendon sheath. AJR Am J Roentgenol 2003;180:1449–53.

39. Bancroft LW, Peterson JJ, Kransdorf MJ. Imaging of soft tissue lesions of the foot and ankle. Radiol Clin North Am 2008;46:1093–103, vii.

40. Flors L, Leiva-Salinas C, Maged IM, et al. MR imaging of soft-tissue vascular malformations: diagnosis, classification, and therapy follow-up. Radiographics 2011;31:1321–40 [discussion: 1340–1].

41. Ly JQ, Sanders TG, Mulloy JP, et al. Osseous change adjacent to soft-tissue hemangiomas of the extremities: correlation with lesion size and proximity to bone. AJR Am J Roentgenol 2003; 180:1695–700.

42. Murphey MD, Carroll JF, Flemming DJ, et al. From the archives of the AFIP: benign musculoskeletal lipomatous lesions. Radiographics 2004;24: 1433–66.

43. Kransdorf MJ, Bancroft LW, Peterson JJ, et al. Imaging of fatty tumors: distinction of lipoma and well-differentiated liposarcoma. Radiology 2002; 224:99–104.

44. Chung E, Enziger FM. Chondroma of soft parts. Cancer 1978;41:1414–24.

45. Hondar Wu HT, Chen W, Lee O, et al. Imaging and pathological correlation of soft-tissue chondroma: a serial five-case study and literature review. Clin Imaging 2006;30:32–6.

46. Papagelopoulos PJ, Savvidou OD, Mavrogenis AF, et al. Extraskeletal chondroma of the foot. Joint Bone Spine 2007;74:285–8.

47. Jo VY, Fletcher CD. WHO classification of soft tissue tumours: an update based on the 2013 (4th) edition. Pathology 2014;46:95–104.

48. Murphey MD, Smith WS, Smith SE, et al. From the archives of the AFIP. Imaging of musculoskeletal neurogenic tumors: radiologic-pathologic correlation. Radiographics 1999;19:1253–80.

49. Suh JS, Abenoza P, Galloway HR, et al. Peripheral (extracranial) nerve tumors: correlation of MR imaging and histologic findings. Radiology 1992;183:341–6.

50. Lin J, Martel W. Cross-sectional imaging of peripheral nerve sheath tumors: characteristic signs on CT, MR imaging, and sonography. AJR Am J Roentgenol 2001;176:75–82.

51. Gielen JL, De Schepper AM, Vanhoenacker F, et al. Accuracy of MRI in characterization of soft tissue tumors and tumor-like lesions. A prospective study in 548 patients. Eur Radiol 2004;14:2320–30.

52. Bakri A, Shinagare AB, Krajewski KM, et al. Synovial sarcoma: imaging features of common and uncommon primary sites, metastatic patterns, and treatment response. AJR Am J Roentgenol 2012;199: W208–15.

53. Murphey MD, Gibson MS, Jennings BT, et al. From the archives of the AFIP: imaging of synovial

sarcoma with radiologic-pathologic correlation. Radiographics 2006;26:1543–65.

54. Jones BC, Sundaram M, Kransdorf MJ. Synovial sarcoma: MR imaging findings in 34 patients. AJR Am J Roentgenol 1993;161:827–30.

55. Nakanishi H, Araki N, Sawai Y, et al. Cystic synovial sarcomas: imaging features with clinical and histopathologic correlation. Skeletal Radiol 2003;32: 701–7.

56. Janzen DL, Peterfy CG, Forbes JR, et al. Cystic lesions around the knee joint: MR imaging findings. AJR Am J Roentgenol 1994;163:155–61.

57. Weishaupt D, Schweitzer ME, Morrison WB, et al. MRI of the foot and ankle: prevalence and distribution of occult and palpable ganglia. J Magn Reson Imaging 2001;14:464–71.

58. Lee KR, Cox GG, Neff JR, et al. Cystic masses of the knee: arthrographic and CT evaluation. AJR Am J Roentgenol 1987;148:329–34.

59. el-Noueam KI, Schweitzer ME, Blasbalg R, et al. Is a subset of wrist ganglia the sequela of internal derangements of the wrist joint? MR imaging findings. Radiology 1999;212:537–40.

60. Kim JY, Jung SA, Sung MS, et al. Extra-articular soft tissue ganglion cyst around the knee: focus on the associated findings. Eur Radiol 2004;14: 106–11.

61. Feldman F, Singson RD, Staron RB. Magnetic resonance imaging of para-articular and ectopic ganglia. Skeletal Radiol 1989;18:353–8.

62. Theumann NH, Pfirrmann CW, Chung CB, et al. Intermetatarsal spaces: analysis with MR bursography, anatomic correlation, and histopathology in cadavers. Radiology 2001;221:478–84.

63. Mutlu H, Sildiroglu H, Pekkafali Z, et al. MRI appearance of retrocalcaneal bursitis and rheumatoid nodule in a patient with rheumatoid arthritis. Clin Rheumatol 2006;25:734–6.

64. Lawrence DA, Rolen MF, Morshed KA, et al. MRI of heel pain. AJR Am J Roentgenol 2013;200:845–55.

65. Studler U, Mengiardi B, Bode B, et al. Fibrosis and adventitious bursae in plantar fat pad of forefoot: MR imaging findings in asymptomatic volunteers and MR imaging-histologic comparison. Radiology 2008;246:863–70.

66. Brown TD, Varney TE, Micheli LJ. Malleolar bursitis in figure skaters. Indications for operative and nonoperative treatment. Am J Sports Med 2000;28: 109–11.

67. Zanetti M, Strehle JK, Zollinger H, et al. Morton neuroma and fluid in the intermetatarsal bursae on MR images of 70 asymptomatic volunteers. Radiology 1997;203:516–20.

68. Waldt S, Rechl H, Rummeny EJ, et al. Imaging of benign and malignant soft tissue masses of the foot. Eur Radiol 2003;13:1125–36.

69. Bencardino J, Rosenberg ZS, Beltran J, et al. Morton's neuroma: is it always symptomatic? AJR Am J Roentgenol 2000;175:649–53.

70. Weishaupt D, Treiber K, Kundert HP, et al. Morton neuroma: MR imaging in prone, supine, and upright weight-bearing body positions. Radiology 2003;226: 849–56.

71. Van Hul E, Vanhoenacker F, Van Dyck P, et al. Pseudotumoural soft tissue lesions of the foot and ankle: a pictorial review. Insights Imaging 2011;2:439–52.

72. Schweitzer ME, Morrison WB. MR imaging of the diabetic foot. Radiol Clin North Am 2004;42: 61–71, vi.

73. Varma DG, Ro JY, Guo SQ, et al. Magnetic resonance imaging appearance of foreign body granulomas of the upper arms. Clin Imaging 1994;18: 39–42.

74. Jabra AA, Taylor GA. MRI evaluation of superficial soft tissue lesions in children. Pediatr Radiol 1993; 23:425–8.

75. Yu JS, Chung C, Recht M, et al. MR imaging of tophaceous gout. AJR Am J Roentgenol 1997;168: 523–7.

76. Girish G, Glazebrook KN, Jacobson JA. Advanced imaging in gout. AJR Am J Roentgenol 2013;201: 515–25.

77. Shmerling RH, Stern SH, Gravallese EM, et al. Tophaceous deposition in the finger pads without gouty arthritis. Arch Intern Med 1988;148:1830–2.

78. Resnick D, Kransdorf MJ. Crystal-induced and related diseases. Chapter 33. In: Resnick D, Kransdorf MJ, editors. Bone and joint imaging. 3rd edition. Philadelphia: Elsevier Saunders; 2005. p. 445–58.

79. Yu KH, Luo SF, Liou LB, et al. Concomitant septic and gouty arthritis–an analysis of 30 cases. Rheumatology (Oxford) 2003;42:1062–6.

80. Sanders TG, Linares R, Su A. Rheumatoid nodule of the foot: MRI appearances mimicking an indeterminate soft tissue mass. Skeletal Radiol 1998;27: 457–60.

MR Imaging of the Diabetic Foot

Eoghan McCarthy, MD, William B. Morrison, MD, Adam C. Zoga, MD*

KEYWORDS

- MR imaging • Diabetic foot • Osteomyelitis • Septic arthritis • Neuropathic osteoarthropathy
- Ulcer • Abscess

KEY POINTS

- Osteomyelitis occurs from direct inoculation in most cases, and identification of a skin defect should be the first step in evaluation of all diabetic feet.
- T2 hyperintensity and T1 hypointensity are required for the diagnosis of osteomyelitis. T2 hyperintensity on its own likely represents osseous stress response.
- Osteomyelitis tends to occur distal to the tarsometatarsal joints and in the malleoli and calcaneus.
- Neuropathic osteoarthropathy tends to be centered at the Lisfranc, Chopart, or metatarsophalangeal joints.
- Imaging findings suggestive of superimposed infection in neuropathic osteoarthropathy are ghosting of bones (indistinct on T1, but present on T2 or T1 postcontrast studies), disappearance of subchondral cysts, and greater-than-expected fluid collections.

INTRODUCTION/CLINICAL PRESENTATION

Diabetic patients develop injury and progressive diseases of the foot from numerous sources, including disease of the peripheral nervous, vascular, and immune systems. There is frequently significant overlap between these issues, with one-third of all diabetic patients having a mixed neuropathic-ischemic foot ulcer.[1] Sensory, motor, and autonomic nervous system problems arise in the setting of chronic hyperglycemia. Sensory neuropathy results in the inability to adapt to mechanical stresses with resultant soft tissue ulceration and articular structural disruption. Autonomic neuropathy deregulates perspiration, skin temperature, and arteriovenous shunting resulting in excessive callus formation and skin cracking. Motor neuropathy results in intrinsic muscle dysfunction or, less commonly, a single nerve defect, most frequently involving the common peroneal nerve. Diabetic patients have both large and small vessel ischemia. This ischemia is worsened by coexisting vascular risk factors, including smoking, hypertension, and hyperlipidemia. It is often refractory to revascularization of the larger vessels because of the extent of microvessel disease. Diabetes also inhibits the activity of polymorphonuclear leukocytes, reducing cellular immune responses. Collagen and keratin formation is also impaired.[2] The primary role of imaging is to identify and delineate the sequelae of these systemic processes, including soft tissue infection, abscess formation, osteomyelitis, and the neuropathic joint. Prompt identification and accurate diagnosis are important for limb-sparing treatment planning.[3]

IMAGING THE DIABETIC FOOT

The first-line examination of the diabetic foot is conventional radiographs, which should be performed in at least 3 planes and optimally 4. Relevant radiographic findings that should be observed include

The authors have nothing to disclose.
Division of Musculoskeletal Imaging, Department of Radiology, Jefferson Medical College, Thomas Jefferson University, 132 South 10th Street, Suite 1096A, Philadelphia, PA 19107, USA
* Corresponding author.
E-mail address: Adam.zoga@jefferson.edu

Magn Reson Imaging Clin N Am 25 (2017) 183–194
http://dx.doi.org/10.1016/j.mric.2016.08.005
1064-9689/17/© 2016 Elsevier Inc. All rights reserved.

soft tissue swelling, radiopaque foreign bodies, cortical disruption/destruction, periostitis, joint incongruity, arterial calcification, and prior amputation. Radiographs can also be a beneficial adjunct in the evaluation of complex midfoot disruption. However, radiographs are insensitive to early osteomyelitis and notoriously underestimate the extent of osseous infection.[4] Ultrasound may be used to evaluate soft tissue processes, such as abscess formation and tenosynovitis, and to locate radiolucent foreign bodies. However, this modality is limited in evaluating underlying bone and is also extremely user dependent. Triple phase bone scans that should be positive on all 3 phases (angiographic, blood pool, and delayed) in the setting of osteomyelitis are sensitive for osseous activity but not specific.[5,6] Scintigraphic studies may be positive in other processes with high bone turnover, such as injury and neuropathic osteoarthropathy, and even osseous stress response.[7] Labeled white blood cell scans have an increased sensitivity over bone scans; but the major limitation of nuclear medicine is the poor anatomic resolution, thus limiting the usefulness of these studies as a preoperative road map.[8] MR imaging has emerged as the dominant imaging modality in the assessment of the diabetic foot, particularly the infected diabetic foot. It has high sensitivity (90%) and specificity (83%) for the diagnosis of osteomyelitis.[9,10] Furthermore, it has the added benefit of providing good anatomic definition, allowing it to serve as an appropriate road map for surgical resection.

MR IMAGING SCAN PROTOCOLS

The MR imaging examination should be tailored to the site of suspected abnormality. The authors divide the diabetic foot examination into either the ankle, including the ankle and hindfoot, or the foot, including the midfoot and forefoot. This designation allows for focused, smaller field-of-view imaging for the precise area of concern. Late-model multichannel ankle/foot receiver coils can provide high-resolution imaging from the ankle through the forefoot with a single acquisition, but prescription of imaging planes becomes difficult in this scenario. Most commercial payers still accept foot and ankle MR imaging examinations as distinct procedures; there are distinct *Current Procedural Terminology* codes: 73,718 and 73,720. The field of view for either examination can easily be tailored to the location of clinical concern.

As a standard protocol, with the use of dedicated extremity receiver coils, 2 sets of acquisitions are obtained in each plane. T1-weighted non–fat-suppressed imaging is performed in at least 2 planes to evaluate the bone marrow and the subcutaneous soft tissues. For these sequences, traditional spin echo is ideal; but multiecho acquisitions with a short echo train are adequate. Fat suppressed, fast spin echo/turbo spin echo T2-weighted images are used to evaluate for edema and fluid signal. A short tau inversion recovery (STIR) sequence is recommended in at least one plane (generally sagittal) to mitigate potential near field homogeneity artifacts. Noncontrast examinations are almost always diagnostic; given the great frequency of renal disease in diabetic patients, contrast is rarely administered. When necessary and feasible, precontrast and postcontrast fat-suppressed, T1-weighted, fast gradient-echo sequences can be used to better delineate sinus tracts and abscess cavities and to identify devitalized/necrotic tissue.[11,12] Dynamic contrast runs can be helpful in some cases, as the rate of enhancement can be measured and compared between normal tissues and devitalized tissues. To date, 1.5 T is still considered the imaging standard. Imaging at 3 T offers theoretic advantages, with shorter imaging times and/or higher resolution; but it is also prone to more artifacts and signal homogeneity issues.

MR IMAGING FINDINGS AND DIAGNOSTIC CRITERIA IN THE DIABETIC FOOT
Soft Tissue Edema, Cellulitis

Skin thickening and edema (T1 hypointensity and T2 hyperintensity) are findings found in both soft tissue edema and cellulitis. Enhancement on postcontrast imaging is a characteristic feature of cellulitis. Furthermore, skin thickening and edema in the vicinity of soft tissue ulcer or abscess should raise suspicion of focal cellulitis rather than bland soft tissue edema.

Callus, Ulcer

Callus is a focal, masslike infiltration of the subcutaneous fat, seen as hypointense T1 and intermediate T2 signal.[13] Callus enhances on T1-weighted postcontrast imaging.[14] Typical locations for callus formation include beneath the first and fifth metatarsal heads and the distal phalanx of the hallux in the forefoot. In the midfoot, callus forms deep to the cuboid in patients with rocker bottom deformities and at the heel in the hind foot.[15,16] Chronic friction at the site of callus can lead to the formation of overlying adventitial bursitis, which appears as a thin, linear, T2 fluid collection.[13] Ulcers typically result from the breakdown of callus. Identifiable skin defects and heaped margins will allow differentiation of these two entities (Fig. 1). Unlike callus, ulcers are T2 hyperintense. This high T2 signal is secondary to granulation tissue at the base and

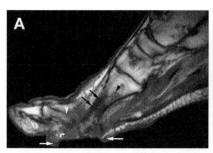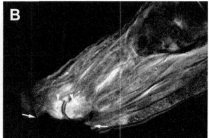

Fig. 1. MR imaging of the right foot of a 59-year-old man with a foul-smelling ulcer underlying the hallux. Consecutive sagittal T1-weighted (*A*) and sagittal STIR (*B*) images of the midfoot and forefoot are shown. There is a large, soft tissue ulceration plantar to the first metatarsophalangeal joint (*white arrows*), which can be seen to be in continuity with the underlying bone on the T2-weighted image (*B*). There is extensive marrow edema (*white arrowheads, B*) on both sides of the joint with T1 marrow replacement (*white arrowhead, A*), a large joint effusion (*curved arrow, A*), and periosteal reaction, cortical thickening, and irregularity of the metatarsal (*black arrows, A*). Features are consistent with osteomyelitis and septic arthritis. Incidental note is made of a bone infarct in the proximal first metatarsal (*black arrowhead, A*).

margins of the lesion. Ulcers also enhance after contrast administration.[16]

Sinus Tract, Abscess

Sinus tracts are tubular or fissurelike conduits extending directly from the skin into the underlying soft tissues, or even into bone, allowing for spread of infection. These tracts may extend to any structure, even articular surfaces and joint spaces, resulting in osteomyelitis or septic arthritis. Identification of sinus tracts is essential. They can be observed on noncontrast fluid sensitive sequences but are more easily visualized on contrast-enhanced imaging as an enhancing connection between skin ulceration and soft tissue abscesses or infiltrated bone. Sinus tracts should be assessed in all 3 planes to accurately map out their full extent.[17,18] Abscesses will be identified as pockets of fluid (areas of increased T2 signal) on fluid-sensitive imaging (**Fig. 2**). Smaller abscesses may be difficult to identify without the aid of contrast. Linear peripheral contrast enhancement along the wall of the fluid collection is diagnostic of an abscess.[12] Accurate delineation of all abscesses is a necessity before any surgical intervention.

Foreign Bodies

Barefoot walking in the presence of sensory neuropathy predisposes diabetic patients to the risk of plantar soft tissue injury and retained foreign bodies. These bodies will incite a local tissue response and can also act as vectors for the introduction of infection. Plain radiographs and particularly sonography are long established as sensitive diagnostic investigations in the evaluation of foreign bodies.[19] MR imaging is generally less useful for detecting foreign bodies. The magnetic resonance (MR) appearance depends on

foreign body composition. Foreign bodies often have low T1 and T2 signal and may be difficult to distinguish from surrounding soft tissues. Metal, air, and some forms of plastic and glass will be visible because of accompanying blooming artifact on gradient echo sequences.[20,21] Surrounding enhancing tissue should be interpreted as reactive local tissue response/granulation tissue. If there is adjacent high T2 signal with an enhancing rim, an abscess can be documented; but it is important to distinguish between reactive soft tissue and adjacent abscess formation.[15]

Muscle Denervation

MR imaging is exquisitely sensitive for muscle atrophy. Early muscle denervation from peripheral neuropathy is seen as high signal T2 linear streaks and patchy T1 hyperintensity in the intrinsic musculature of the forefoot, either diffusely or along neurotomal distribution.[22] With advanced disease, there is fatty atrophy of these muscles. The muscle fibers become completely replaced by fat, appearing as bright signal on both T1 and T2 sequences and low signal on fat-suppressed imaging (**Fig. 3**). Diabetic vasculopathy most frequently leads to the diffuse pattern of forefoot muscle atrophy, in contrast to posttraumatic and impingement processes that are more often neurotomal, along distributions of the medial or lateral plantar nerves. Forefoot muscle atrophy is associated with neuropathic arthropathies in the foot and, even at a preclinical stage, should be observed on MR imaging.[23]

Necrotizing Fasciitis, Pyomyositis, Gangrene

Necrotizing fasciitis is a rapidly progressive medical emergency with mortality rates reported as high as 70% to 80%.[24] Usually a polymicrobial

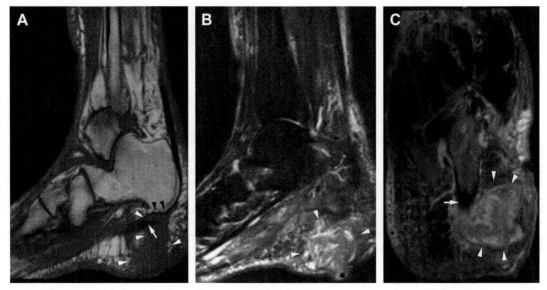

Fig. 2. MR imaging of the right foot of a 63-year-old diabetic woman with a focal, discharging ulcer on the medial plantar aspect of the foot, underlying the calcaneus. Sagittal T1 (*A*), sagittal STIR (*B*), and coronal fat-suppressed T2 (*C*) images all demonstrate a large heterogeneous abscess in the plantar soft tissues (*white arrowheads*) with the focal skin defect/ulcer evident on the STIR imaging (*black asterisk, B*). The abscess is intimately associated with central cord of the plantar fascia (*white arrow, A, C*) and can be seen to track around the superior aspect of the fascia (*most superior white arrowhead, A*). There is, however, no osteomyelitis. There was no abnormal T2 marrow edema in the plantar aspect of the calcaneus (not shown) and no T1 marrow replacement. The cortical margin of the plantar aspect of the calcaneus is normal, without breach or periosteal reaction (*black arrowheads, A*).

infection, it starts in the superficial fascia extending to the deep fascia, resulting in necrosis by microvascular occlusion.[24] MR imaging will demonstrate circumferential dermal and soft tissue thickening with smooth or fusiform thickening of the superficial and deep fascia. In advanced cases, fluid collections and gas formation occurs in the fascial planes. Gas bubbles appear as signal voids on all conventional sequences. If gas is suspected, but not visualized on conventional sequences, gradient sequences can be added to identify subtle areas of blooming artifact.[15] The muscle immediately adjacent the fascia may ultimately become necrotic and demonstrate reduced enhancement when compared with the adjacent fascia.[24–26] Although MR imaging is usually superior to computed tomography (CT) for demonstrating the extent of the infection, CT is

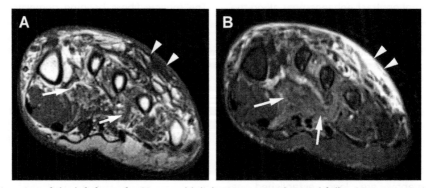

Fig. 3. MR imaging of the left foot of a 65-year-old diabetic woman obtained following a traumatic foot injury. Axial T1-weighted (*A*) and axial, fat-suppressed T2-weighted (*B*) imaging through the forefoot demonstrates moderate neurogenic atrophy of the intrinsic musculature of the forefoot as T1 and T2 streaky high signal (*white arrows, A, B*). Nonspecific subcutaneous soft tissue edema is noted overlying the dorsolateral forefoot (*white arrowheads, A, B*).

often preferred when necrotizing fasciitis is suspected as the CT examination can be completed more rapidly, thus, facilitating urgent treatment.[24] Air bubbles may also be more readily appreciated on CT.

The formation of ring-enhancing abscesses in muscle is a characteristic of pyomyositis and is less common in necrotizing fasciitis. Pyomyositis typically involves one muscle; however, in up to 40% of cases, multiple sites can be involved.[27] Furthermore, thick irregular contrast enhancement of the deep fascia is more commonly seen in pyomyositis, compared with the smooth thickening of necrotizing fasciitis.[28] The findings of early necrotizing fasciitis are not specific, and careful clinical correlation is required.

Diabetic myonecrosis or muscle infarction is not generally a diagnostic consideration in the foot, occurring more commonly in the thigh and calf. Diabetic myonecrosis displays nonspecific MR findings of inflammation interspersed with necrotic foci.[29,30]

Gangrene results from tissue ischemia and can be described as either dry (noninfected) or wet (superinfected). Soft tissue devascularization will be identified as nonenhancing regions on postcontrast imaging. The margins of these regions may enhance secondary to reactive hyperemia. In areas of wet gangrene, marginal abscesses or foci of air may be evident in the adjacent tissues.[15]

Tenosynovitis

Tendons in the foot and ankle are separated from the skin by minimal overlying soft tissue and are intimately related to the bones below. Direct extension of ulceration can lead to involvement of the tendon. The forefoot flexor, peroneal and Achilles tendons are most commonly involved (Fig. 4).[15] Tendon thickening, T2 hyperintensity, and enhancement on postcontrast imaging may indicate septic tenosynovitis; however, these findings are not specific and can be seen in a variety of pathologies, most notably in inflammatory arthropathies or after trauma.[31] It is important to evaluate the entirety of the involved tendon. This evaluation is particularly important for flexor hallucis longus, evaluating for extension to the flexor digitorum longus at the intersection of both tendons (knot of Henry).

Osteomyelitis/Septic Arthritis

In most cases, bone infection in the diabetic foot is the result of direct inoculation via skin ulceration, underlying more than 90% of cases of pedal osteomyelitis.[32,33] It is, therefore, imperative to identify a skin/soft tissue defect, with either a sinus tract or

abscess extending in contiguity through the soft tissues to the bone or joint below. Osteomyelitis is characterized by loss of the normal fat signal on T1-weighted images (T1 replacement) and edema on T2/STIR imaging (Fig. 5). Bone marrow edema on fluid-sensitive sequences but no T1 replacement should not be overcalled as true osteomyelitis. Frank cortical destruction and/or periosteal elevation (periostitis) are common MR findings in osteomyelitis (see Fig. 1). Cortical destruction should be easily identified as interruption of normal thick dark cortical line on T1-weighted imaging. On MR imaging, periosteal reaction appears as linear edema and enhancement along the outer cortex of a bone, wrapping around the bone.[15,34] Where joints are involved, a complex joint effusion with outpouchings is commonly seen. However, it should be noted that joint effusions might decompress via sinuses to the skin surface or to underlying tendon sheaths. Close evaluation of adjacent structures is required when septic arthritis is considered but joint fluid is absent. Other imaging findings, such as marginal erosions and reactive subchondral edema, may be seen. Osteomyelitis can occur anywhere in the foot but is most common at weight-bearing locations close to skin surfaces, including the distal toes, the plantar-lateral cuboid, and the medial eminence of the first metatarsal.

When faced with the conundrum of deciding whether or not to call early osteomyelitis in a diabetic foot, the non–fat-suppressed T1-weighted sequence is the imager's most reliable tool.[35,36] Osseous hyperintensity on T2-weighted fat-suppressed images could reflect osseous stress response (exceedingly common in the weight-bearing insensate foot) or a reaction in the bone marrow to surrounding soft tissue inflammation. When there is focal or diffuse replacement of normal marrow fat on T1-weighted images and a site of direct inoculation, a diagnosis of osteomyelitis can be made confidently. Infected bone can demonstrate geographic enhancement on T1 postcontrast-enhanced images (Fig. 6); however, contrast is rarely required as the T1 images should be diagnostic.[37,38] It is important to remember that intraosseous (Brodie) abscesses will not enhance centrally as they represent devitalized, necrotic bone. When osteomyelitis is considered, care should also be taken to correlate with any recent sites of bone debridement or resection, where changes in the marrow could mimic osteomyelitis.

Neuropathic Osteoarthropathy

Neuropathic osteoarthropathy of the foot is the result of repetitive trauma to an insensate foot.

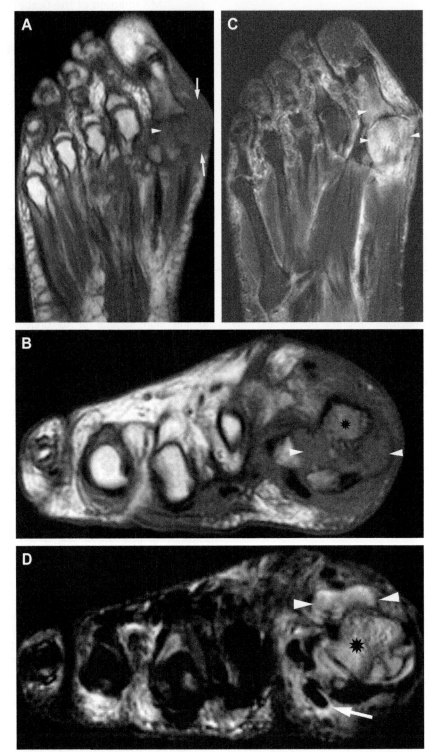

Fig. 4. MR imaging of the left foot of a 42-year-old woman with a focal ulcer on the tibial aspect of the first metatarsal head with clinical concern for osteomyelitis. Coronal and axial T1-weighted (A, B) and coronal and axial fat-suppressed T2-weighted images (C, D) are shown. There is a skin defect with extensive soft tissue infiltration/callus overlying the medial eminence of the first metatarsal (*white arrows, A*). The white arrowheads on the coronal images and the black asterisk on the axial images demonstrate extensive marrow edema and T1 marrow replacement on both sides of the joint. Axial images (B, D) demonstrate a moderate-sized, septic first metatarsophalangeal (MTP) joint effusion (*white arrowheads*). The white arrow in (D) demonstrates mild flexor hallucis longus tenosynovitis. Imaging is consistent with osteomyelitis/septic arthritis of the first MTP joint, with associated septic tenosynovitis of the flexor hallucis longus.

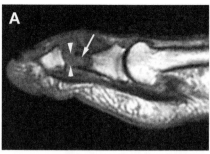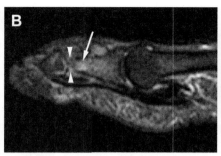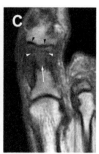

Fig. 5. MR imaging of the right forefoot (with magnification of the phalanges of the hallux) in a 45-year-old diabetic man with an ulcer overlying the interphalangeal joint. Sagittal T1 (*A*), sagittal STIR (*B*), and coronal T1 (*C*) images are demonstrated. The white arrow demonstrates focal marrow edema (*B*) and T1 marrow replacement (*A, C*) in the distal aspect of the proximal phalanx. There is loss of a clear cortical margin at the distal aspect of the proximal phalanx (*white arrowheads, A–C*) when compared with the intact cortex on the distal phalangeal aspect of the interphalangeal joint (*black arrowhead, C*). These findings, contiguity with a skin ulcer, T1 marrow replacement in the setting of marrow edema, and cortical erosion, are all associated with osteomyelitis.

An initial injury results in localized fracture and the disruption of ligamentous attachments. Continued weight bearing results in the progressive involvement of surrounding structures, which usually only becomes evident when significant destruction has occurred.[39] Acute neuropathic foot presents as a warm, erythematous, swollen foot/ankle. There may be minimally elevated inflammatory markers (erythrocyte sedimentation or C-reactive protein). Common MR findings in the acute phase include soft tissue edema, disruption of the Lisfranc ligament, joint effusions and subchondral marrow edema, and potentially any osseous or articular disorganization. T1 postcontrast imaging may demonstrate enhancement of the subchondral marrow, and patchy regions of bone marrow edema on fluid sensitive sequences are common.[40–42] In the chronically neuropathic, insensate foot, there has been resolution of the erythema and warmth on clinical examination, though the soft tissue edema can persist. On MR imaging, the marrow edema and enhancement has reduced. Subchondral cysts are seen as T1 hypointensities and T2 hyperintensities with bone proliferation, deformity (subluxation/dislocation), and fragmentation (intra-articular bodies). Linear areas of subchondral sclerosis (T1 hypointensity) will also be evident (**Fig. 7**).[42]

Occasionally, patients with undiagnosed diabetes undergo MR imaging for chronic pain or abnormal radiographs. Disruption of the Lisfranc interval without a known history of trauma almost certainly indicates an insensate foot and should raise a primary concern for diabetic neuropathy (**Fig. 8**). Similarly, displaced fractures and dislocations not commensurate with reported trauma should raise concern for an insensate neuropathic arthropathy.

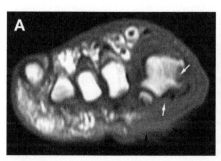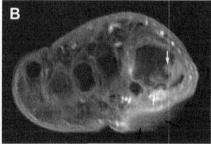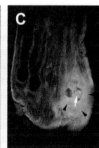

Fig. 6. MR imaging of the forefoot of a 28-year-old man. Axial T1 (*A*), axial T2 fat-suppressed, (*B*) and coronal, postcontrast T1 fat-suppressed (*C*) images are displayed. There is a large plantar skin defect (*black arrows, A, B*) with infiltration and enhancement of the plantar soft tissues (*black arrowheads, C*). There is cortical erosion, bone marrow edema, and T1 marrow replacement of the tibial sesamoid and medial eminence of the first metatarsal head (*white arrows, A, B*) with enhancement of the sesamoid marrow (*white arrow, C*) consistent with osteomyelitis.

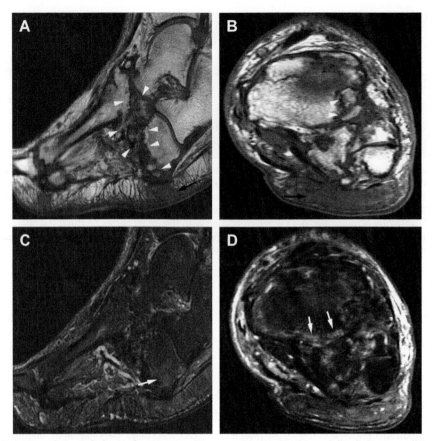

Fig. 7. MR imaging of the left foot of a 49-year-old man with insulin-dependent diabetes mellitus and long-standing foot pain and swelling. Sagittal and axial T1-weighted (*A, B*) and sagittal STIR and axial fat-suppressed T2-weighted (*C, D*) images of the midfoot and forefoot are shown. There is extensive destruction, fragmentation, disorganization, and deformity of the midfoot, centered at the tarsometatarsal articulations but also involving the cuboid and navicular bones (*white arrowheads, A, B*). There is only minimal, marginal marrow edema (*white arrows, C, D*). Soft tissue thickening/callus formation is noted on the plantar surface, deep to this destruction (*black arrow, A, B*). No fluid collections, skin ulcerations, or sinus tracts are identified. Imaging findings are consistent with neuropathic (Charcot) osteoarthropathy.

Differentiating Osteomyelitis/Septic Arthritis from Neuropathic Osteoarthropathy

Herein lies the importance of accurate MR interpretation. As previously stated, most cases of osteomyelitis originate from direct inoculation. The first stage in the evaluation of the diabetic foot should always be careful examination of the skin and subcutaneous fat for localized defects extending to the underlying bones and joints. The location of marrow abnormality can also help distinguish osteomyelitis from a neuropathic joint. Osteomyelitis tends to occur distal to the tarsometatarsal joints and in the malleoli and calcaneus. Neuropathic osteoarthropathy tends to be centered at the Lisfranc (tarsometatarsal), Chopart (talonavicular and calcaneocuboid), or metatarsophalangeal joints. Bone marrow changes in neuropathic osteoarthropathy can be extensive but are

joint centered and, thus, tend to occur relatively symmetrically on either side of the joint. Marrow changes in osteomyelitis, in the absence of superimposed septic arthritis, tend to be limited to one side of a joint, that is, single bone involvement as compared with neuropathy, which typically involves multiple bones and joints.

Of course, a neuropathic joint can become secondarily infected. When evaluating a possible infected neuropathic joint, the authors look for total obliteration of the adjacent soft tissue fat signal and larger-than-expected soft tissue fluid collections. Interval loss of subchondral cysts or the disappearance of intra-articular bodies suggests superimposed infection.[43] Bones with indistinct cortical margins on T1-weighted MR images with distinct margins on T2-weighted images or with distinct margins after the administration of

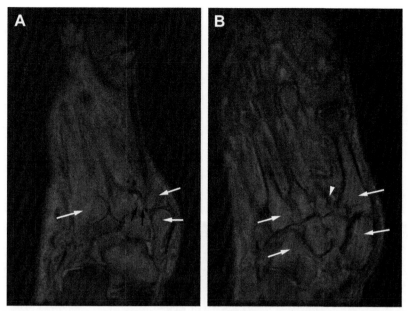

Fig. 8. Coronal T2 fat-suppressed MR imaging of the right foot of 46-year-old woman. There is extensive marrow edema on both sides of the tarsometatarsal articulations (*white arrows, A, B*). There is edema of the Lisfranc interval (*black arrows, A*). The second metatarsal attachment of the plantar Lisfranc ligament is evident (*white arrowhead, B*). The ligament was deemed intact but sprained on other sequences. The diffuse nature of the edema across the TMT (tarsal-metatarsal) articulations combined with the Lisfranc sprain and interval edema were concerning for evolving Charcot arthropathy.

contrast material (ghosting) likely have superimposed osteomyelitis. In the sterile neuropathic foot, the bones are destroyed and, as such, will not ghost the margins, such that the margins will be indistinct on both T1 and T2 sequences.[15] Ultimately, accurate differentiation of bland and infected Charcot foot may require aspiration of joint fluid or percutaneous biopsy. Biopsy of bone in this situation should be performed using a path remote from skin and subcutaneous infection in order to avoid introducing infection into noninfected bone, especially given the setting of poor vascular supply. In addition, it is important to note that culture may be unreliable because of contamination from the overlying soft tissues.

Postoperative MR Imaging

Follow-up after limb-sparing surgery in diabetic patients can be a clinical conundrum. These patients can represent with wound breakdown, recurrent ulceration, persistent swelling, or erythema. Wound breakdown can be caused by either recurrent/residual infection or tissue ischemia. MR imaging is extremely sensitive in diagnosing recurrent/residual infection. There is usually very little marrow edema after amputation. T2 hyperintensity can be postoperative in nature or may result from stress secondary to altered biomechanics. Similar

criteria should be used when diagnosing osteomyelitis in both virgin and postoperative marrow. T1 replacement adjacent the resection margin should be a prerequisite when calling osteomyelitis (**Fig. 9**).[13] Correlation with preoperative MR imaging can be of benefit to distinguish between recurrent and residual infection.[34] Soft tissue abnormalities, such as sinus tracts or abscesses, are often identifiable on nonenhanced imaging sequences. Addition of intravenous Gadolinium based contrast agents at an on label dose is often helpful if images are being reviewed during scanning; however, this is rarely feasible. Increased soft tissue enhancement at the margins of the resection site should be identified as a reactive/hypervascular reactive phenomenon. Ischemic tissue will not enhance.

Ultimately, at sites of resection and amputation, the most convincing findings to indicate osteomyelitis are a skin defect with a fistula extending directly to a site of abnormal bone and bone marrow replacement by low signal on T1-weighted images.

PEARLS, PITFALLS, AND VARIANTS

- The tissues of the diabetic foot are relatively devascularized. Therefore, hematogenous spread of infection is extremely rare. Direct

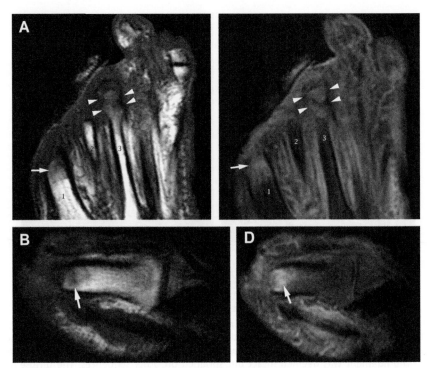

Fig. 9. MR imaging of the left foot of a 50-year-old man with a history of osteomyelitis and resection of the first and second rays at the metatarsal level. The patient presented with foot pain and swelling at the amputation site with raised inflammatory markers and clinical concern for recurrent osteomyelitis. Coronal and sagittal T1-weighted (A, B) and coronal fat-suppressed T2 and sagittal STIR-weighted (C, D) images of the forefoot are shown. The sharp resection margins are clearly identified at the distal ends of both the first (1) and second (2) metatarsals. Marrow edema (C, D) and T1 marrow replacement (A, B) is identified proximal to the resection margin at the first metatarsal (white arrows) consistent with recurrent osteomyelitis at this site. No marrow edema or replacement is noted at the resection margin of the second metatarsal. Furthermore, marrow edema (C), T1 marrow replacement, and cortical irregularity (arrowheads, A) is identified in the third (3) metatarsal head consistent with osteomyelitis.

inoculation is the most common path of spread of infection in these patients. Look for the ulcer and sinus tract.

- Diffuse atrophy of the intrinsic foot muscles is suggestive of diabetic neuropathy. Isolated muscle atrophy is not.
- Postoperative margins, whether through bones or joints, do not generally result in significant marrow edema at theses margins. The presence of marrow edema is concerning, however. As in virgin bone, T1 marrow replacement should be evident to confidently diagnose osteomyelitis.

WHAT REFERRING PHYSICIANS NEED TO KNOW

- Delineation of skin ulceration and all subcutaneous/soft tissue abscesses.
- Differentiation between osteomyelitis, septic arthritis, and neuropathic osteoarthropathy.
- Determination of extent of joint involvement and in particular the status of the Lisfranc ligament.

- Accurate delineation of ischemic tissue to plan surgical tissue flap formation.

SUMMARY

MR imaging is the standard imaging modality for both bone and soft tissue infection in the preoperative assessment of the diabetic foot, combining great sensitivity with strong specificity. With MR, the imager is capable of delineating the full extent of soft tissue and bone abnormalities in a fashion allowing for appropriate incision and drainage or limited amputation when necessary. Bone marrow replacement with low signal on T1-weighted images and sinus tracts extending from skin to a site of abnormal bone are the most reliable imaging findings for the diagnosis of osteomyelitis.

REFERENCES

1. Laing P. The development and complications of diabetic foot ulcers. Am J Surg 1998;176:11s–9s.
2. Calhoun JH, Lipsky BA, Manring MN. Diabetic foot infections. Chapter 20. In: Cierny G III, McLaren AC,

Wongworawat MD, editors. Orthopedic knowledge update, musculoskeletal infection. Rosemont (IL): American Academy of orthopedic surgeons; 2009. p. 227–41.

3. Loredo RA, Garcia G, Chhaya S. Medical imaging of the diabetic foot. Clin Podiatr Med Surg 2007;24: 397–424.

4. Donovan A, Schweitzer ME. Current concepts in imaging diabetic pedal osteomyelitis. Radiol Clin North Am 2008;46:1105–24.

5. Palestro C, Love C. Nuclear medicine and diabetic foot infections. Semin Nucl Med 2009;39:53–65.

6. Schauwecker DS. The scintigraphic diagnosis of osteomyelitis. AJR Am J Roentgenol 1992;158:9–18.

7. Boutin RD, Brossmann J, Sartoris DJ, et al. Update on imaging of orthopedic infections. Orthop Clin North Am 1998;29:41–66.

8. Morrison WB, Ledermann HP. Diabetic pedal infection. Chapter 65. In: Pope TL, Bloem HL, Beltran J, et al, editors. Imaging of the musculoskeletal system, vol. II. Philadelphia: Saunders, Elsevier; 2008. p. 1291–309.

9. Schweitzer ME, Daffner RH, Weissman BN, et al. ACR Appropriateness Criteria on suspected osteomyelitis in patients with diabetes mellitus. J Am Coll Radiol 2008;5(8):881–6.

10. Kapoor A, Page S, Lavelley M, et al. Magnetic resonance imaging for diagnosing foot osteomyelitis: a meta-analysis. Arch Intern Med 2007;167(2):125–32.

11. Ledermann HP, Schweitzer ME, Morrison WB. Non-enhancing tissue on MR imaging of pedal infection: characterization of necrotic tissue and associated limitations for diagnosis of osteomyelitis and abscess. AJR Am J Roentgenol 2002;178:215–22.

12. Ledermann HP, Morrison WB, Schweitzer ME. Pedal abscesses in patient suspected of having pedal osteomyelitis: analysis with MR imaging. Radiology 2002;224:649–55.

13. Schweitzer ME, Morrison WB. MR imaging of the diabetic foot. Radiol Clin North Am 2004;42(1):61–71.

14. Russell J, Peterson J, Bancroft L. MR imaging of the diabetic foot. Magn Reson Imaging Clin N Am 2008; 16(1):59–70.

15. Donovan A, Schweitzer ME. Use of MR imaging in diagnosing diabetes-related pedal osteomyelitis. Radiographics 2010;30:723–36.

16. Ledermann HP, Morrison WB, Schweitzer ME. MR image analysis of pedal osteomyelitis: distribution, patterns of spread and frequency of associated ulceration and septic arthritis. Radiology 2002; 223(3):747–55.

17. Morrison WB, Schweitzer ME, Bock GW, et al. Diagnosis of osteomyelitis: utility of fat-suppressed contrast-enhanced MR imaging. Radiology 1993; 189(1):251–7.

18. Morrison WB, Schweitzer ME, Batte WG, et al. Osteomyelitis of the foot: relative importance of primary and secondary MR imaging signs. Radiology 1998;207(3):625–32.

19. Horton LK, Jacobson JA, Powell A, et al. Sonography and radiography of soft tissue foreign bodies. AJR AM J Roentgenol 2001;176:1155–9.

20. Ingraham CR, Mannelli L, Robinson JD, et al. Radiology of foreign bodies: how do we image them? Emerg Radiol 2015;22(4):425–30.

21. Hunter TB, Taljanovic MS. Foreign bodies. Radiographics 2003;23(3):731–57.

22. Kamath S, Venkatanarasimha N, Walsh MA, et al. MRI appearance of muscle denervation. Skeletal Radiol 2008;37(5):397–404.

23. Andersen H, Gjerstad MD, Jakobsen J. Atrophy of foot muscles: a measure of diabetic neuropathy. Diabetes Care 2004;27(10):2382–5.

24. Chaudhry AA, Baker KS, Gould ES, et al. Necrotizing fasciitis and its mimics: what radiologists need to know. AJR AM J Roentgenol 2015;204: 128–39.

25. Turecki MB, Taljanovic MS, Stubbs AY, et al. Imaging of musculoskeletal soft tissue infections. Skeletal Radiol 2010;39:957–71.

26. Yu JS, Habib P. MR imaging of urgent inflammatory and infectious conditions affecting the soft tissues of the musculoskeletal system. Emerg Radiol 2009;16: 267–76.

27. Bickels J, Ben-Sira L, Kessler A, et al. Primary pyomyositis. J Bone Joint Surg Am 2002;84: 2277–86.

28. Seok JH, Jee WH, Chun KA, et al. Necrotizing fasciitis versus pyomyositis: discrimination with using MR imaging. Korean J Radiol 2009;10:121–8.

29. Mazoch MJ, Bajaj G, Nicholas R, et al. Diabetic myonecrosis: likely an underrecognized entity. Orthopedics 2014;37:e936–9.

30. Jelinek JS, Murphey MD, Aboulafia AJ, et al. Muscle infarction in patients with diabetes mellitus: MR imaging findings. Radiology 1999;211:241–7.

31. Ledermann HP, Morrison WB, Schweitzer ME, et al. Tendon involvement in pedal infection: MR analysis of frequency, distribution and spread of infection. AJR Am J Roentgenol 2002;179(4):939–47.

32. Lipsky BA, Pecoraro RE, Wheat LJ. The diabetic foot: soft tissue and bone infection. Infect Dis Clin North Am 1990;4(3):409–32.

33. Thomas MB, Patel M, Marwin SE, et al. The diabetic foot. Br J Radiol 2000;73:443–50.

34. Morrison WB, Sanders TG. Section III problem solving: disease categories, Ch 5 infection of the musculoskeletal system. In: Morrison WB, Sanders TG, editors. Problem solving in musculoskeletal imaging. Philadelphia: Mosby Elsevier; 2008. p. 183–250.

35. Johnson PW, Collins MS, Wenger DE. Diagnostic utility of T1-weighted MRI characteristics in evaluation of osteomyelitis of the foot. AJR Am J Roentgenol 2009;192(1):96–100.

36. Collins MS, Schaar MM, Wenger DE, et al. T1-weighted MRI characteristics of pedal osteomyelitis. AJR Am J Roentgenol 2005;185(2):386–93.

37. Umans H, Haramati N, Flusser G. The diagnostic role of gadolinium enhanced MRI in distinguishing between acute medullary bone infarct and osteomyelitis. Magn Reson Imaging 2000;18(3):255–62.

38. Kan JH, Young RS, Yu C, et al. Clinical impact of gadolinium in the MRI diagnosis of musculoskeletal infection in children. Pediatr Radiol 2010;40(7):1197–205.

39. Frykberg RG, Belczyk R. Epidemiology of the Charcot foot. Clin Podiatr Med Surg 2008;25(1):17–28.

40. Morrison WB, Ledermann HP. Work up of the diabetic foot. Radiol Clin North Am 2002;40:1171–92.

41. Marcus CD, Ladam-Marcus VJ, Leone J, et al. MR imaging of osteomyelitis and neuropathic osteoarthropathy in the feet of diabetics. Radiographics 1996;16:1337–48.

42. Ergen FB, Sanverdi SE, Oznur A. Charcot foot in diabetes and an update on imaging. Diabet Foot Ankle 2013;4:21884.

43. Ahmadi ME, Morrison WB, Carrino JA, et al. Neuropathic arthropathy of the foot with and without superimposed osteomyelitis: MR imaging characteristics. Radiology 2006;238(2):622–31.

Postoperative Foot and Ankle MR Imaging

Samuel D. Madoff, MD*, Jeffrey Kaye, MD, Joel S. Newman, MD

KEYWORDS

- Tendon reconstruction • Ligament repair • Morton neuroma • Tarsal coalition • Osteomyelitis
- Ankle surgery

KEY POINTS

- MR imaging of postoperative tendon repair, reconstruction, and augmentation are potentially challenging examinations to interpret. Clinical history is important when interpreting these cases.
- Postoperative tendon appearance varies by time from surgery.
- There are a variety of operative approaches for lateral collateral ligament reconstruction.
- Abnormal findings on postoperative imaging may not correlate with symptoms.
- A variety of MR imaging sequences is used to differentiate osteomyelitis from other entities; in particular, the T1 sequence increases specificity.

INTRODUCTION

MR imaging of the postoperative ankle and foot can be challenging. The anatomy is compact with a variety of structures in close proximity. Additionally, postoperative changes may considerably alter expected anatomic relationships. Factors that inform imaging interpretation often stem from the primary diagnosis, subsequent management, intended therapeutic consequences, complications, and the current presenting symptoms. This article touches on a selection of surgical approaches to common ankle and foot problems, and their expected outcome. Possible complications will also be discussed. Although radiography is the principal imaging modality for postoperative imaging, MR imaging allows problem-solving in symptomatic and refractory cases, particularly when soft tissue disease is suspected. This discussion focuses on fundamentals of MR imaging technique and applications in the postoperative ankle and foot.

MR IMAGING

MR imaging is the favored imaging modality for evaluating the ankle and foot following surgery because of the excellent contrast resolution. In particular, MR imaging is sensitive in evaluating postoperative bone marrow response and in evaluating surrounding soft tissues, including the tendons and ligaments.

MR imaging artifacts generated from implanted metallic objects in the magnetic field are a significant obstacle to obtaining clinically relevant postsurgical MR imaging. Magnetic field susceptibilities created by metals of varying properties, sizes, and orientations lead to signal shift away from the true position, in the form of signal loss, signal pile-up, and geometric distortion.[1–3] This manifested artifact may obscure clinically relevant surrounding structures. Optimizing MR imaging technique to limit this artifact is, therefore, essential.

The authors have nothing to disclose.
Department of Radiology, New England Baptist Hospital, Tufts University School of Medicine, 125 Parker Hill Avenue, Boston, MA 02120, USA
* Corresponding author.
E-mail address: smadoff@nebh.org

Magn Reson Imaging Clin N Am 25 (2017) 195–209
http://dx.doi.org/10.1016/j.mric.2016.08.008
1064-9689/17/© 2016 Elsevier Inc. All rights reserved.

Many techniques exist to minimize metallic artifact, the simplest of which include selecting the appropriate field strength, selecting the appropriate sequences, and imaging in multiple planes. Because the degree of distortion increases with magnetic field strength, lower field strength magnets are advantageous. Fast (turbo) spin echo imaging is less susceptible to magnetic field inhomogeneity when compared with gradient echo imaging and is the foundation for most postoperative sequencing. Short tau inversion recovery imaging (STIR) is less susceptible to magnetic field inhomogeneity than frequency selective fat-suppression techniques, which often fail to uniformly fat suppress in the presence of metal.[1] The utility of multiplanar imaging should not be underestimated; MR imaging metallic artifacts are not isotropic, meaning that artifact in 1 plane may be considerably less than in another.[3]

Increasing receiver bandwidth to an acceptable level of signal-to-noise, using shorter echo spacing, reducing slice thickness, and implementing view angle tilting can each help further diminish metal-induced artifact. Multispectral techniques, such as multiacquisition variable-resonance image combination (MAVRIC) and slice-encoding magnetic artifact compensation (SEMAC), can be used at the trade-off of longer scan times, which can be shortened when combined with parallel imaging acceleration.[4]

Routine postoperative imaging is generally performed without contrast. Postcontrast imaging with intravenous gadolinium can be incorporated into the MR examination for the appropriate clinical indications, which would include suspicion of mass or infection.

Separate imaging protocols tailored to evaluate the ankle, midfoot and metatarsals, and distal forefoot are preferred due to different optimal imaging planes for each region and due to postoperative clinical concerns that are unique to each region. The preferred short-axis imaging plane is directed through the talar dome at the ankle, through the metatarsals at the midfoot, and through the MTP joints or plantar plates at the forefoot. These protocols and imaging planes can be adjusted to address the clinical question and region of highest clinical interest.

Patients are imaged in the supine position, feet first, with slight passive plantar flexion.[5] Standard MR examination of the ankle, midfoot, and forefoot is detailed using a high-definition foot and ankle array coil (Invivo, Gainesville, FL) on a 1.5 T GE (Boston, MA) magnet. The sequences and relevant sequence criteria are included in **Tables 1–3** for the respective ankle, midfoot, and forefoot. In the setting of known postoperative metal or implants or failed fat-saturation at the time of imaging, the fat-saturated sequences included in the protocol are substituted with STIR sequences. In addition, the receiver bandwidth for the proton density (PD) sequences is doubled.

TENDON REPAIR AND RECONSTRUCTION

There are many tendon procedures involving the foot and ankle, many of which are named. MR imaging findings may be confusing, particularly if the surgical history is limited. A few principles help guide MR imaging interpretation. Tendons may be repaired directly, reconstructed with tendon graft, and/or augmented by nearby tendons. Augmentations may be the most difficult to evaluate on imaging because tendons may be rerouted, divided, and/or anchored at new locations to support the failed tendon.

Table 1
Ankle MR imaging protocol

Sequence	FOV (cm)	Slice Thickness (mm)	Slice Spacing (mm)	Matrix	NEX	TE	TR	TI	ETL	Receiver Bandwidth
Axial T2	12	3	1.0	256 × 192	2	100	3617	—	23	20.83
Axial PD	12	3	1.0	256 × 224	2	18	2050	—	13	31.25
Coronal PD FS	14	3	1.0	256 × 192	2	20	2234	—	11	20.83
Sagittal T1	18	3	1.0	512 × 256	2	Min Full	500	—	—	20.83
Sagittal IR	16	4	0.5	320 × 192	2	50	4125	150	8	20.83
Coronal PD	10	4	0.0	512 × 256	3	36	1584	—	13	31.25
Axial T2 FS	12	3	1.0	256 × 192	2	100	3434	—	19	20.83

Abbreviations: ETL, echo train length; FOV, field of view; FS, fat-saturation; IR, inversion recovery; NEX, number of excitations; PD, proton density; TE, echo time; TR, repetition time; TI, inversion time.

Table 2
Midfoot MR imaging protocol

Sequence	FOV (cm)	Slice Thickness (mm)	Slice Spacing (mm)	Matrix	NEX	TE	TR	TI	ETL	Receiver Bandwidth
Coronal PD FS	14	3	1.0	320 × 192	2	Min Full	3417	—	6	20.83
Axial T1	14	3	0.5	320 × 192	2	Min Full	617	—	—	15.63
Axial IR	14	3	0.5	256 × 192	2	50	4800	150	8	22.73
Sagittal T2	14	3	0.5	320 × 192	4	102	2767	—	23	25.00
Sagittal IR	1	3	0.5	256 × 192	2	50	4800	150	8	22.73

Achilles and posterior tibialis reconstructions are relatively commonly performed. Augmentations and transfers may be accomplished with a variety of native tendons, including the flexor hallucis longus, flexor digitorum longus (FDL), and the peroneal tendons. Surgery on the anterior tibialis or extensor tendons constitutes a minority of cases, most often for lacerations or acute trauma.[6,7]

Three characteristics that distinguish injured or postoperative tendons from their normal counterparts are signal heterogeneity, signal intensity, and size. The MR imaging appearance of the postoperative tendon may never completely normalize.[8] Typically, the heterogeneous signal seen in the postoperative tendon will become more uniform by 4 to 8 weeks. Postoperative tendon usually displays intermediate to hyperintense PD or T2 signal. Signal intensity should diminish with time, often stabilizing at intermediate to low-signal intensity. By 12 weeks, repaired tendon or graft may closely approximate the signal of the adjacent nonoperative tendon.[9] It is unusual for a reconstructed tendon in the immediate postoperative period to match the size of a noninjured,

preoperative tendon. The reconstituted tendon is most often enlarged, though the size may decrease over time. In general, compared with the preoperative injured tendon, a healed postoperative tendon exhibits less signal heterogeneity, lower signal intensity, and is smaller. Compared with an uninjured tendon, the postoperative tendon may retain modest signal heterogeneity, intermediate (but not high) PD-T2 signal, and enlargement.[10,11]

Thus, it may be difficult to differentiate postoperative changes from tendinosis. In a study of Achilles tendon ruptures, Möller and colleagues[11] reported poor correlation between clinical findings and those observed on postoperative ultrasound or MR imaging. The only significant imaging finding between operative and nonoperative groups was identified with ultrasound and this did not correlate to clinical measures of strength or range of motion.

Tendinosis is degeneration due to structural breakdown of collagen and other tendon components.[12,13] The term tendinopathy is often used interchangeably with tendinosis. MR imaging

Table 3
Forefoot MR imaging protocol

Sequence	FOV (cm)	Slice Thickness (mm)	Slice Spacing (mm)	Matrix	NEX	TE	TR	TI	ETL	Receiver Bandwidth
Axial IR	14	3	0.5	320 × 160	2	50	4425	150	8	20.83
Axial T1	14	3	0.5	320 × 192	2	Min Full	450	—	—	15.63
Coronal T2 FS	14	3	1.0	320 × 192	2	102	3117	—	6	19.23
Coronal T1	14	3	1.0	320 × 160	2	Min Full	367	—	—	17.86
Sagittal T2	14	3	0.5	320 × 192	4	102	3017	—	23	25.00
Sagittal IR	14	3	0.5	320 × 160	2	50	4425	150	8	20.83

findings in tendinosis include signal heterogeneity, tendon enlargement, and intermediate PD-T2 signal (**Fig. 1**). Separately, the encasing tissues of a tendon may be abnormal. Most tendons in the ankle and foot have a synovial sheath, such as the flexor hallucis longus and FDL tendons. Tenosynovitis is inflammation of this sheath and is apparent on MR imaging as sheath thickening. There is typically abnormal fluid within the tendon sheath and surrounding edema. The Achilles tendon is distinct in the ankle because it possesses a paratenon, rather than a synovial sheath. The paratenon encloses the Achilles along its dorsal, medial, and lateral margins, and facilitates tendon gliding.[14] Paratenonitis is invoked when there is thickening and edema signal of the paratenon.

Achilles Tendon

The Achilles is the largest tendon in the body. The bulk of Achilles surgery is undertaken for tendon rupture repair. Ruptures are typically spontaneous, occur during recreational sports, and may be attributed to eccentric loading while the gastrocnemius and soleus are maximally

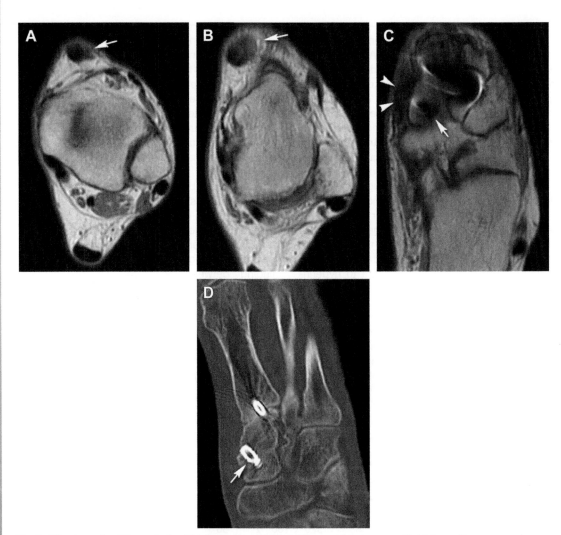

Fig. 1. Direct repair of the anterior tibialis tendon (ATT). A 68-year-old woman with history of surgery and symptoms remote from the prior operative site. Axial PD images demonstrate (*A*) thickening of the ATT proximally (*arrow*), (*B*) signal heterogeneity and marked tendon enlargement at the level of the talus (*arrow*), and (*C*) continued tendon enlargement and deformity at the medial cuneiform repair site (*arrowheads*) with susceptibility artifact from the tendon anchor (*arrow*) and fusion hardware. (*D*) Long-axis CT depicts the tendon anchor in the medial cuneiform (*arrow*). Hardware transfixes the great toe metatarsophalangeal joint more distally, unrelated to the ATT repair.

stretched (ankle dorsiflexed and the knee extended). Rupture is more frequent in men than women. Peak occurrence is in active 30- to 50-year-olds who are otherwise healthy.[15]

Treatment is controversial with divergent reports supporting both operative and nonoperative approaches.[16,17] The December 2009 workgroup of the American Academy of Orthopedic Surgery cites limited strength of recommendation for both operative and nonoperative treatment. The workgroup did reach a consensus recommendation that, when considering surgical repair, caution is warranted in patients with comorbidities such as diabetes, obesity, age above 65 years, sedentary lifestyle, and peripheral vascular disease.[18] Young individuals and athletes are more likely to receive operative treatment.

Operative treatment depends on the acuity of the injury, the degree of tendon retraction, and resultant tendon gap. Acute tears with a small gap (less than 2 or 3 cm) may be amenable to end-to-end repair. In contrast, a chronic tear with a larger gap may require augmentation using nearby structures, such as the plantaris tendon or a flap from the gastrocnemius soleus complex.[19] One technique uses a turn-down of gastrocnemius fascia, which is interwoven to span the torn tendon segment.[20] There are multiple variations to this approach. A variety of tendon transfer procedures use nearby tendons, such as the flexor hallucis longus and peroneus brevis.[21]

In either conservative or operative treatment scenarios, MR imaging reliably depicts tendon changes, from a healthy, uniformly low-signal structure to a thickened band with heterogeneous signal. Thickening may be diffuse or focal, most often in a fusiform configuration on sagittal sequences. Signal alterations change over time.

Peritendinous edema is atypical after a few months postsurgery. If present, this may indicate reinjury or ongoing tendinosis. Tendon defects or retears are evident as focal discontinuity of fibers and areas of hyperintense signal on fluid-sensitive sequences. Ossification within the tendon may be associated with retear and should be documented in the radiology report. This is represented by abnormal signal within the tendon substance that is isointense with marrow.[22]

Haglund syndrome is another cause of posterior ankle pain involving the Achilles tendon and occasionally necessitates operative treatment. A prominent posterior calcaneal tuberosity and extrinsic compression via constrictive footwear, such as high heels, results in retrocalcaneal bursitis and insertional Achilles tendinosis.[23] Surgical repair of Haglund syndrome involves osteotomy of the posterior calcaneus protuberance and resection of the

inflamed retrocalcaneal bursa. The distal Achilles may be debrided and reanchored to the calcaneus.[24] Postoperative tendon thickening and signal heterogeneity may be apparent on subsequent MR imaging, with anchors present within the calcaneus (**Fig. 2**).

Posterior Tibialis Tendon

The posterior tibialis tendon (PTT) and muscle are principal dynamic stabilizers of the medial longitudinal arch. The PPT also works to generate inversion and/or plantar flexion. The tendon has multiple distal components, with the main portion inserting onto the medial aspect of the tarsal navicular. The PTT at and just distal to the medial malleolus is particularly vulnerable to degeneration and tearing due to poor blood supply. This watershed area is within 6 cm of the navicular insertion.[25,26]

PTT dysfunction and tears are treated operatively via primary repair or augmentation. The most common approach to augmentation uses the FDL tendon. The FDL is released distally and either sutured to the PTT or anchored directly to the tarsal navicular (**Fig. 3**).[27] The flexor hallucis longus tendon is less frequently used because it requires a more extensive dissection and loss of its function is considered less desirable.

An alternative augmentation technique, termed the Cobb procedure, relies on the tibialis anterior (TA) tendon. The distal TA from the ankle down to the medial cuneiform is longitudinally divided. The medial half is released proximally, passed through an osseous tunnel in the medial cuneiform (or navicular), and sutured to the PTT. Distally, the medial cuneiform insertion is maintained and the remaining nonreleased half of the TA continues to provide some of its native function.[28–30]

PTT insufficiency is a primary cause of adult-acquired flat foot deformity (pes planus). Therefore, operative repair of the PTT is often part of a larger attempt to restore the medial longitudinal arch and correct hindfoot malalignment. A 4-part staging system is commonly used to guide operative treatment. Relevant factors for staging include extent of hindfoot malalignment, loss of the longitudinal arch, and talar head uncovering.[31]

Early stage disease (stage I or IIa) prompts PTT transfer and tenosynovectomy. Cotton osteotomy and/or medial calcaneal slide osteotomy are considered. Intermediate stages IIb and III include, in addition to these, consideration of hindfoot fusion and lateral column lengthening. Stage IV considerations are ankle fusion and ankle arthroplasty.

The goal of a Cotton osteotomy is to plantar flex the medial column, thereby restoring the medial

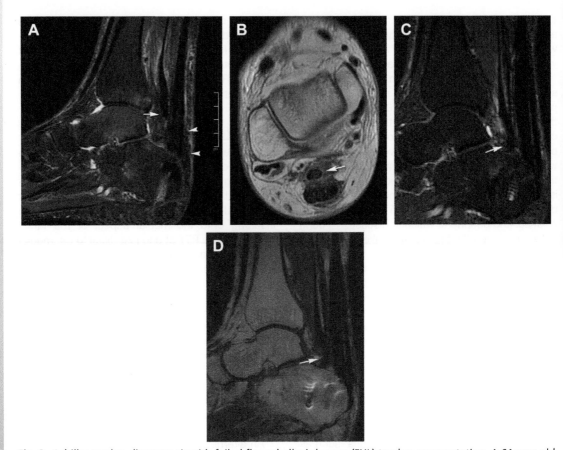

Fig. 2. Achilles tendon direct repair with failed flexor hallucis longus (FHL) tendon augmentation. A 64-year-old woman with history of surgery and new onset pain. (*A*) Sagittal STIR image demonstrates thickened Achilles tendon status after repair (*arrowheads*) with susceptibility artifact from anchors in the calcaneus. Anterior to the repaired Achilles, the FHL (*arrow*), which was used for Achilles augmentation, is thickened and discontinuous, retracted several centimeters proximally from the calcaneus anchor site. There is surrounding soft tissue edema. Hyperintense reactive signal is also present in the tibial plafond, talus, and calcaneus. (*B*) Axial PD image confirms the thickened FHL tendon (*arrow*) used for Achilles augmentation with surrounding soft tissue edema and postoperative changes. (*C, D*) Status post revision, sagittal STIR and T1 images display reanchored, intact FHL (*arrows*) with modest surrounding soft tissue edema. The repaired Achilles remains intact.

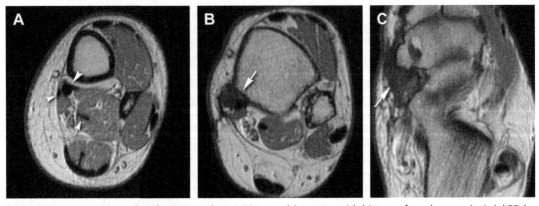

Fig. 3. PTT augmentation using the FDL tendon. A 58-year-old woman with history of tendon repair. Axial PD images progressing distally demonstrate (*A*) 3 separate flexor tendons proximally: PTT (*large arrowhead*), FDL (*small arrowhead*), and FHL (*arrow*), (*B*) poor PTT definition and enlargement with postoperative changes and intimate association with the FDL (*arrow*) and (*C*) enlarged, postoperative tendon with FDL augment (*arrow*) at the navicular insertion with bone anchor.

longitudinal arch. The procedure involves a medial cuneiform opening wedge osteotomy with a dorsally based wedge.[32] On imaging, it is worthwhile to confirm the osteotomy has healed because malunion or nonunion are common indications for revision surgery.[33,34]

ANKLE LATERAL COLLATERAL LIGAMENTS

Ankle inversion injuries may result in damage to the lateral collateral ligaments, most commonly the anterior talofibular ligament, followed by the calcaneofibular ligament. The posterior talofibular ligament is nearly always spared. Treatment of a single event is nonoperative, involving rest, rehabilitation, and bracing. With repeated injuries, ligamentous laxity and instability may develop, necessitating operative intervention.[35]

Many procedures and modifications for lateral collateral ligament reconstruction have been reported. Two common approaches may be grouped into either direct repair or soft-tissue augmentation with the peroneus brevis tendon (PBT). The classic direct approach involves debriding the residual ligaments, approximating the ends, and suturing them together (Broström procedure). Occasionally a bone anchor may be placed in the lateral malleolus. Other modifications include using the lateral extensor retinaculum or periosteal flaps to fortify the repair.[36] MR imaging may reveal susceptibility artifact from an anchor or postoperative changes at the anterior aspect of the lateral malleolus.

Soft-tissue augmentation with the PBT is used for marked laxity, long-standing ligament insufficiency, and salvage.[37] Procedures include PBT rerouting, PBT loop, and PBT split with rerouting. The PBT is transected, redirected through a tunnel in the fibula, and reattached. The reattachment sites vary. In rerouting, the tendon is reattached proximally to the original peroneus brevis transection site. MR imaging may reveal susceptibility artifact and postoperative changes at the reattachment site several centimeters proximal to the lateral malleolus. In PBT loop, the tendon is circled around to reattach to the distal PBT. Proximally, the residual PBT stump is sutured to the peroneus longus tendon. Both sites of tendon attachment will be evident on MR imaging. In PBT split with rerouting, the tunneled PBT segment is attached to both the talus and calcaneus via periosteal flaps and reattached to the distal PBT (just like the PBT loop). The advantage of this latter procedure is that it maintains some of the natural function of the PBT. At first glance, the MR imaging appearance may be confusing, with extensive postoperative changes just distal to the lateral malleolus. The PBT should be identified and carefully traced through its surgical course to evaluate for tendon tear or discontinuity and resultant failure (**Figs. 4** and **5**).

ANKLE MEDIAL COLLATERAL LIGAMENTS

The deltoid ligament complex stabilizes the medial ankle. The deltoid is less frequently injured

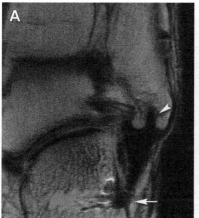
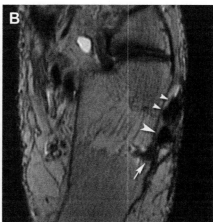

Fig. 4. Chrisman-Snook procedure for lateral collateral ligament reconstruction. A 57-year-old woman with history of lateral ligament surgery. (*A*) Coronal PD image demonstrates PBT graft running anterior to posterior in a tunnel in the lateral malleolus (*arrowhead*) (to replace the anterior talofibular ligament) and continuing down to the calcaneal anchor (*arrow*) (to replace the calcaneofibular ligament). (*B*) Axial PD image at the level of the calcaneal anchor displays the origin of the PB surgically divided tendon with a bilobed tendon configuration (*small arrowheads*). The peroneus longus tendon is located just posterior (*large arrowhead*). The PB graft is anchored at the calcaneus with resultant susceptibility artifact (*arrow*).

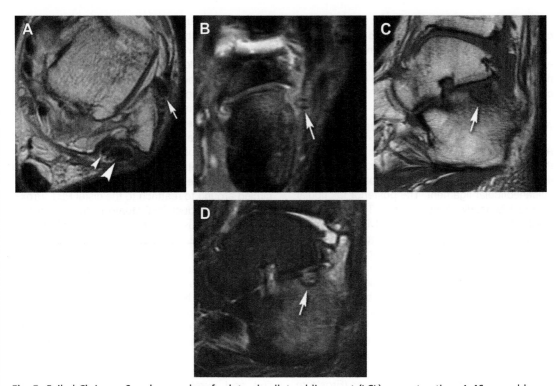

Fig. 5. Failed Chrisman-Snook procedure for lateral collateral ligament (LCL) reconstruction. A 46-year-old man with prior ligament surgery and recent recurrence of symptoms. (*A*) Axial PD image demonstrates the split section of PB (*arrow*) for the LCL reconstruction located anterior to the lateral malleolus and the remaining PB (*small arrowhead*) located posterior to the lateral malleolus along the peroneus longus tendon (*large arrowhead*). (*B*) Coronal PD fat-saturation image demonstrates a cylindrical anchor fragment (*arrow*) that has migrated out of the calcaneus into the lateral soft tissues with surrounding soft tissue edema. (*C, D*) Sagittal T1 and STIR images demonstrate calcaneal anchor site (*arrows*) with violation of the subchondral bone plate along the posterior sub-talar joint and marked surrounding osseous edema.

compared with the lateral collateral complex. Physical examination and radiographs are limited for detecting deltoid ligament injuries, whereas MR imaging can be quite helpful.[38] Although individual ligaments may be delineated on anatomic studies, for practical surgical (and imaging) purposes, the deltoid ligament complex is divided into superficial and deep components. The superficial deltoid is often damaged, either alone or in combination with the deep deltoid.[39,40] A small fraction of injuries are confined to the deep deltoid alone.[39] Superficial injuries typically involve detachment of the superficial deltoid origin and/or the medial fascial sleeve. The flexor retinaculum is also damaged in about one-third of cases. For superficial deltoid injuries, the reported sensitivity and specificity of MR imaging are 83% and 94%, respectively. Likewise, MR imaging for deep deltoid injuries has a sensitivity and specificity greater than 95%.[40] Anteromedial and posteromedial impingement syndromes may be concomitantly identified, along with other soft tissue or osseous injuries.

Treatment of acute injuries is typically nonoperative, involving rest, ice, compression, and elevation. Physical therapy is occasionally used. If symptoms are refractory or instability is identified, operative management is considered. Instability cases nearly always manifest as rotational instability due to superficial deltoid and/or fascial sleeve tear. A subset of instability cases results in coronal tibiotalar instability with valgus stress due to deep deltoid tear. The integrity of the deep deltoid allows categorization of instability into 2 groups.[41]

If the deep deltoid ligament is intact, rotational instability alone is present. For most cases, a direct repair of the superficial deltoid is elected. Postoperative MR imaging findings may reveal a suture anchor (or susceptibility artifact) in the anterior aspect of the medial malleolus for reattachment of the superficial deltoid origin.[41]

If the deep deltoid ligament is incompetent, rotational instability is accompanied by coronal tibiotalar instability with valgus stress. The scope of injury is larger and may include PTT dysfunction and/or hindfoot valgus deformity. Often, deltoid ligament reconstruction, rather than direct repair, is required. One technique involves proximally translating the osseous origin of the superficial ligament and securing it with an anchor.[41] Additional procedures to address concomitant abnormalities may include a variety of procedures for PTT dysfunction, such as peroneus longus rerouting via talar and medial malleolus bone tunnels, or flexor hallucis longus tendon transfer. Hindfoot valgus correction may be performed with calcaneus-lengthening osteotomy or tibiocalcaneal arthrodesis.

MORTON NEUROMA-INTERDIGITAL PERINEURAL FIBROSIS

Morton neuroma reflects interdigital perineural fibrosis in the plantar aspect of the intermetatarsal space, deep to the transverse metatarsal ligament, and near the common plantar digital nerve, perhaps due to entrapment and repetitive irritation. Interdigital fibrosis occurs most of the time at the third interspace with perhaps one-third of cases located at the second interspace.[42] Occurrence in either the first or fourth interspace is rare, likely due to the larger size of these spaces and/or the mechanics of ambulation.[43]

MR imaging has a reported sensitivity of 87% and specificity of 100% for detecting interdigital fibrosis.[44] In a series, MR imaging resulted in an altered treatment plan for 57% of cases.[45] Although readily identified on MR imaging, findings of interdigital fibrosis may be present in up to one-third of asymptomatic patients.[46] Larger lesions (greater than 5 mm) are more likely to be symptomatic.[47]

First-line treatment of interdigital perineural fibrosis is nonoperative. Footwear adjustments, padding, orthoses, and/or steroid injections are typically effective. Recalcitrant symptoms prompt operative intervention. The fibrotic region, encompassing the common plantar digital nerve, is resected, along with transection of the intermetatarsal ligament.[48]

If symptoms persist after surgery, an expanded differential diagnosis includes stress fracture, intermetatarsal bursitis, and metatarsophalangeal joint synovitis.[45] Operative failures have been attributed to partial resection, failure to divide the transverse metatarsal ligament, and too distal transection of the common plantar digital nerve.[49] Failure rates are variably reported up to 25%.[50,51]

A subset of postresection patients develops a stump neuroma with consequent toe dysesthesias. Attempted nerve regeneration after injury, whether traumatic or operative, can result in a disorderly regenerative response, leading to a clump of poorly organized tissue termed a stump neuroma.[52] Preventive measures to avoid stump neuromas include minimizing scar tissue and facilitating the retraction of the common digital nerve far proximally once transected. Only a fraction of stump neuromas are symptomatic. Nonoperative therapies such as steroid injection and footwear modifications are often successful. Occasionally, additional surgery may be required.[53]

Although recurrence of interdigital perineural fibrosis does occur, MR imaging should be interpreted with caution. Espinosa and colleagues[42] reported about one-quarter of postoperative patients were symptomatic. MR imaging findings of interdigital fibrosis was observed in 26% of asymptomatic patients compared with 50% of symptomatic patients. Scars and intermetatarsal bursitis were also identified in both symptomatic and asymptomatic groups. This high degree of overlap between symptomatic and asymptomatic groups on postoperative MR imaging warrants careful clinically directed decision-making regarding additional treatment and possible repeat surgery.

COALITION

Almost all tarsal bone coalitions are either calcaneonavicular or talocalcaneal coalitions. Although most calcaneonavicular coalitions present in children (8–12 year olds), talocalcaneal coalitions are commonly identified in young adults (teens to early 20s).[54] In the authors' experience, many coalitions are detected incidentally in adults even at middle-age or older during MR imaging and computed tomography (CT) evaluation, often for unrelated problems. For imaging purposes, coalitions are categorized as either osseous or nonosseous. Nonosseous coalitions are cartilaginous, fibrous, or a combination of both (Fig. 6).[55]

Clinical evaluation and radiographs typically establish the diagnosis. Coalitions occur bilaterally about 50% of the time. Initial treatment is nonoperative, using activity modification, bracing, and orthotics. Immobilization with casting may be considered in refractory cases. If symptoms persist, surgery may be indicated.[56]

Operative planning involves resection versus arthrodesis. Resection is preferred in young and active patients without arthropathy. The goal is to relieve symptoms and improve range of motion. To prevent recurrence, interposition of adipose tissue, bone wax, fascia lata allograft, or flexor hallucis longus tendon into the surgical defect may be performed.[57,58] Arthrodesis is elected in the setting of degenerative joint disease and/or failed resection. Triple arthrodesis is typical.

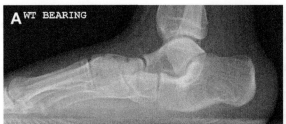
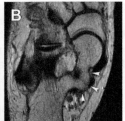
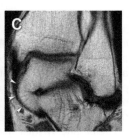
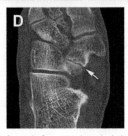

Fig. 6. Coalition. A 14-year-old girl with flatfoot deformity (*A, B*). (*A*) Lateral radiograph displays marked pes pla-nus. (*B*) Axial T2 image demonstrates osseous talocalcaneal coalition (*arrowheads*). Treatment included triple arthrodesis with coalition resection and flatfoot correction. A 33-year-old woman with chronic hindfoot pain (*C, D*). (*C*) Coronal PD image displays osseous talocalcaneal coalition (*arrowheads*). Age of presentation is older than typical. (*D*) Axial CT image demonstrates a nonosseous cuboid-navicular coalition (*arrow*) in the same foot. This type of coalition is quite rare. Treatment involved resection of both coalitions and fusion.

For calcaneonavicular coalitions, it is valuable to identify other deformities, such as pes planus, equinus, and cavus. Some investigators advocate correcting these deformities along with the coali-tion site for better long-term results.[59] Adjunctive procedures include calcaneal osteotomies, subta-lar arthrodesis, medial column arthrodesis, and posterior muscle group lengthening.[60]

Preoperative MR imaging is useful to charac-terize the coalition, evaluate nearby articular degenerative changes, and assess tendon patho-logic conditions, such as the PTT or peroneal ten-dons, because these may impact operative planning. Postoperative MR imaging may be used to evaluate integrity of soft tissue repairs and for osseous stress injury in the setting of arthrodesis. CT scan is more commonly per-formed and demonstrates the maturity of fusion sites and hardware integrity.

COMPLICATIONS
Stress Injury or Fracture

Altered biomechanics following ankle and foot sur-gery result in new weightbearing stresses on adja-cent bones, particularly in the forefoot. This may result in a stress injury or fracture near operative sites.[61] MR imaging is helpful for delineating stress reactions and early fractures that may remain occult on radiographs.[62] Intramedullary and periosteal edema, either alone or in combination, indicate a stress injury (**Fig. 7**). Hyperintense

intracortical signal on fluid-sensitive sequences most likely corresponds to impending fracture. A fracture line will be delineated by a low-signal linear focus on both T1 and fluid-sensitive sequences.[63,64]

Osteomyelitis

Osteomyelitis is an uncommon postoperative complication. Its occurrence in the ankle or foot is of clinical concern given the relatively compact anatomy and ease of spread to nearby structures. Radiography is excellent at depicting advanced cases of osteomyelitis or when treatment has been delayed. Osseous erosion and destruction may be apparent, along with periosteal reaction.[65] In the setting of surgery, it may be helpful to compare immediate postoperative radiographs with subsequent follow-up examinations to eval-uate for changes. However, radiography is not sensitive for the detection of early osteomyelitis.[66]

MR imaging is the principal imaging modality for osteomyelitis detection, particularly early on. Sensitivity and specificity have been reported at 90% and 83%, respectively.[67,68] MR imaging also allows accurate preoperative planning so that surgical margins encompass infected bone and soft tissue, while sparing as much nearby un-affected tissue as possible. Diagnosis relies on 3 types of MR imaging sequences: T1-weighted, T2-weighted, and postcontrast. A fluid-sensitive sequence with fat-suppression technique, such

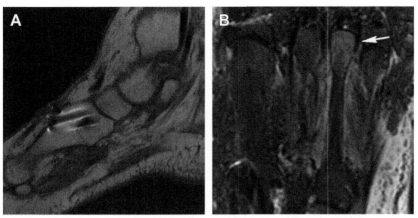

Fig. 7. Stress injury. A 61-year-old woman 5 months status postsurgery presenting with forefoot pain. (*A*) Sagittal PD image depicts fusion hardware transfixing the first tarsometatarsal joint. (*B*) Long-axis STIR image reveals hyperintense marrow signal throughout the third metatarsal head (*arrow*), compatible with stress injury. Extensive surrounding soft tissue edema. No fracture line is present as yet.

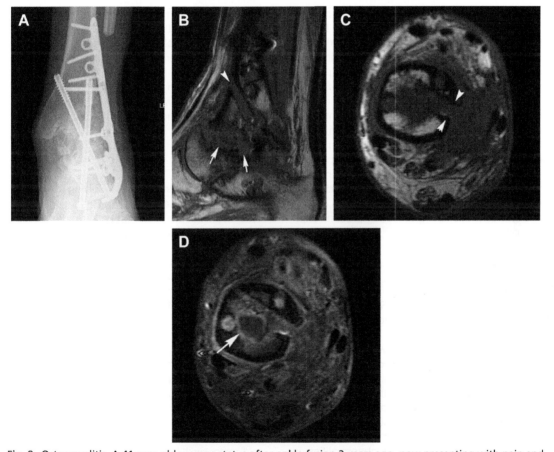

Fig. 8. Osteomyelitis. A 41-year-old woman status after ankle fusion 2 years ago, now presenting with pain and swelling. (*A*) Frontal radiograph demonstrates plate and screws transfixing the tibiotalar and subtalar joints. The distal fibula has been resected. (*B*) Sagittal T1 image status after hardware removal demonstrates intermediate signal throughout the hardware tracts (*arrowhead*) and occupying the bone along the margins of the tibiotalar joint (*arrows*). There is bone loss and deformity of the distal tibia, talus, and calcaneus. (*C*) Axial T1 image displays intermediate signal in the lateral soft tissues communicating to the intramedullary space through a cortical defect (*arrowheads*), representing soft tissue, fluid, or a combination of the two. (*D*) Axial T1 fat-saturation post-contrast image demonstrates a rim-enhancing tibial intramedullary collection (*arrow*) with surrounding heterogeneous enhancement, compatible with abscess and osteomyelitis.

as an STIR or T2 with fat-saturation sequence, is an efficient way to diagnose infected bone. The hyperintense signal identified on these sequences is highly sensitive for medullary abnormalities, though not specific for osteomyelitis.[69,70]

Similarly, medullary enhancement on postcontrast sequences corroborates abnormal areas identified on the fluid-sensitive sequences but does not increase specificity for osteomyelitis.

T1 sequences are the most specific sequence for identifying osteomyelitis. Johnson and colleagues[71] report a 91% specificity, 95% sensitivity, 79% positive predictive value, and 98% negative predictive value. A confluent intramedullary region of intermediate to low T1 signal with geographic margins strongly indicates osteomyelitis (Fig. 8).[72]

Not all types of abnormal T1 signal are representative of osteomyelitis. Intermediate or low T1 medullary signal may occur with reactive marrow edema, osteitis, stress reaction, altered biomechanics, and neuropathic osteoarthropathy.[73,74] The abnormal T1 signal will typically be reticulated and hazy in contrast to a confluent, geographically marginated region present in osteomyelitis.[72]

Multiple secondary findings support the diagnosis of osteomyelitis, including adjacent sinus tracts, periosteal reaction, cellulitis, phlegmon, abscess, cortical bone destruction, foreign body, septic arthritis, and tenosynovitis. Postoperative diabetic patients warrant special attention given their higher vulnerability to infection and delayed healing. In the diabetic patient, soft tissue ulcerations and skin thickening are often present adjacent to sites of deep infection.[70,75]

Multifocal Bone Marrow Edema

On occasion, postoperative MR imaging reveals multiple bones with abnormal signal intensity that suggests bone marrow edema, typically hyperintense on fluid-sensitive or T2-weighted fat-suppressed sequences. Several common causes include altered biomechanics, immobilization, and complex regional pain syndrome (CRPS).[76]

Altered biomechanics is attributed to modified gait and/or weightbearing after surgery. The metatarsals and calcaneus bear most of the stress with ambulation.[77] Therefore, signal abnormalities in these bones particularly suggest a cause of altered biomechanics.[73] Although striking on MR imaging, the patient may be asymptomatic and almost all cases resolve with time. A small fraction of cases can worsen due to impaired or delayed healing and continued use, resulting in stress injury or stress fracture.

Immobilization can also result in scattered foci of bone marrow edema-like signal. Correlation with clinical history is important in these cases. Patients are typically asymptomatic and MR imaging findings typically resolve or stabilize within 18 weeks.[78]

CRPS, previously designated reflex sympathetic dystrophy, may also present with a multifocal pattern of bone marrow edema-like foci. Unlike the previous 2 conditions associated with multifocal bone marrow edema, CRPS is symptomatic.[76] Autonomic dysfunction results in pain (throbbing or burning), sensitivity to temperature or touch, joint stiffness, decreased mobility of the affected body part, and muscle weakness or atrophy. Skin edema, thickening, labile temperature changes, and labile color changes may also be present. These symptoms allow differentiation of multifocal marrow edema due to CRPS from that due to altered biomechanics and immobilization. CRPS has several stages, each of which may affect symptomatology and imaging findings.[79] Bone marrow edema-like findings may be less prevalent than soft tissue abnormalities.[80] Further imaging evaluation may be performed with 3-phase bone scan, which displays a typical pattern of activity depending on the time since the inciting injury.

SUMMARY

MR imaging is a useful problem-solving tool for the postoperative foot and ankle. MR imaging readily depicts operative sequela across a range of surgical procedures and related pathologic conditions, including tendon and ligament reconstruction, tarsal coalition, and interdigital perineural fibrosis. Surgical complications may be identified as well. MR imaging provides valuable information for guiding the care of postoperative foot and ankle patients.

REFERENCES

1. Hargreaves BA, Worters PW, Pauly KB, et al. Metal-induced artifacts in MRI. AJR Am J Roentgenol 2011;197:547–55.
2. Olsen RV, Munk PL, Lee MJ, et al. Metal artifact reduction sequence: early clinical applications. Radiographics 2000;20:699–712.
3. Lee MJ, Kim S, Lee SA, et al. Overcoming artifacts from metallic orthopedic implants at high-field-strength MR imaging and multi-detector CT. Radiographics 2007;27:791–803.
4. Hargreaves BA, Chen W, Lu W, et al. Accelerated slice encoding for metal artifact correction. J Magn Reson Imaging 2010;31:987–96.

5. Weishaupt D, Treiber K, Kundert HP, et al. Morton neuroma: MR imaging in prone, supine, and upright weight-bearing body positions. Radiology 2003;226: 849–56.

6. Patten A, Pun WK. Spontaneous rupture of the tibialis anterior tendon: a case report and literature review. Foot Ankle Int 2000;21(8):697–700.

7. Ouzounian TJ, Anderson R. Anterior tibial tendon rupture. Foot Ankle Int 1995;16(7):406–10.

8. Karjalainen PT, Ahovuo J, Pihlajamäki HK, et al. Postoperative MR imaging and ultrasonography of surgically repaired Achilles tendon ruptures. Acta Radiol 1996;37(3P2):639–46.

9. Platt MA. Tendon repair and healing. Clin Podiatr Med Surg 2005;22(4):553–60.

10. Fujikawa A, Kyoto Y, Kawaguchi M, et al. Achilles tendon after percutaneous surgical repair: serial MRI observation of uncomplicated healing. AJR Am J Roentgenol 2007;189(5):1169–74.

11. Möller M, Kälebo P, Tidebrant G, et al. The ultrasonographic appearance of the ruptured Achilles tendon during healing: a longitudinal evaluation of surgical and nonsurgical treatment, with comparisons to MRI appearance. Knee Surg Sports Traumatol Arthrosc 2002;10(1):49–56.

12. Maffulli N. Overuse tendon conditions: time to change a confusing terminology. Arthroscopy 1998;14(8):840–3.

13. Kader D, Saxena A, Movin T, et al. Achilles tendinopathy: some aspects of basic science and clinical management. Br J Sports Med 2002;36(4):239–49.

14. Karjalainen PT, Soila K, Aronen HJ, et al. MR imaging of overuse injuries of the Achilles tendon. AJR Am J Roentgenol 2000;175(1):251–60.

15. Leppilahti J, Puranen J, Orava S. Incidence of Achilles tendon rupture. Acta Orthop Scand 1996;67(3): 277–9.

16. Willits K, Amendola A, Bryant D, et al. Operative versus nonoperative treatment of acute Achilles tendon ruptures. J Bone Joint Surg Am 2010;92(17):2767–75.

17. Khan RJ, Fick D, Keogh A, et al. Treatment of acute Achilles tendon ruptures. J Bone Joint Surg Am 2005;87(10):2202–10.

18. Chiodo CP, Glazebrook M, Bluman EM, et al. Diagnosis and treatment of acute Achilles tendon rupture. J Am Acad Orthop Surg 2010;18(8):503–10.

19. Lynn TA. Repair of the torn Achilles tendon, using the plantaris tendon as a reinforcing membrane. J Bone Joint Surg Am 1966;48(2):268–72.

20. Bosworth DM. Repair of defects in the tendo achillis. J Bone Joint Surg Am 1956;38(1):111–4.

21. Pérez TA. Traumatic rupture of the Achilles Tendon. Reconstruction by transplant and graft using the lateral peroneus brevis. Orthop Clin North Am 1974;5(1):89–93.

22. Kannus PE, Jozsa L. Histopathological changes preceding spontaneous rupture of a tendon. A controlled study of 891 patients. J Bone Joint Surg Am 1991;73(10):1507–25.

23. Haglund P. Beitrag zur klinik der achillessehne. Zeitschr Orthop Chir 1928;49:49–58.

24. Sammarco GJ, Taylor AL. Operative management of Haglund's deformity in the nonathlete: a retrospective study. Foot Ankle Int 1998;19(11):724–9.

25. Petersen W, Hohmann G, Stein V, et al. The blood supply of the posterior tibial tendon. J Bone Joint Surg Br 2002;84(1):141–4.

26. Frey CA, Shereff M, Greenidge N. Vascularity of the posterior tibial tendon. J Bone Joint Surg Am 1990; 72(6):884–8.

27. Myerson MS. Adult acquired flatfoot deformity: treatment of dysfunction of the posterior tibial tendon. Instr Course Lect 1996;46:393–405.

28. Knupp M, Hintermann B. The Cobb procedure for treatment of acquired flatfoot deformity associated with stage II insufficiency of the posterior tibial tendon. Foot Ankle Int 2007;28(4):416–21.

29. Janis LR, Wagner JT, Kravitz RD, et al. Posterior tibial tendon rupture: classification, modified surgical repair, and retrospective study. J Foot Ankle Surg 1992;32(1):2–13.

30. Helal B. Cobb repair for tibialis posterior tendon rupture. J Foot Surg 1989;29(4):349–52.

31. Deland JT. Adult-acquired flatfoot deformity. J Am Acad Orthop Surg 2008;16(7):399–406.

32. Cotton FJ. Foot statics and surgery. N Engl J Med 1936;214(8):353–62.

33. Rush SM. Reconstructive options for failed flatfoot surgery. Clin Podiatr Med Surg 2007;24(4):779–88.

34. Sofka CM. Postoperative magnetic resonance imaging of the foot and ankle. J Magn Reson Imaging 2013;37(3):556–65.

35. Karlsson J, Bergsten TO, Lansinger OL, et al. Reconstruction of the lateral ligaments of the ankle for chronic lateral instability. J Bone Joint Surg Am 1988;70(4):581–8.

36. Colville MR. Surgical treatment of the unstable ankle. J Am Acad Orthop Surg 1998;6(6):368–77.

37. Baumhauer JF, O'brien T. Surgical considerations in the treatment of ankle instability. J Athl Train 2002; 37(4):458.

38. Chhabra A, Subhawong TK, Carrino JA. MR imaging of deltoid ligament pathologic findings and associated impingement syndromes. Radiographics 2010;30(3):751–61.

39. Chun KY, Choi YS, Lee SH, et al. Deltoid ligament and tibiofibular syndesmosis injury in chronic lateral ankle instability: magnetic resonance imaging evaluation at 3T and comparison with arthroscopy. Korean J Radiol 2015;16(5): 1096–103.

40. Crim J, Longenecker LG. MRI and surgical findings in deltoid ligament tears. AJR Am J Roentgenol 2015;204(1):W63–9.

41. Beals TC, Crim J, Nickisch F. Deltoid ligament injuries in athletes: techniques of repair and reconstruction. Oper Tech Sports Med 2010;18(1):11–7.

42. Espinosa N, Schmitt JW, Saupe N, et al. Morton neuroma: MR imaging after resection—postoperative MR and histologic findings in asymptomatic and symptomatic intermetatarsal spaces. Radiology 2010;255(3):850–6.

43. Alexander IJ, Johnson KA, Parr JW. Morton's neuroma: a review of recent concepts. Orthopedics 1987;10(1):103–6.

44. Zanetti M, Ledermann T, Zollinger H, et al. Efficacy of MR imaging in patients suspected of having Morton's neuroma. AJR Am J Roentgenol 1997 Feb;168(2):529–32.

45. Zanetti M, Strehle JK, Kundert HP, et al. Morton neuroma: effect of MR imaging findings on diagnostic thinking and therapeutic decisions. Radiology 1999;213(2):583–8.

46. Bencardino J, Rosenberg ZS, Beltran J, et al. Morton's neuroma: is it always symptomatic? AJR Am J Roentgenol 2000;175(3):649–53.

47. Zanetti M, Strehle JK, Zollinger H, et al. Morton neuroma and fluid in the intermetatarsal bursae on MR images of 70 asymptomatic volunteers. Radiology 1997;203(2):516–20.

48. Coughlin MJ, Pinsonneault T. Operative treatment of interdigital neuroma. J Bone Joint Surg Am 2001;83(9):1321–8.

49. Johnson JE, Johnson KA, Unni KK. Persistent pain after excision of an interdigital neuroma. Results of reoperation. J Bone Joint Surg Am 1988;70(5):651–7.

50. Stamatis ED, Myerson MS. Treatment of recurrence of symptoms after excision of an interdigital neuroma. J Bone Joint Surg Br 2004;86(1):48–53.

51. Stamatis ED, Karabalis C. Interdigital neuromas: current state of the art—surgical. Foot Ankle Clin 2004;9(2):287–96.

52. Thordarson DB, Shean CJ. Nerve and tendon lacerations about the foot and ankle. J Am Acad Orthop Surg 2005;13(3):186–96.

53. Wolfort SF, Dellon AL. Treatment of recurrent neuroma of the interdigital nerve by implantation of the proximal nerve into muscle in the arch of the foot. J Foot Ankle Surg 2001;40(6):404–10.

54. Cowell HR, Elener V. Rigid painful flatfoot secondary to tarsal coalition. Clin Orthop Relat Res 1983;177:54–60.

55. Newman JS, Newberg AH. Congenital tarsal coalition: multimodality evaluation with emphasis on CT and MR imaging. Radiographics 2000;20(2):321–32.

56. Varner KE, Michelson JD. Tarsal coalition in adults. Foot Ankle Int 2000;21(8):669–72.

57. Lemley F, Berlet G, Hill K, et al. Current concepts review: tarsal coalition. Foot Ankle Int 2006;27(12):1163–9.

58. Mubarak SJ, Patel PN, Upasani VV, et al. Calcaneonavicular coalition: treatment by excision and fat graft. J Pediatr Orthop 2009;29(5):418–26.

59. Giannini S, Ceccarelli F, Vannini F, et al. Operative treatment of flatfoot with talocalcaneal coalition. Clin Orthop Relat Res 2003;411:178–87.

60. Kernbach KJ, Blitz NM, Rush SM. Bilateral single-stage middle facet talocalcaneal coalition resection combined with flatfoot reconstruction: a report of 3 cases and review of the literature. Investigations involving middle facet coalitions—part 1. J Foot Ankle Surg 2008;47(3):180–90.

61. Weatherall JM, Chapman CB, Shapiro SL. Postoperative second metatarsal fractures associated with suture-button implant in hallux valgus surgery. Foot Ankle Int 2013;34(1):104–10.

62. Spitz DJ, Newberg AH. Imaging of stress fractures in the athlete. Magn Reson Imaging Clin N Am 2003;11(2):323–39.

63. Stafford SA, Rosenthal DI, Gebhardt MC, et al. MRI in stress fracture. Am J Roentgenol 1986;147(3):553–6.

64. Fredericson M, Bergman AG, Hoffman KL, et al. Tibial stress reaction in runners correlation of clinical symptoms and scintigraphy with a new magnetic resonance imaging grading system. Am J Sports Med 1995;23(4):472–81.

65. Kothari NA, Pelchovitz DJ, Meyer JS. Imaging of musculoskeletal infections. Radiol Clin North Am 2001;39(4):653–71.

66. Pineda C, Espinosa R, Pena A. Radiographic imaging in osteomyelitis: the role of plain radiography, computed tomography, ultrasonography, magnetic resonance imaging, and scintigraphy. Semin Plast Surg 2009;23(2):80.

67. Kapoor A, Page S, LaValley M, et al. Magnetic resonance imaging for diagnosing foot osteomyelitis: a meta-analysis. Arch Intern Med 2007;167(2):125–32.

68. Schweitzer ME, Daffner RH, Weissman BN, et al. ACR appropriateness criteria on suspected osteomyelitis in patients with diabetes mellitus. J Am Coll Radiol 2008;5(8):881–6.

69. Chatha DS, Cunningham PM, Schweitzer ME. MR imaging of the diabetic foot: diagnostic challenges. Radiol Clin North Am 2005;43(4):747–59.

70. Donovan A, Schweitzer ME. Use of MR imaging in diagnosing diabetes-related pedal osteomyelitis. Radiographics 2010;30(3):723–36.

71. Johnson PW, Collins MS, Wenger DE. Diagnostic utility of T1-weighted MRI characteristics in evaluation of osteomyelitis of the foot. AJR Am J Roentgenol 2009;192(1):96–100.

72. Collins MS, Schaar MM, Wenger DE, et al. T1-weighted MRI characteristics of pedal osteomyelitis. AJR Am J Roentgenol 2005;185(2):386–93.

73. Schweitzer ME, White LM. Does altered biomechanics cause marrow edema? Radiology 1996;198(3):851–3.

74. Jones KM, Unger EC, Granstrom P, et al. Bone marrow imaging using STIR at 0.5 and 1.5 T. Magn Reson Imaging 1992;10(2):169–76.

75. Unger E, Moldofsky P, Gatenby R, et al. Diagnosis of osteomyelitis by MR imaging. AJR Am J Roentgenol 1988;150(3):605–10.

76. Rios AM, Rosenberg ZS, Bencardino JT, et al. Bone marrow edema patterns in the ankle and hindfoot: distinguishing MRI features. AJR Am J Roentgenol 2011;197(4):W720–9.

77. Ogilvie-Harris DJ, Roscoe MA. Reflex sympathetic dystrophy of the knee. J Bone Joint Surg Br 1987; 69(5):804–6.

78. Elias I, Zoga AC, Schweitzer ME, et al. A specific bone marrow edema around the foot and ankle following trauma and immobilization therapy: pattern description and potential clinical relevance. Foot Ankle Int 2007;28(4):463–71.

79. Crozier F, Champsaur P, Pham T, et al. Magnetic resonance imaging in reflex sympathetic dystrophy syndrome of the foot. Joint Bone Spine 2003;70(6): 503–8.

80. Schweitzer ME, Mandel S, Schwartzman RJ, et al. Reflex sympathetic dystrophy revisited: MR imaging findings before and after infusion of contrast material. Radiology 1995;195(1):211–4.

New Techniques in MR Imaging of the Ankle and Foot

Won C. Bae, PhD[a,b], Thumanoon Ruangchaijatuporn, MD[c],
Christine B. Chung, MD[a,b],*

KEYWORDS

- MR imaging • 3D isotropic MR imaging • MR neurography • Diffusion-weighted imaging
- Sodium MR • Ultrashort TE • Quantitative MR imaging • Ankle

KEY POINTS

- Isotropic three-dimensional MR imaging provides comprehensive joint assessment by offering exquisite, submillimeter anatomic detail while maintaining soft tissue contrast comparable with conventional two-dimensional sequences.
- MR neurography leverages fast spin echo and diffusion-weighted imaging techniques to provide high-resolution, nerve-selective images for assessing peripheral nerve injuries of the foot and ankle.
- Advanced tools for characterizing the structural integrity of cartilage, tendon, and bone include ultrashort echo time MR imaging, quantitative MR imaging, and diffusion tensor imaging.
- Sodium imaging with ultrahigh-field-strength MR imaging holds promise for assessing structural properties such as the glycosaminoglycan content of articular cartilage.

INTRODUCTION

Disorders of the foot and ankle, both in the setting of acute diagnosis and follow-up of lesions, are an important part of any musculoskeletal imaging practice. The incidence of foot and ankle injuries has been reported to represent as high as 10% of all trauma cases.[1] Costs related to diabetic foot ulcer care are greater than $1 billion annually and increasing, with neuropathy and infection accounting for 90% of related admissions.[2] Although only 3% of osseous neoplasms are found in the foot and ankle, 8% of benign soft tissue tumors and 5% of malignant soft tissue tumors are localized to these regions.[3] Similarly, as reflected in this issue, the breadth of disorders that affect the foot and ankle is substantial. Coupled with the anatomic complexity of the foot and ankle, this presents challenges to clinicians and imagers alike. MR imaging has become established as an invaluable tool for the noninvasive diagnosis and characterization of foot and ankle evaluation because of its soft tissue contrast resolution, high spatial resolution, and multiplanar capabilities. This article discusses the state-of-the-art techniques (**Table 1**) that are currently available on MR vendor platforms, presenting applications that may aid in diagnosis or characterization of disease. In addition, translational techniques (see **Table 1**) are presented that offer insight into

Disclosure: The authors have nothing to disclose.
[a] Radiology Service, Veterans Affairs San Diego Healthcare System, 3350 La Jolla Village Drive, MC 114, San Diego, CA 92161, USA; [b] Department of Radiology, UCSD MSK Imaging Research Lab, University of California, San Diego, 9427 Health Sciences Drive, La Jolla, CA 92093-0997, USA; [c] Department of Diagnostic and Therapeutic Radiology, Faculty of Medicine, Ramathibodi Hospital, Mahidol University, 270 Rama VI Road, Ratchatewi, Bangkok 10400, Thailand
* Corresponding author.
E-mail address: cbchung@ucsd.edu

1064-9689/17/© 2016 Elsevier Inc. All rights reserved.

Table 1
Currently available and novel translational techniques in MR imaging of the ankle and foot

MR Techniques	Reference
Currently Available	
Isotropic 3D FSE for 3D rendering	6–9,18,19
MR neurography	20–22
Diffusion-weighted imaging	20,23,24
Diffusion tensor imaging	31,34,35
Novel Translational	
Ultrashort TE for invisible tissues	40–46
Quantitative MR Biomarkers	
Collagen Sensitive	
SE T2	60,61,64,65
UTE T2*	47,72–77,84
Proteoglycan Sensitive	
T1rho	85–87
Sodium	94–98
Functional Assessment	
Kinematic MR imaging	99–103

Abbreviations: 3D, three-dimensional; FSE, fast spin echo; SE, spin echo; TE, echo time; UTE, ultrashort echo time.

potential future applications that indicate that the true destiny of MR will exceed gross structural evaluation of tissue.

APPLICATIONS OF CURRENTLY AVAILABLE SEQUENCES

Isotropic Three-Dimensional Fast Spin Echo Acquisition for Three-Dimensional Rendering

Historically, most musculoskeletal MR imaging protocols have relied heavily on two-dimensional (2D) multislice acquisitions, reserving three-dimensional (3D) volumetric sequences for instances in which thinner slice thickness, higher in-plane resolution, reduced volume averaging, and the ability to reconstruct in other planes were desired. The major disadvantages of these sequences were suboptimal soft tissue contrast and long acquisition times.[4,5] More recently, 3D fast spin echo (FSE) sequences have been developed that achieve tissue contrast similar to 2D FSE sequences, in clinically feasible scan times.[6,7] Some version of an isotropic 3D FSE sequence is available on the major MR vendor platforms.

Two major advantages have been leveraged in the literature with regard to implementation of the isotropic 3D FSE sequences. First, the approximation of tissue contrast that approaches 2D FSE techniques provides the possibility for a comprehensive joint assessment with markedly decreased overall scan times (scan once and reformat in any plane).[8,9] Second, the submillimeter, high-resolution source images allow detailed evaluation of small, complex anatomic structures.[10–13]

Although computed tomography (CT) has traditionally been the imaging method used for the evaluation of bone, both qualitatively and for generating 3D reconstructions, recent developments related to 3D MR imaging sequences suggest a potential new role for MR imaging in this regard. Studies are emerging in the literature that establish that MR provides resolution and contrast that allow equal or superior ability compared with CT to detect osseous disorders such as occult fracture, as well as characterization of fractures required for preoperative planning.[14–17] A few recent studies have addressed the use of 3D MR sequences to generate 3D renderings of bones,[18,19] and this is clearly an area of potential development in joints such as the ankle, in which complex trauma, articular surface evaluation, and bone alignment, among other things, may benefit from 3D visualization of bones (**Fig. 1**). The capability to provide this added information from the MR imaging study establishes a sort of one-stop shop, where the patient can avoid the delay of an added imaging study and the exposure to ionizing radiation, and that also represents a better use of health care dollars.

Magnetic Resonance Neurography

General MR protocols to evaluate peripheral nerves require the ability to detect alteration in nerve signal intensity and morphology, necessitating a combination of sequences that provides high-resolution and sensitivity to mobile water. Acquiring a high-quality peripheral nerve MR study that is clinically helpful requires time and attention to detail. Protocols should be planned with all available clinical information as well as electrodiagnostic test results. In many cases, the field of view must be tailored to cover a broader area initially for the purposes of screening, followed by smaller field of view 2D and 3D imaging targeted to areas of identified abnormalities. Protocols based on a combination of T2 and diffusion-weighted imaging (DWI) neurographic sequences have been proposed. These sequences include T1 FSE, T2 adiabatic inversion recovery, proton density, 3D inversion recovery, and 3D diffusion-weighted reversed fast imaging with steady state precession (DW-PSIF) hybrid pulse sequences.[20–22] The DW-PSIF hybrid pulse sequences provide nerve-selective images, with suppression of adjacent vascular structures,

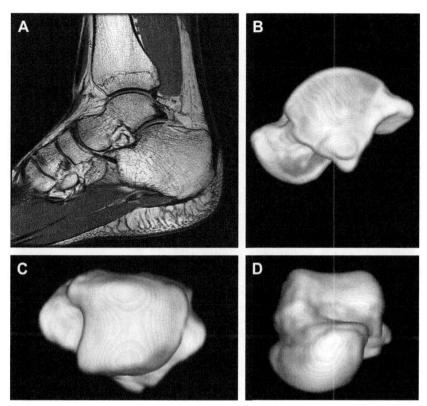

Fig. 1. (A) High-resolution 3D FSE image of an ankle in the sagittal plane, taken at field of view = 140 mm, matrix = 320 × 320, slice = 0.5 mm, repetition time (TR) = 800 milliseconds, TE = 19 milliseconds, echo train length = 28. The talus was segmented to render a 3D model shown in (B) sagittal, (C) axial, and (D) coronal views.

which can be particularly helpful in the foot and ankle (**Fig. 2**). Diffusion tensor imaging (DTI) is another technique that has been implemented in peripheral nerve evaluation. It exploits the anisotropic properties of axonal fiber tracts, allowing fiber tract mapping as well as calculation of quantitative parameters such as the absolute diffusion coefficient (ADC).[23] This technique is technically demanding, and has not been broadly adapted for clinical use, but shows great promise for lesion characterization.[20,24] The ADC is a quantitative descriptor of diffusivity and fractional anisotropy (**Fig. 3**). The mean diffusivity quantifies the average displacement of water molecules, and fractional anisotropy measures the directional preference of the diffusion of the water molecules. If the fractional anisotropy measurement is zero, diffusion is isotropic and can go in any direction (unrestricted), or can go nowhere (completely restricted). If the fractional anisotropy is 1, it means diffusion occurs along only 1 axis and is fully restricted in all other directions. Neuropathic conditions often result in a decreased fractional anisotropy (increased ADC), in which recovering axons often show increased fractional anisotropy (decreased ADC).[23]

Peripheral nerve injury in the foot and ankle is common and can be related to acute trauma, chronic repetitive microtrauma, entrapment syndromes within fibro-osseous tunnels, and postprocedural iatrogenic lesions.[25–27] Nerve sheath tumors and systemic neuropathies can also affect the nerves of the foot and ankle.[28–30] MR criteria (**Box 1**) for distinguishing a normal versus abnormal nerve include size (using adjacent vascular structures as an internal standard), signal intensity (isointense to skeletal muscle on T1 and T2; may be minimally hyperintense to muscle with T2 fat suppression or inversion recovery), preservation of fascicular pattern, smooth course without deviation, preserved perineural fat, normal diffusion tensor tracts, normal fractional anisotropy values (>0.4–0.5), and symmetric brightness on diffusion tensor images.[31]

Diffusion-Weighted Imaging

As indicated earlier, DWI has been studied in the peripheral nervous system, and even more robustly in the central nervous system, for some time.[32] Tissue analysis using DWI is based on assumptions that magnitude and direction of local

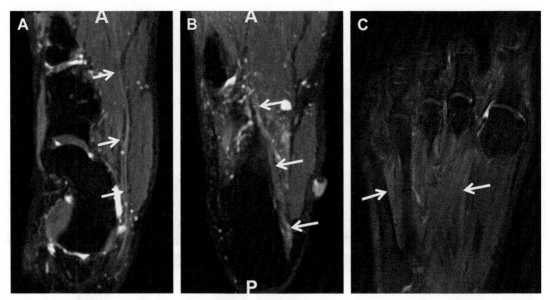

Fig. 2. Ankle MR neurography. Man with medial ankle pain following plantar fascial release. (*A*) Coronal 3D DW-PSIF maximal intensity projection (MIP) image shows normal intermediate signal appearance of the medial plantar nerve (*arrows*). (*B*) More plantar image shows irregular contoured and thickened lateral plantar nerve (*arrows*) with distal hyperintensity in keeping with Sunderland class III injury. (*C*) Horizontal long-axis T2 Spectral attenuated inversion recovery (SPAIR) image shows lateral compartment edemalike signal in keeping with muscle denervation changes (*arrows*). A, anterior; P, posterior. (*Courtesy of* Dr Vibhor Wadhwa, Radiology Intern, and Dr Avneesh Chhabra, Associate Professor Radiology & Orthopedic Surgery, University of Texas Southwestern Medical Center, Dallas, TX.)

diffusivity in tissue are influenced by the macromolecular environment of diffusing bulk water. Information on tissue structural property is provided by measuring spatial restriction of diffusivity (in contrast with unrestricted diffusion in free water) according to tissue ultrastructure.[33] With conventional DWI, diffusion-sensitizing gradients are applied in a single direction with the subsequent total diffusion movement registration limited to that direction. By combining DWI with DTI, several diffusion-sensitizing gradient pairs in different noncoplanar directions are applied, allowing determination of degree of diffusional anisotropy as well as main directions of local diffusion in a tissue.[34] DTI is based on the fact that the magnitude and molecular motion of water are restricted by structural elements within the tissue, theoretically lending itself to the evaluation of ordered structures such as cartilage and tendon. It has already been implemented in skeletal muscle, bone, and musculoskeletal soft tissues.[35] DTI has been proposed as a biomarker for cartilage composition and structure because of its sensitivity to proteoglycan content through mean diffusivity and to collagen architecture through the fractional anisotropy. It has recently been used to assess postoperative tendon quality in patients with Achilles tendon rupture, providing information regarding the trajectory and tendinous fiber continuity in the repair tissue.[36]

The advantages of DTI as a potential MR biomarker for assessment of articular cartilage are that it evaluates both proteoglycan and collagen without the need for exogenous contrast material and it does so at a higher resolution than sodium (^{23}Na)-based MR imaging (**Fig. 4**). In addition, DTI has the ability to assess collagen and proteoglycan independently of each other. The configuration of the collagen fibril network induces anisotropy (measured with fractional anisotropy) of the water molecules. However, the proteoglycan molecules do not show preferred orientation and therefore restrict motion of water molecules equally in all directions. For this reason, proteoglycan content affects only mean diffusivity. However, diffusion cannot provide a quantitative estimation of the absolute proteoglycan or collagen composition. Further, translation of DWI to the musculoskeletal system has proved difficult for 2 reasons. First, the short T2 of articular cartilage (20–40 milliseconds) causes low signal-to-noise ratio in standard DWI techniques that require long echo times (TEs). Second, the sensitivity of DWI to patient motion makes it difficult to achieve the high spatial resolution required for cartilage evaluation.[37] Several

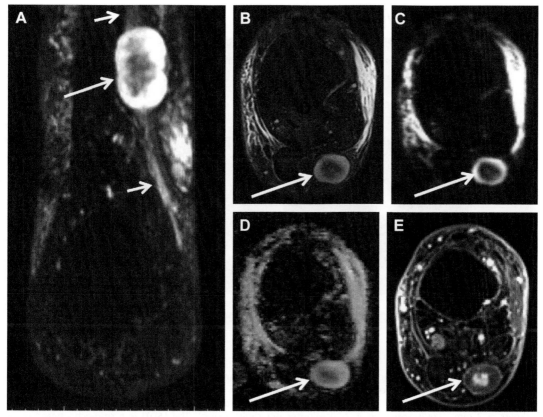

Fig. 3. MR neurography with DTI. (*A*) Coronal 3D DW-PSIF MIP image shows sural nerve (*small arrows*) with associated peripheral nerve sheath tumor (pathology-proven neurofibroma, *large arrow*). (*B*) Axial T2 SPAIR, (*C*) trace image (reflects global diffusion magnitude calculated from diffusion images obtained with diffusion gradients in at least 3 different spatial directions), (*D*) ADC image, and (*E*) postcontrast image. Note the target appearance on all images (*long arrows*) with high ADC = 2.0×10^{-3} mm^2/s, consistent with a benign lesion. (*Courtesy of* Dr Vibhor Wadhwa, Radiology Intern, and Dr Avneesh Chhabra, Associate Professor Radiology & Orthopedic Surgery, University of Texas Southwestern Medical Center, Dallas, TX.)

Box 1 **Criteria for a normal nerve on diffusion tensor MR images**
MR criteria for a normal nerve
Size, using adjacent vascular structures as an internal standard
Signal intensity isointense to skeletal muscle on T1 and T2 (may be minimally hyperintense to muscle with T2 fat-suppressed or inversion recovery)
Preservation of fascicular pattern
Smooth course without deviation
Preservation of perineural fat
Normal diffusion tensor tracts
Normal fractional anisotropy values greater than 0.4 to 0.5
Symmetric brightness on diffusion tensor images

recent publications suggest promise for overcoming these technical challenges in patient cohorts.[38,39]

NOVEL MAGNETIC RESONANCE PULSE SEQUENCES
Ultrashort Echo Time MR Imaging

Ultrashort TE (UTE) MR imaging is represented by a group of pulse sequences capable of providing TE values of less than 1 millisecond.[40,41] Conventional MR imaging sequences use long TEs, resulting in limited opportunity to encode decaying signal of short-T2 tissues before that signal reaches zero. For this reason, biological tissues with intrinsic transverse relaxation times (T2, T2*) that are short (generally considered <10 milliseconds, although subclassification exists within the short category) appear black; that is, void of signal on standard MR pulse sequences. By decreasing

MD   FA

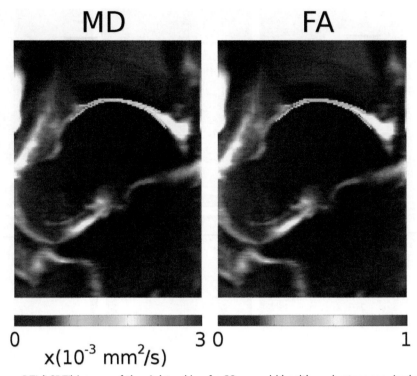

0   3 0   1

$x(10^{-3} \text{ mm}^2/s)$

Fig. 4. Line scan DTI (LSDTI) images of the right ankle of a 28-year-old healthy volunteer acquired at 7 T using a custom-built 8-channel carotid coil (TE/TR/TR_{eff} = 46/180/2880 milliseconds, matrix = 256 × 128, in-plane resolution = 0.5 × 0.5 mm^2, rotation angle = 20°, b-values = 5450 mm^2/s, 6 diffusion directions, thickness = 3 mm, acquisition time = 2:30 minutes per sagittal slice). The LSDTI is a spin-echo–based pulse sequence, in which only 1 line is excited and acquired per TR, avoiding phase encoding (ie, motion artifact). Mean diffusivity (MD) and fractional anisotropy (FA) maps of the tibiotalar cartilage are shown in color over the LSDTI b_0-image. Averaged over 7 volunteers, FA/ADC values were (0.44 ± 0.09)/(1.49 ± 0.18) × 10^{-3} mm^2/s and (0.48 ± 0.11)/(1.26 ± 0.12) × 10^{-3} mm^2/s for the tibial and talar cartilages, respectively. (*Courtesy of* Dr Jose Raya, Assistant Professor of Radiology, NYU Langone Medical Center, Department of Radiology, New York, NY.)

the TE to the range of the intrinsic T2/T2* value of short-T2 tissues, signal can be acquired from these tissues, allowing morphologic evaluation. Moreover, UTE sequences can be used for quantitative evaluation of short-T2 tissues (this capability is addressed later).

The application of UTE MR imaging to the musculoskeletal system has been revolutionary, largely because of the short T2 nature of many musculoskeletal tissues. These tissues include the calcified layer of cartilage, fibrocartilaginous structures, ligaments, tendons, and bone.[42–46] The ability to acquire signal and characterize the infrastructure of short T2 tissues presents a paradigm shift in diagnosis and characterization of structural alteration. Rather than being limited to diagnosis of disorders at a point in time when the short T2 tissue has failed through traumatic tearing or severe degeneration, effectively transforming it into a long T2 tissue, UTE MR imaging affords the opportunity to identify pathologic changes at an

earlier stage, which provides the chance for earlier intervention and controlled treatment. The UTE MR imaging sequences currently have limited availability on vendor platforms, but promising results have been introduced in the literature for clinical application of these sequences in the setting of meniscal repair, cartilage repair, and osteoarthrosis.[47–49]

Potential applications for UTE MR imaging include evaluation of osteochondral injury, assessment of degenerative changes, and monitoring of tissue healing. Ankle sprains have an estimated daily occurrence of 27,000 in the United States, with 50% leading to osteochondral lesions.[50] UTE MR imaging allows assessment of the calcified layer of cartilage at the talar dome, helping to characterize osteochondral junction injury acutely and in follow-up (**Fig. 5**). Further, bone marrow–stimulating techniques (abrasion, drilling, microfracture) are used to treat chondral defects.[51] In such procedures, it is important to assess the presence and nature of fill tissue at

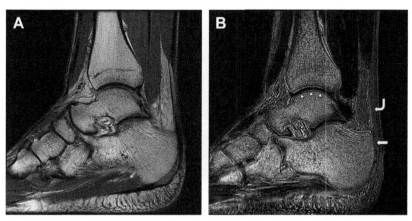

Fig. 5. Comparison of conventional proton density–weighted spin echo image (TE = 19 milliseconds) (A) versus novel UTE echo subtraction image (TE = 0.05 milliseconds minus TE = 8 milliseconds) (B). UTE image (B) shows the deepest layer (including calcified layer) of talar dome cartilage (arrowheads), the Achilles tensile tendon (curved arrow), and Achilles enthesis (arrow) with high signal intensity. These areas all appear as black signal voids on the conventional proton density–weighted spin echo image (A), because of rapid T2 shortening of the tendon and deep layers of hyaline cartilage. These structures have already lost signal by the time they are measured at the conventional TEs and require UTE measurement to show intrasubstance signal.

the repair site, as well to assess the reconstitution of the cartilage-bone interface.[52]

In addition, UTE MR imaging is well suited to evaluating ankle tendons, both tensile components and entheseal attachments to bone (see Fig. 5; Fig. 6). Achilles tendinopathy is the most common cause of posterior heel pain, and is often caused by mechanical stress related to overload or overuse of the muscle-tendon unit.[53] Recently, overuse conditions in the Achilles tendon have been associated with nonuniform mechanical loading of the triceps surae (lateral gastrocnemius, medial gastrocnemius, soleus).[54] UTE MR imaging offers the ability to identify the distribution of the relative contributions of the Achilles tendon, as well as the ability to identify structural alteration through loss of the normal fascicular appearance of the tendon (Fig. 7).

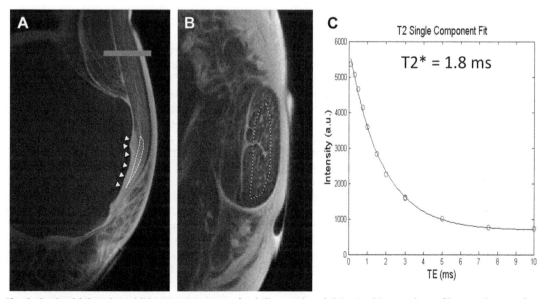

Fig. 6. Sagittal (A) and axial (B) UTE MR images of Achilles tendon. (A) Sagittal image shows fibrocartilage surface of calcaneus (arrowheads) as well as fibrocartilaginous nodule within the tendon (dotted area). In an axial cross section (A, thick line; B), tensile tendon with normal fascicular appearance can be seen. (C) UTE T2* quantification performed on axial images revealed a short T2* value of 1.8 milliseconds, within the normal range.

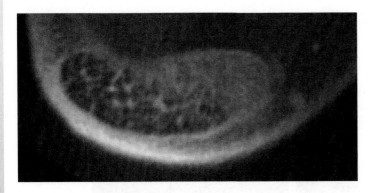

Fig. 7. Axial UTE MR image of Achilles tensile tendon shows differential microstructure of the tendon with geographic effacement of the normal fascicular appearance within the tendon representing intrasubstance degeneration.

The entheseal attachment of the Achilles tendon also has great interest from a clinical standpoint. It is suggested in the literature that there is a significant cohort of seronegative patients with spondyloarthropathy who have subclinical disease involving the lower limb.[55,56] UTE MR imaging is well suited to characterizing the normal appearance of the Achilles tendon synovioentheseal complex, as well as alterations that may reflect early changes of subclinical entheseal disease[57] (see **Fig. 5**).

QUANTITATIVE MR IMAGING BIOMARKERS

MR-based techniques have been developed that allow characterization and quantification of the biochemical composition of tissue. This ability has been a revolutionary step forward in musculoskeletal MR, allowing noninvasive assessment of biochemical and structural tissue status at very early stages of disease as well as in repair tissue. The quantitative nature offers an objective data point that will undoubtedly prove important in guiding treatment, developing new treatment options, and perhaps serving as a surrogate for tissue material property.

Most quantitative biomarkers in the musculoskeletal system have been designed for collagen and proteoglycan evaluation, because they are major structural elements in most musculoskeletal tissues. Further, much of the initial biomarker work was performed in articular cartilage, and has expanded rapidly to applications in other musculoskeletal tissues. For the purposes of potential applications of quantitative biomarkers in the foot and ankle, the focus here is on evaluation of tendon and cartilage. In tendons, quantitative assessment has focused on collagen content, rather than proteoglycan evaluation, because proteoglycans represent a small percentage of the overall dry weight of tendons

(0.2%–5%) compared with articular cartilage (12%).[58,59]

Collagen Evaluation

T2 mapping

T2 relaxation times represent the rate of constant proton dephasing after an initial radiofrequency pulse is delivered. The T2 relaxation value of articular cartilage reflects water content, collagen content, and collagen fiber orientation in the extracellular matrix, with longer T2 relaxation values representing cartilage degeneration.[60,61] T2 relaxation data are acquired using a constant repetition time (TR) variable TE technique, in which signal intensities from regions of interest are plotted against TE, resulting in a map of T2 relaxation times within the tissue. A zonal variation in T2 values has been shown in articular cartilage caused by the densely packed nature of the collagen fibers in the deeper layers of articular cartilage. This variation limits the mobility of protons, and results in a lower T2 value in the deeper cartilage layers.[62] Further, at the junction of cartilage and bone, the calcified layer of cartilage has a very short T2 relaxation time, making T2 measurements unreliable in this region.[42,63]

A T2 mapping pulse sequence is available on most vendor platforms. Extensive studies have shown this form of T2 quantification to be reproducible and have shown the validity of the measurements.[60,64,65] The technique has been used in many clinical studies that have explored articular cartilage in the context of osteoarthrosis, malalignment, and trauma.[60,66] T2 mapping has been also been widely used in the evaluation of ankle articular cartilage (**Fig. 8**). Studies performed in the ankle, similar to those performed in the knee, have focused on structure, posttraumatic changes, evaluation of repair tissue, and exploration of novel techniques such as traction in the foot and ankle to improve visualization and thereby improve quantification.[67–71]

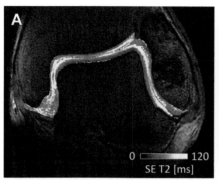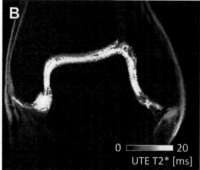

Fig. 8. Color maps of the tibiotalar articular cartilage obtained from conventional multiecho spin echo (SE) T2 (*A*) and UTE T2* (*B*) techniques show the short and long T2 components of articular cartilage. T2 (*A*) map shows the normal zonal variation in T2 values with shorter T2 relaxation times (*red band*) closer to the subchondral bone, and longer T2 relaxation times (*yellow*) at the articular surface. In the UTE T2* map (*B*), the linear short T2* (*red*) region adjacent to the subchondral bone interface represents the normal, intact calcified layer of cartilage. The shorter T2* range does not offer evaluation of the integrity of zonal variation in the longer T2 tissue of the more superficial layers of articular cartilage.

Ultrashort echo time T2 mapping*

T2* relaxation time depends on interactions between spins, tissue hydration, and susceptibility.[41] Similar to T2 mapping, quantification is performed with a constant TR and variable TE technique. However, T2* mapping uses UTE sequences, allowing much shorter TE ranges to be exploited (lowest TE in the microsecond to 1 millisecond range). Studies applying UTE T2* mapping suggest that the evaluation of short T2 tissues by methods that operate in a short T2 range offer more sensitive evaluation of structural alteration. UTE T2* mapping is most effectively applied to short T2 tissues (see **Fig. 8**). To date, clinical feasibility has been shown in the evaluation of articular cartilage in the knee and hip.[47,72–77]

Quantitative T2* mapping of tendon, specifically the Achilles tendon, has been performed in animal models and in ex vivo and in vivo human tissue.[78–83] Much of this work has been performed with T2* or UTE T2* techniques that allow identification of long and short T2 tissue fractions. The tendon seems to have a complex composition, with significant long and short T2 components, necessitating care in interpretation of the quantitative data (see **Fig. 6**). Exciting work suggests that

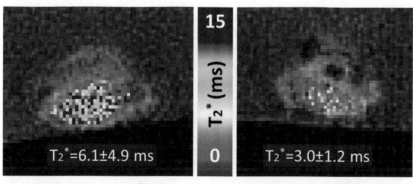

Prior to Loading   **After Loading**

Fig. 9. Tissue evaluation after loading. T2* maps of rabbit patellar tendon before and after 45 N of cyclic loading for 100 cycles. T2* values before loading are increased and have greater variability than corresponding T2* values after loading. Changes in values before and after loading may indicate level of tissue organization and collagen fibril disruption. Evaluation of tissue preload and postload may ultimately give insight into tissue function and point of failure. (*Courtesy of* Dr Matthew F. Koff, Associate Scientist, and Dr Hollis Potter, Professor of Radiology, Department of Radiology and Imaging, Hospital for Special Surgery.)

quantitative measures may have the potential to serve as a reference standard for mechanical property of tissue.[84] From a practical standpoint, the prediction of tissue material property and function over time may prove far more important than the detection of structural alteration (**Fig. 9**).

Proteoglycan Evaluation

T1 rho MR imaging

T1 rho (the spin-lattice relaxation time in the rotating frame), is a technique that has been used to assess low-frequency interactions between hydrogen and macromolecules in free water. It uses clusters of radiofrequency pulses to lock magnetization in the transverse plane, followed by additional radiofrequency pulses to drive longitudinal recovery.[85] T1 rho probes slow-motion interactions between motion-restricted water molecules and their local macromolecular environment. In vitro studies showed that depletion of proteoglycan resulted in increased T1 rho values, suggesting that T1 rho estimates proteoglycan content.[86,87] There is some evidence that other factors, including collagen fiber orientation and concentration of other macromolecules, may contribute to T1 rho values.[88] However, T1 rho may be more sensitive than T2 mapping for differentiating between normal cartilage and early-stage osteoarthritis (OA).[89] This raises the possibility that proteoglycan loss may precede collagen degradation in OA, and further suggests that T1 rho may provide a better measure.

T1 rho has been used extensively in patient cohorts, primarily focusing on the knee. Studies have emphasized T1 rho as a biomarker in articular cartilage representing early degenerative changes in the joint, a potential surrogate for altered meniscal function, and altered mechanical axis of load distribution in weight bearing in the ACL-reconstructed knee.[90–93] Although this technique has not been described in the ankle articular cartilage, clearly it holds similar potential to the knee (**Fig. 10**).

Sodium MR imaging and ultrahigh field MR imaging (7 T)

MR imaging at ultrahigh field (7 T) offers high signal/noise ratio, which can be used beneficially in several different musculoskeletal applications. Spatial resolution in morphologic imaging of small structures, such as those found in the foot and ankle, can be significantly improved. In addition, imaging techniques that have low signal/noise ratio and low sensitivity can offset these disadvantages through partnering with ultrahigh field MR. Sodium (^{23}Na) MR imaging is one such technique (**Fig. 11**). As its name implies, ^{23}Na MR imaging is based on the detection of sodium ions in tissues (requiring a radiofrequency coil tuned to sodium), allowing quantification of their concentration. In musculoskeletal tissues, sodium ions balance the fixed negative charge of the glycosaminoglycan side chains of proteoglycan molecules, making sodium ion concentration a biomarker for proteoglycan concentration. One major strength of this technique is its strong correlation with glycosaminoglycan concentration in cartilage.[94]

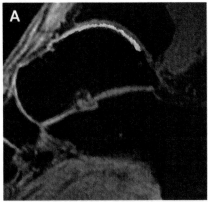 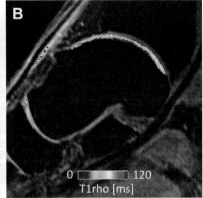

Fig. 10. T1rho mapping of (*A*) lateral and (*B*) medial talar dome cartilage, obtained with the following parameters: TR = 8 milliseconds; TE = 2 milliseconds; matrix = 256 × 128; slice = 4 mm; spin lock times = 0, 10, 40, 80 milliseconds. Some evidence suggests that T1rho mapping reflects proteoglycan content and possibly also collagen fiber orientation and other macromolecules, and that it may be more sensitive than T2 mapping in identifying early hyaline cartilage degradation. (*Courtesy of* Dr Richard Souza, Associate Professor, Department of Physical Therapy and Rehabilitation Science, Department of Radiology and Biomedical Imaging, University of California, San Francisco, CA.)

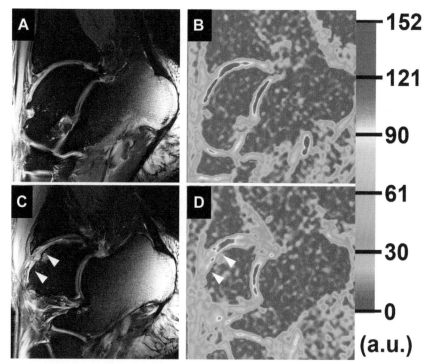

Fig. 11. Seven-Tesla images of the ankle joint in a 35-year-old man who received microfracture (MFX) treatment 54 months earlier. Images of the medial side (*upper row*) and of the lateral side (*lower row*) of the ankle joint. The repair tissue is situated between arrowheads. Proton density–weighted, fat-suppressed, 2D TSE images (*A, C*) and corresponding color-coded sodium images (*B, D*) of reference cartilage and repair tissue. (*Courtesy of* Dr Gregory Chang, Associate Professor, and Dr Ravinder Regatte, Professor of Radiology, NYU Langone Medical Center, Department of Radiology.)

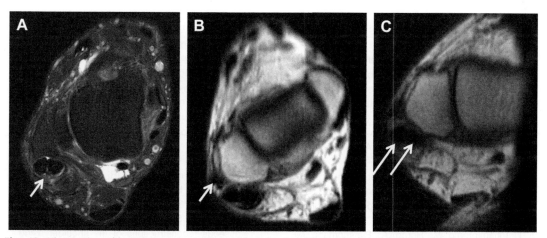

Fig. 12. Kinematic ankle MR imaging. Man with lateral ankle pain and popping sensation. (*A*) Axial fat-suppressed proton density image shows intrasubstance split tears of the peroneal tendons and ill-defined superior peroneal retinaculum (*short arrow*). (*B, C*) Kinematic MR imaging obtained during real-time dorsiflexion (*B*) and plantar flexion (*C*) maneuvers show torn and retracted superior peroneal retinaculum (*short arrow*) and subluxed peroneal tendons on dorsiflexion (*long arrows*). (*Courtesy of* Dr Vibhor Wadhwa, Radiology Intern, and Dr Avneesh Chhabra, Associate Professor Radiology & Orthopedic Surgery, UT Southwestern Medical Center, Dallas, TX.)

In vivo application of ^{23}Na imaging has been performed in articular cartilage, skeletal muscle, and tendon.[95–98]

FUNCTIONAL ASSESSMENT OF TISSUE
Kinematic MR Imaging

MR application in the musculoskeletal system has evolved significantly to emerge as a noninvasive imaging study that can provide a global structural evaluation. As noted, pulse sequence development provides not only excellent soft tissue analysis but rivals CT for the evaluation of bone. Quantitative imaging techniques may offer insight into tissue biochemistry and even material property. An additional frontier to address with regard to musculoskeletal MR is the dynamic nature of the system. Patients are imaged in static positions, whereas injury is incurred dynamically. Further, joint instability is not likely to be apparent in static images.

Methodology has developed and applied to the musculoskeletal system to allow real-time evaluation through range of motion using ultrafast MR imaging scans (**Fig. 12**). The degree of motion is limited by the physical constraints of the scanner, but studies have been described in various joints, including the ankle.[99–103] The ability to dynamically evaluate a joint, while visualizing static and dynamic stabilizers, would be a valuable tool in providing targeted and effective diagnosis and ultimate treatment.

REFERENCES

1. Sharma GK, Dhillon MS, Dhatt SS. The influence of foot and ankle injury patterns and treatment delays on outcomes in a tertiary hospital; a one-year prospective observation. Foot (Edinb) 2016;26:48.
2. Hicks CW, Selvarajah S, Mathioudakis N, et al. Burden of infected diabetic foot ulcers on hospital admissions and costs. Ann Vasc Surg 2016;17:17.
3. Kennedy JG, Ross KA, Smyth NA, et al. Primary tumors of the foot and ankle. Foot Ankle Spec 2016; 9:58.
4. Gold GE, Busse RF, Beehler C, et al. Isotropic MRI of the knee with 3D fast spin-echo extended echo-train acquisition (XETA): initial experience. AJR Am J Roentgenol 2007;188:1287.
5. Notohamiprodjo M, Horng A, Pietschmann MF, et al. MRI of the knee at 3T: first clinical results with an isotropic PDfs-weighted 3D-TSE-sequence. Invest Radiol 2009;44.505.
6. Busse RF, Brau AC, Vu A, et al. Effects of refocusing flip angle modulation and view ordering in 3D fast spin echo. Magn Reson Med 2008;60:640.
7. Busse RF, Hariharan H, Vu A, et al. Fast spin echo sequences with very long echo trains: design of variable refocusing flip angle schedules and generation of clinical T2 contrast. Magn Reson Med 2006;55:1030.
8. Kijowski R, Davis KW, Woods MA, et al. Knee joint: comprehensive assessment with 3D isotropic resolution fast spin-echo MR imaging–diagnostic performance compared with that of conventional MR imaging at 3.0 T. Radiology 2009;252:486.
9. Rosas H, Kijowski R. Volumetric magnetic resonance imaging of the musculoskeletal system. Semin Roentgenol 2013;48:140.
10. Notohamiprodjo M, Kuschel B, Horng A, et al. 3D-MRI of the ankle with optimized 3D-SPACE. Invest Radiol 2012;47:231.
11. Park HJ, Lee SY, Park NH, et al. Three-dimensional isotropic T2-weighted fast spin-echo (VISTA) ankle MRI versus two-dimensional fast spin-echo T2-weighted sequences for the evaluation of anterior talofibular ligament injury. Clin Radiol 2016;71:349.
12. Sutherland JK, Nozaki T, Kaneko Y, et al. Initial experience with 3D isotropic high-resolution 3 T MR arthrography of the wrist. BMC Musculoskelet Disord 2016;17:30.
13. Yi J, Cha JG, Lee YK, et al. MRI of the anterior talofibular ligament, talar cartilage and os subfibulare: comparison of isotropic resolution 3D and conventional 2D T2-weighted fast spin-echo sequences at 3.0 T. Skeletal Radiol 2016;45(7): 899–908.
14. Yin ZG, Zhang JB, Kan SL, et al. Diagnostic accuracy of imaging modalities for suspected scaphoid fractures: meta-analysis combined with latent class analysis. J Bone Joint Surg Br 2012;94:1077.
15. Hakkarinen DK, Banh KV, Hendey GW. Magnetic resonance imaging identifies occult hip fractures missed by 64-slice computed tomography. J Emerg Med 2012;43:303.
16. Collin D, Geijer M, Gothlin JH. Computed tomography compared to magnetic resonance imaging in occult or suspect hip fractures. A retrospective study in 44 patients. Eur Radiol 2016. Epub ahead of print].
17. Gyftopoulos S, Hasan S, Bencardino J, et al. Diagnostic accuracy of MRI in the measurement of glenoid bone loss. AJR Am J Roentgenol 2012;199:873.
18. Gyftopoulos S, Yemin A, Mulholland T, et al. 3DMR osseous reconstructions of the shoulder using a gradient-echo based two-point Dixon reconstruction: a feasibility study. Skeletal Radiol 2013;42:347.
10. Glaoor C, D'Anastasi M, Theisen D, et al. Understanding 3D TSE sequences: advantages, disadvantages, and application in MSK imaging. Semin Musculoskelet Radiol 2015;19:321.

20. Chhabra A, Andreisek G, Soldatos T, et al. MR neurography: past, present, and future. AJR Am J Roentgenol 2011;197:583.

21. Chhabra A, Lee PP, Bizzell C, et al. 3 Tesla MR neurography–technique, interpretation, and pitfalls. Skeletal Radiol 2011;40:1249.

22. Chhabra A, Soldatos T, Subhawong TK, et al. The application of three-dimensional diffusion-weighted PSIF technique in peripheral nerve imaging of the distal extremities. J Magn Reson Imaging 2011; 34:962.

23. Burge AJ, Gold SL, Kuong S, et al. High-resolution magnetic resonance imaging of the lower extremity nerves. Neuroimaging Clin N Am 2014;24:151.

24. Simon NG, Lagopoulos J, Gallagher T, et al. Peripheral nerve diffusion tensor imaging is reliable and reproducible. J Magn Reson Imaging 2016; 43:962.

25. Thordarson DB, Shean CJ. Nerve and tendon lacerations about the foot and ankle. J Am Acad Orthop Surg 2005;13:186.

26. Lopez-Ben R. Imaging of nerve entrapment in the foot and ankle. Foot Ankle Clin 2011;16:213.

27. Chhabra A, Williams EH, Wang KC, et al. MR neurography of neuromas related to nerve injury and entrapment with surgical correlation. AJNR Am J Neuroradiol 2010;31:1363.

28. Carvajal JA, Cuartas E, Qadir R, et al. Peripheral nerve sheath tumors of the foot and ankle. Foot Ankle Int 2011;32:163.

29. Pham M, Oikonomou D, Hornung B, et al. Magnetic resonance neurography detects diabetic neuropathy early and with proximal predominance. Ann Neurol 2015;78:939.

30. Kollmer J, Hund E, Hornung B, et al. In vivo detection of nerve injury in familial amyloid polyneuropathy by magnetic resonance neurography. Brain 2015;138:549.

31. Chhabra A. Peripheral MR neurography: approach to interpretation. Neuroimaging Clin N Am 2014; 24:79.

32. Pierpaoli C, Jezzard P, Basser PJ, et al. Diffusion tensor MR imaging of the human brain. Radiology 1996;201:637.

33. Glaser C. New techniques for cartilage imaging: T2 relaxation time and diffusion-weighted MR imaging. Radiol Clin North Am 2005;43:641.

34. Le Bihan D, Mangin JF, Poupon C, et al. Diffusion tensor imaging: concepts and applications. J Magn Reson Imaging 2001;13:534.

35. Bhojwani N, Szpakowski P, Partovi S, et al. Diffusion-weighted imaging in musculoskeletal radiology-clinical applications and future directions. Quant Imaging Med Surg 2015;5:740.

36. Sarman H, Atmaca H, Cakir O, et al. Assessment of postoperative tendon quality in patients with Achilles tendon rupture using diffusion tensor imaging

and tendon fiber tracking. J Foot Ankle Surg 2015;54:782.

37. Miller KL, Hargreaves BA, Gold GE, et al. Steady-state diffusion-weighted imaging of in vivo knee cartilage. Magn Reson Med 2004;51:394.

38. Apprich S, Trattnig S, Welsch GH, et al. Assessment of articular cartilage repair tissue after matrix-associated autologous chondrocyte transplantation or the microfracture technique in the ankle joint using diffusion-weighted imaging at 3 Tesla. Osteoarthritis Cartilage 2012;20:703.

39. Raya JG, Dettmann E, Notohamiprodjo M, et al. Feasibility of in vivo diffusion tensor imaging of articular cartilage with coverage of all cartilage regions. Eur Radiol 2014;24:1700.

40. Bydder GM. Review. The Agfa Mayneord lecture: MRI of short and ultrashort T(2) and T(2)* components of tissues, fluids and materials using clinical systems. Br J Radiol 2011;84:1067.

41. Chang EY, Du J, Chung CB. UTE imaging in the musculoskeletal system. J Magn Reson Imaging 2015;41:870.

42. Bae WC, Dwek JR, Znamirowski R, et al. Ultrashort echo time MR imaging of osteochondral junction of the knee at 3 T: identification of anatomic structures contributing to signal intensity. Radiology 2010; 254:837.

43. Gatehouse PD, He T, Puri BK, et al. Contrast-enhanced MRI of the menisci of the knee using ultrashort echo time (UTE) pulse sequences: imaging of the red and white zones. Br J Radiol 2004; 77:641.

44. Sanal HT, Bae WC, Pauli C, et al. Magnetic resonance imaging of the temporomandibular joint disc: feasibility of novel quantitative magnetic resonance evaluation using histologic and biomechanical reference standards. J Orofac Pain 2011;25:345.

45. Han M, Larson PE, Liu J, et al. Depiction of Achilles tendon microstructure in vivo using high-resolution 3-dimensional ultrashort echo-time magnetic resonance imaging at 7 T. Invest Radiol 2014;49:339.

46. Bae WC, Chen PC, Chung CB, et al. Quantitative ultrashort echo time (UTE) MRI of human cortical bone: correlation with porosity and biomechanical properties. J Bone Miner Res 2012;27:848.

47. Sneag DB, Shah P, Koff MF, et al. Quantitative ultrashort echo time magnetic resonance imaging evaluation of postoperative menisci: a pilot study. HSS J 2015;11:123.

48. Chu CR, Williams AA, West RV, et al. Quantitative magnetic resonance imaging UTE-T2* mapping of cartilage and meniscus healing after anatomic anterior cruciate ligament reconstruction. Am J Sports Med 1847;2014:42.

49. McWalter EJ, Gold GE. UTE T2 * mapping detects sub-clinical meniscus degeneration. Osteoarthritis Cartilage 2012;20:471.

50. Savage-Elliott I, Ross KA, Smyth NA, et al. Osteo-chondral lesions of the talus: a current concepts review and evidence-based treatment paradigm. Foot Ankle Spec 2014;7:414.

51. Domayer SE, Welsch GH, Stelzeneder D, et al. Microfracture in the ankle: clinical results and MRI with T2-mapping at 3.0 T after 1 to 8 years. Cartilage 2011;2:73.

52. Chen H, Chevrier A, Hoemann CD, et al. Characterization of subchondral bone repair for marrow-stimulated chondral defects and its relationship to articular cartilage resurfacing. Am J Sports Med 2011;39:1731.

53. Berner J, Zufferey P. Achilles tendinopathy. Rev Med Suisse 2015;11:606 [in French].

54. Toumi H, Larguech G, Cherief M, et al. Implications of the calf musculature and Achilles tendon architectures for understanding the site of injury. J Biomech 2016;49(7):1180–5.

55. Bandinelli F, Prignano F, Bonciani D, et al. Ultrasound detects occult entheseal involvement in early psoriatic arthritis independently of clinical features and psoriasis severity. Clin Exp Rheumatol 2013;31:219.

56. Gisondi P, Tinazzi I, El-Dalati G, et al. Lower limb enthesopathy in patients with psoriasis without clinical signs of arthropathy: a hospital-based case-control study. Ann Rheum Dis 2008;67:26.

57. Du J, Chiang AJ, Chung CB, et al. Orientational analysis of the Achilles tendon and enthesis using an ultrashort echo time spectroscopic imaging sequence. Magn Reson Imaging 2010;28:178.

58. Sophia Fox AJ, Bedi A, Rodeo SA. The basic science of articular cartilage: structure, composition, and function. Sports Health 2009;1:461.

59. Amiel D, Frank C, Harwood F, et al. Tendons and ligaments: a morphological and biochemical comparison. J Orthop Res 1984;1:257.

60. Nissi MJ, Rieppo J, Toyras J, et al. T(2) relaxation time mapping reveals age- and species-related diversity of collagen network architecture in articular cartilage. Osteoarthritis Cartilage 2006;14:1265.

61. Mosher TJ, Smith H, Dardzinski BJ, et al. MR imaging and T2 mapping of femoral cartilage: in vivo determination of the magic angle effect. AJR Am J Roentgenol 2001;177:665.

62. Carballido-Gamio J, Blumenkrantz G, Lynch JA, et al. Longitudinal analysis of MRI T(2) knee cartilage laminar organization in a subset of patients from the osteoarthritis initiative. Magn Reson Med 2010;63:465.

63. Bae WC, Biswas R, Chen K, et al. UTE MRI of the osteochondral junction. Curr Radiol Rep 2014;2:35.

64. Dunn TC, Lu Y, Jin H, et al. T2 relaxation time of cartilage at MR imaging: comparison with severity of knee osteoarthritis. Radiology 2004;232:592.

65. Mosher TJ, Zhang Z, Reddy R, et al. Knee articular cartilage damage in osteoarthritis: analysis of MR image biomarker reproducibility in ACRIN-PA 4001 multicenter trial. Radiology 2011;258:832.

66. Friedrich KM, Shepard T, Chang G, et al. Does joint alignment affect the T2 values of cartilage in patients with knee osteoarthritis? Eur Radiol 2010; 20:1532.

67. Juras V, Zbyn S, Mlynarik V, et al. The compositional difference between ankle and knee cartilage demonstrated by T2 mapping at 7 Tesla MR. Eur J Radiol 2016;85:771.

68. Lim Y, Cha JG, Yi J, et al. Topographical and sex variations in the T2 relaxation times of articular cartilage in the ankle joints of healthy young adults using 3.0T MRI. J Magn Reson Imaging 2016;43:455.

69. Golditz T, Steib S, Pfeifer K, et al. Functional ankle instability as a risk factor for osteoarthritis: using T2-mapping to analyze early cartilage degeneration in the ankle joint of young athletes. Osteoarthritis Cartilage 2014;22:1377.

70. Kubosch EJ, Erdle B, Izadpanah K, et al. Clinical outcome and T2 assessment following autologous matrix-induced chondrogenesis in osteochondral lesions of the talus. Int Orthop 2016;40:65.

71. Jungmann PM, Baum T, Schaeffeler C, et al. 3.0T MR imaging of the ankle: axial traction for morphological cartilage evaluation, quantitative T2 mapping and cartilage diffusion imaging–A preliminary study. Eur J Radiol 2015;84:1546.

72. Williams A, Qian Y, Bear D, et al. Assessing degeneration of human articular cartilage with ultra-short echo time (UTE) T2* mapping. Osteoarthritis Cartilage 2010;18:539.

73. Williams A, Qian Y, Chu CR. UTE-T2 * mapping of human articular cartilage in vivo: a repeatability assessment. Osteoarthritis Cartilage 2011;19:84.

74. Williams A, Qian Y, Golla S, et al. UTE-T2 * mapping detects sub-clinical meniscus injury after anterior cruciate ligament tear. Osteoarthritis Cartilage 2012;20:486.

75. Bittersohl B, Hosalkar HS, Hughes T, et al. Feasibility of T2* mapping for the evaluation of hip joint cartilage at 1.5T using a three-dimensional (3D), gradient-echo (GRE) sequence: a prospective study. Magn Reson Med 2009;62:896.

76. Bittersohl B, Miese FR, Hosalkar HS, et al. T2* mapping of hip joint cartilage in various histological grades of degeneration. Osteoarthritis Cartilage 2012;20:653.

77. Miese FR, Zilkens C, Holstein A, et al. Assessment of early cartilage degeneration after slipped capital femoral epiphysis using T2 and T2* mapping. Acta Radiol 2011;52:106.

78. Fukawa T, Yamaguchi S, Watanabe A, et al. Quantitative assessment of tendon healing by using MR

T2 mapping in a rabbit Achilles tendon transection model treated with platelet-rich plasma. Radiology 2015;276:748.

79. Wang N, Xia Y. Anisotropic analysis of multi-component T2 and T1rho relaxations in Achilles tendon by NMR spectroscopy and microscopic MRI. J Magn Reson Imaging 2013;38:625.

80. Filho GH, Du J, Pak BC, et al. Quantitative characterization of the Achilles tendon in cadaveric specimens: T1 and T2* measurements using ultrashort-TE MRI at 3 T. AJR Am J Roentgenol 2009;192:W117.

81. Juras V, Apprich S, Pressl C, et al. Histological correlation of 7 T multi-parametric MRI performed in ex-vivo Achilles tendon. Eur J Radiol 2013;82:740.

82. Chang EY, Du J, Statum S, et al. Quantitative bi-component T2* analysis of histologically normal Achilles tendons. Muscles Ligaments Tendons J 2015;5:58.

83. Juras V, Apprich S, Szomolanyi P, et al. Bi-exponential T2 analysis of healthy and diseased Achilles tendons: an in vivo preliminary magnetic resonance study and correlation with clinical score. Eur Radiol 2013;23:2814.

84. Koff MF, Pownder SL, Shah PH, et al. Ultrashort echo imaging of cyclically loaded rabbit patellar tendon. J Biomech 2014;47:3428.

85. Potter HG, Black BR, Chong le R. New techniques in articular cartilage imaging. Clin Sports Med 2009;28:77.

86. Akella SV, Regatte RR, Gougoutas AJ, et al. Proteoglycan-induced changes in T1rho-relaxation of articular cartilage at 4T. Magn Reson Med 2001;46:419.

87. Guermazi A, Alizai H, Crema MD, et al. Compositional MRI techniques for evaluation of cartilage degeneration in osteoarthritis. Osteoarthritis Cartilage 2015;23:1639.

88. Mlynarik V, Trattnig S, Huber M, et al. The role of relaxation times in monitoring proteoglycan depletion in articular cartilage. J Magn Reson Imaging 1999;10:497.

89. Stahl R, Luke A, Li X, et al. T1rho, T2 and focal knee cartilage abnormalities in physically active and sedentary healthy subjects versus early OA patients–a 3.0-Tesla MRI study. Eur Radiol 2009;19:132.

90. Bolbos RI, Zuo J, Banerjee S, et al. Relationship between trabecular bone structure and articular cartilage morphology and relaxation times in early OA of the knee joint using parallel MRI at 3 T. Osteoarthritis Cartilage 2008;16:1150.

91. Zarins ZA, Bolbos RI, Pialat JB, et al. Cartilage and meniscus assessment using T1rho and T2 measurements in healthy subjects and patients with osteoarthritis. Osteoarthritis Cartilage 2010;18:1408.

92. Nishioka H, Hirose J, Nakamura E, et al. Detecting ICRS grade 1 cartilage lesions in anterior cruciate ligament injury using T1rho and T2 mapping. Eur J Radiol 2013;82:1499.

93. Souza RB, Feeley BT, Zarins ZA, et al. T1rho MRI relaxation in knee OA subjects with varying sizes of cartilage lesions. Knee 2013;20:113.

94. Madelin G, Poidevin F, Makrymallis A, et al. Classification of sodium MRI data of cartilage using machine learning. Magn Reson Med 2015;74:1435.

95. Zbyn S, Mlynarik V, Juras V, et al. Evaluation of cartilage repair and osteoarthritis with sodium MRI. NMR Biomed 2016;29:206.

96. Newbould RD, Miller SR, Tielbeek JA, et al. Reproducibility of sodium MRI measures of articular cartilage of the knee in osteoarthritis. Osteoarthritis Cartilage 2012;20:29.

97. Madelin G, Regatte RR. Biomedical applications of sodium MRI in vivo. J Magn Reson Imaging 2013; 38:511.

98. Juras V, Zbyn S, Pressl C, et al. Sodium MR imaging of Achilles tendinopathy at 7 T: preliminary results. Radiology 2012;262:199.

99. Borotikar BS, Sheehan FT. In vivo patellofemoral contact mechanics during active extension using a novel dynamic MRI-based methodology. Osteoarthritis Cartilage 1886;2013:21.

100. Borotikar BS, Sipprell WH 3rd, Wible EE, et al. A methodology to accurately quantify patellofemoral cartilage contact kinematics by combining 3D image shape registration and cine-PC MRI velocity data. J Biomech 2012;45:1117.

101. Draper CE, Besier TF, Santos JM, et al. Using real-time MRI to quantify altered joint kinematics in subjects with patellofemoral pain and to evaluate the effects of a patellar brace or sleeve on joint motion. J Orthop Res 2009;27:571.

102. Fei Z, Fan C, Ngo S, et al. Dynamic evaluation of cervical disc herniation using kinetic MRI. J Clin Neurosci 2011;18:232.

103. Clarke EC, Martin JH, d'Entremont AG, et al. A non-invasive, 3D, dynamic MRI method for measuring muscle moment arms in vivo: demonstration in the human ankle joint and Achilles tendon. Med Eng Phys 2015;37:93.

Index

Note: Page numbers of article titles are in **boldface** type.

Magn Reson Imaging Clin N Am 25 (2017) 227–230
http://dx.doi.org/10.1016/S1064-9689(16)30107-6
1064-9689/17

Printed and bound by CPI Group (UK) Ltd, Croydon, CR0 4YY

08/05/2025

01864696-0008